Pocket Companion to
OBSTETRICS
NORMAL & PROBLEM PREGNANCIES

Pocket Companion to
OBSTETRICS
NORMAL & PROBLEM PREGNANCIES

Third Edition

Steven G. Gabbe, M.D.
Professor and Chairman
Department of Obstetrics and Gynecology
University of Washington School of Medicine
Seattle, Washington

Jennifer R. Niebyl, M.D.
Professor and Head
Department of Obstetrics and Gynecology
University of Iowa College of Medicine
Iowa City, Iowa

Joe Leigh Simpson, M.D.
Ernst W. Bertner Professor and Chairman
Department of Obstetrics and Gynecology
Professor of Molecular and Human Genetics
Baylor College of Medicine
Houston, Texas

Illustrated by Mikki Senkarik, M.S., A.M.I.

CHURCHILL LIVINGSTONE

A Division of Harcourt Brace & Company
New York, Edinburgh, London, Madrid, Melbourne, San Francisco, Tokyo

CHURCHILL LIVINGSTONE
A Division of Harcourt Brace & Company

The Curtis Center
Independence Square West
Philadelphia, Pennsylvania 19106

Library of Congress Cataloging-in-Publication Data

Pocket companion to Obstetrics: normal & problem
pregnancies, third edition / [edited by] Steven G. Gabbe
  Jennifer R. Niebyl, Joe Leigh Simpson :
  Illustrated by Mikki Sankarik.
    p. cm.
    Companion v. to: Obstetrics: normal & problem
  pregnancies. 3rd ed.
  1996.
    ISBN 0-443-07982-X
    1. Obstetrics—Handbooks, manuals, etc.
  2. Pregnancy—Complications—Handbooks, manuals,
etc. I. Gabbe, Steven G.
II. Niebyl, Jennifer R.   III. Simpson, Joe Leigh,
IV. Obstetrics.
    [DNLM: 1. Pregnancy handbooks. 2. Pregnancy
  Complications
handbooks. 3. Perinatal Care handbooks.
WQ 39 P7378 1999]
RG531.P63 1999
618.2—dc21
DNLM/DLC   98–41893

POCKET COMPANION TO OBSTETRICS
ISBN 0-443-07982-X

Last digit is the print number: 9 8 7 6 5 4 3 2 1

Contributors

THOMAS J. BENEDETTI, M.D.
Professor and Vice Chairman, Department of
Obstetrics and Gynecology, University of Washington
School of Medicine, Seattle, Washington
Obstetric Hemorrhage

RICHARD L. BERKOWITZ, M.D.
Professor and Chairman, Department of Obstetrics,
Gynecology, and Reproductive Sciences, Mount Sinai
School of Medicine of the City University of New
York; Director of Obstetrics and Gynecology, Mount
Sinai Hospital, New York, New York
Multiple Gestations

IRA BERNSTEIN, M.D.
Associate Professor, Department of Obstetrics and
Gynecology, University of Vermont College of
Medicine; Attending Physician, Fletcher and Allen
Health Care, Burlington, Vermont
Intrauterine Growth Restriction

WATSON A. BOWES, JR., M.D.
Clinical Professor of Obstetrics and Gynecology,
University of North Carolina at Chapel Hill School
of Medicine; University of North Carolina Hospitals,
Chapel Hill, North Carolina
Postpartum Care

D. WARE BRANCH, M.D.
Associate Professor, Department of Obstetrics and
Gynecology, University of Utah School of Medicine,
Salt Lake City, Utah
Rhesus Isoimmunization in Pregnancy

ROBERT C. CEFALO, M.D., PH.D.

Professor, Department of Obstetrics and Gynecology, University of North Carolina at Chapel Hill School of Medicine, Chapel Hill, North Carolina

Labor and Delivery

FRANK A. CHERVENAK, M.D.

Professor and Vice Chairman, Cornell University Medical College; Director of Obstetrics, Director of Maternal-Fetal Medicine, The New York Hospital, New York, New York

Obstetric Ultrasound: Assessment of Fetal Growth and Anatomy

DAVID H. CHESTNUT, M.D.

Professor and Chairman of Anesthesiology, University of Alabama School of Medicine, Birmingham, Alabama

Obstetric Anesthesia

USHA CHITKARA, M.D.

Associate Professor, Department of Gynecology and Obstetrics, Division of Maternal-Fetal Medicine, Stanford University School of Medicine, Stanford, California

Multiple Gestations

LARRY J. COPELAND, M.D.

Professor and Chair, Department of Obstetrics and Gynecology, The Ohio State University College of Medicine, Columbus, Ohio

Malignant Diseases and Pregnancy

RICHARD DEPP, M.D.

Paul A. and Eloise Bowers Professor of Obstetrics and Gynecology; Chairman, Department of Obstetrics and Gynecology, Jefferson Medical College of Thomas Jefferson University, Philadelphia, Pennsylvania

Cesarean Delivery

MAURICE L. DRUZIN, M.D.

Professor of Gynecology and Obstetrics, Stanford University School of Medicine; Chief, Division of Maternal-Fetal Medicine, Director of the Perinatal Diagnostic Center, Stanford University Medical Center, Stanford, California

Antepartum Fetal Evaluation

PATRICK DUFF, M.D.

Professor and Residency Program Director, Department of Obstetrics and Gynecology, University of Florida, Gainesville, Florida

Maternal and Perinatal Infection

PAMELA M. FOY, B.S., R.D.M.S.

Clinical Coordinator of Ultrasound Services, Department of Obstetrics and Gynecology, The Ohio State University College of Medicine, Columbus, Ohio

Appendices: Obstetric Ultrasound Measurement Tables

ROGER K. FREEMAN, M.D.

Professor, Department of Obstetrics and Gynecology, University of California, Irvine, College of Medicine, Irvine, California; Medical Director of Obstetrics and Gynecology, Women's Services, Long Beach Memorial Medical Center, Long Beach, California

Postdate Pregnancy

STEVEN G. GABBE, M.D.

Professor and Chairman, Department of Obstetrics and Gynecology, University of Washington School of Medicine, Seattle, Washington

Obstetric Ultrasound: Assessment of Fetal Growth and Anatomy; Antepartum Fetal Evaluation; Intrapartum Fetal Evaluation; Intrauterine Growth Restriction

CHARLES P. GIBBS, M.D.

Professor and Chairman, Department of Anesthesiology, University of Colorado Health Sciences Center, Denver, Colorado

Obstetric Anesthesia

MICHAEL C. GORDON, M.D.

Staff Perinatologist, Chief, Outpatient Services, Department of Obstetrics and Gynecology, Wilford Hall Medical Center, Lackland AFB, Texas

Dermatologic Disorders

JOY L. HAWKINS, M.D.

Professor of Anesthesiology, Director of Obstetric Anesthesiology, University of Colorado School of Medicine, Denver, Colorado

Obstetric Anesthesia

JAY D. IAMS, M.D.

Frederick P. Zuspan Professor of Obstetrics and Gynecology; Director, Division of Maternal-Fetal Medicine, The Ohio State University College of Medicine, Columbus, Ohio

Preterm Birth

MARC JACKSON, M.D.

Assistant Professor, Department of Obstetrics and Gynecology, University of Pennsylvania Medical Center, Philadelphia, Pennsylvania

Rhesus Isoimmunization in Pregnancy

TIMOTHY R.B. JOHNSON, M.D.

Professor and Chair, Department of Obstetrics and Gynecology, University of Michigan, Ann Arbor, Michigan

Preconception and Prenatal Care

DAVID C. LAGREW, JR., M.D.

Assistant Professor, Department of Obstetrics and Gynecology, University of California, Irvine, College of Medicine, Irvine, California; Medical Director, Women's Hospital, Saddleback Memorial Medical Center, Laguna Hills, California

Postdate Pregnancy

Mark B. Landon, M.D.

Associate Professor, Division of Maternal-Fetal Medicine, Department of Obstetrics and Gynecology, The Ohio State University College of Medicine, Columbus, Ohio

Medical Complications; Cardiac and Pulmonary Disease; Diabetes Mellitus and Other Endocrine Diseases; Hepatic and Gastrointestinal Disorders; Malignant Diseases and Pregnancy; Dermatologic Disorders

William C. Mabie, M.D.

Professor, Division of Maternal–Fetal Medicine, Department of Obstetrics and Gynecology, University of Tennessee, Memphis College of Medicine; Director of Obstetric Intensive Care Unit, Department of Obstetrics and Gynecology, Regional Medical Center, Memphis, Tennessee

Critical Care Obstetrics

Jennifer R. Niebyl, M.D.

Professor and Head, Department of Obstetrics and Gynecology, The University of Iowa College of Medicine; Head, Department of Obstetrics and Gynecology, University of Iowa Hospitals and Clinics, Iowa City, Iowa

Preconception and Prenatal Care; Drugs in Pregnancy and Lactation

William F. O'Brien, M.D.

Professor, Department of Obstetrics and Gynecology; Director, Division of Obstetrics, University of South Florida College of Medicine, Tampa, Florida

Labor and Delivery

Roy H. Petrie, M.D., Sc.D.*

Professor and Chairman, Department of Obstetrics and Gynecology, St. Louis University School of Medicine, St. Louis, Missouri

Intrapartum Fetal Evaluation

---

*Deceased.

ROSEMARY E. REISS, M.D.
Associate Professor of Clinical Obstetrics
and Gynecology, Department of Obstetrics
and Gynecology, The Ohio State University; Director
of Clinical Obstetrics, Ohio State University Hospital,
Columbus, Ohio
Intrapartum Fetal Evaluation

ADAM A. ROSENBERG, M.D.
Professor of Pediatrics, University of Colorado
School of Medicine; Director of Newborn Services,
University Hospital, Denver, Colorado
The Neonate

PHILIP SAMUELS, M.D.
Associate Professor, Division of Maternal-Fetal
Medicine, Department of Obstetrics and Gynecology,
The Ohio State University College of Medicine,
Columbus, Ohio
*Medical Complications; Cardiac and Pulmonary Disease;
Renal Disease; Hematologic Complications of Pregnancy;
Collagen Vascular Diseases; Hepatic and Gastrointestinal
Disorders; Neurologic Disorders*

JOHN W. SEEDS, M.D.
Professor and Chair, Medical College of Virginia of
Virginia Commonwealth University, Richmond,
Virginia
Malpresentations

BAHA M. SIBAI, M.D.
Professor, University of Tennessee, Memphis; Chief,
Division of Maternal-Fetal Medicine, University of
Tennessee Medical Group, Memphis, Tennessee
Hypertension in Pregnancy

JOE LEIGH SIMPSON, M.D.
Ernst W. Bertner Professor and Chairman,
Department of Obstetrics and Gynecology and
Professor of Molecular and Human Genetics, Baylor
College of Medicine, Houston, Texas
Genetic Counseling and Prenatal Diagnosis; Fetal Wastage

MARLENE A. WALKER, RNC, N.P.

Nurse Practitioner, Department of Obstetrics and Gynecology, The Johns Hopkins Hospital, Baltimore, Maryland

Preconception and Prenatal Care

MARGARET WALSH, M.D.

Private Practice, Southside Women's Health Care, PC, Colonial Heights, Virginia

Malpresentations

Preface

The first edition of our *Pocket Companion* has been written in response to requests from readers of our textbook, *Obstetrics: Normal and Problem Pregnancies*. Today, we find ourselves providing obstetric care in many, many settings–private offices, in-hospital clinics, labor and delivery floors, operating rooms, antepartum and postpartum floors, outreach clinics and, in some cases, through telephone, television, and computer consult lines. Our readers have asked for a comprehensive, yet condensed form of our textbook that would be available to them at any site of care; thus, the publication of our *Pocket Companion*. The material for our *Pocket Companion* has been prepared by the three editors of our textbook and is based on the outstanding chapters written by our contributors to whom we are extremely grateful. We have added new, important information to the *Pocket Companion* that has appeared since the publication of the 3rd Edition of our textbook in 1996. Readers will find that we have included many of the tables, flow diagrams, and illustrations from the textbook so information can be easily obtained. The *Pocket Companion* is a clinical guide, and, therefore, we have included anatomy, physiology, and basic science material when relevant to clinical care. The important points which were added to the end of each of the chapters in our 3rd Edition are included in the *Pocket Companion*, again summarizing the key information on each subject. We have also included tables of ultrasound biometry as a resource for the interpretation of these studies. Readers will note that the reference numbers from our textbook have been included in the *Pocket Companion* but the references have been omitted. Including the references would have made the *Pocket Companion* too large, but, with the reference numbers available, readers will be able to refer to the textbook if they want to find the original sources.

Years ago, there was a popular detective show on television. One of the leading characters would always tell witnesses, he wanted the facts, just the facts. Our *Pocket Companion* contains the facts, presented in a way we hope will be helpful to all who provide obstetric care.

Steven G. Gabbe, M.D.
Jennifer R. Niebyl, M.D.
Joe Leigh Simpson, M.D.

Notice about references

Please note that superscript reference numbers appearing throughout **Pocket Companion** refer to references in equivalent chapters of *Obstetrics: Normal and Problem Pregnancies* (third edition).

Contents

NOTICE

Obstetrics is an ever-changing field. Standard safety precautions must be followed, but as new research and clinical experience broaden our knowledge, changes in treatment and drug therapy become necessary or appropriate. The editors of this work have carefully checked the generic and trade drug names and verified drug dosages to ensure that the dosage information in this work is accurate and in accord with the standards accepted at the time of publication. Readers are advised, however, to check the product information currently provided by the manufacturer of each drug to be administered to be certain that changes have not been made in the recommended dose or in the contraindications for administration. This is of particular importance in regard to new or infrequently used drugs. It is the responsibility of the treating physician, relying on experience and knowledge of the patient, to determine dosages and the best treatment for the patient. The editors cannot be responsible for misuse or misapplication of the material in this work.

THE PUBLISHER

SECTION 1
Prenatal Care

Preconception and Prenatal Care

Timothy R. B. Johnson,
Marlene A. Walker, and
Jennifer R. Niebyl

Prenatal care is an excellent example of preventive medicine. The goal of prenatal care is to help the mother maintain her well-being and achieve a healthy outcome for herself and her infant. Education about pregnancy, childbearing, and childrearing is an important part of prenatal care, as are detection and treatment of abnormalities. This process is best realized when begun even before pregnancy at a preconceptional visit. Another important component of prenatal care is establishment of gestational age.

Prenatal Care

The fetus has emerged as a patient in utero, and prevention of morbidity as well as mortality is now the goal. At the same time, pregnancy is basically a physiologic process, and the normal pregnant patient may not benefit from advanced technology.

There have been no prospective controlled trials demonstrating efficacy of prenatal care overall. However, many individual components have been shown to be effective (e.g., treatment with corticosteroids to prevent respiratory distress syndrome and screening for and treating asymptomatic bacteriuria for prevention of pyelonephritis).[16] In retrospective studies, however, patients with increased numbers of visits have improved maternal and fetal outcomes. This may be because of self-selection of patients for care who are motivated to take care of themselves in other ways, as women with no prenatal care often come from underprivileged socioeconomic groups.

Preconceptional Education

The best time to see a woman for prenatal care is when she is considering pregnancy. At gynecologic visits, patients should be asked about their plans for pregnancy. If there are questions about the history, such as family history of fetal anomaly or previous cesarean delivery, further details can be obtained from family members or the appropriate medical facility. This is the time to draw a rubella titer and immunize the susceptible patient. Hepatitis B immunization can be given to appropriate patients and human immunodeficiency virus (HIV) testing offered.

Before pregnancy is the time to screen appropriate populations for genetic disease carrier states such as Tay-Sachs disease or hemoglobinopathies. Resolution of these issues is much less harried without the time limits placed by an advancing pregnancy. Medical conditions such as anemia, urinary tract infection, or hypothyroidism can be fully evaluated and the woman medically treated before pregnancy. If the patient is obese, weight reduction should be attempted before pregnancy.

For some conditions, such as diabetes mellitus and phenylketonuria, medical disease management before conception can positively influence pregnancy outcome. This is also the time to review drug usage and other practices, such as alcohol ingestion and smoking (see Ch. 2). Advice can be given about avoiding medications in the first trimester, and general advice can be given concerning diet, exercise, and occupational exposures.

Periconceptional supplements with folic acid can reduce the incidence of neural tube defects and other anomalies. The Centers for Disease Control and Prevention recommends that all women of childbearing age who are capable of becoming pregnant should consume 0.4 mg of folic acid daily, which is most easily achieved by taking a supplement. For women with a previously affected child, the recommendation is that they take 4 mg daily from 4 weeks before conception through the first 3 months of pregnancy.

The Initial Preconceptional or Prenatal Visit

Social and Demographic Risks

Extremes of age are obstetric risk factors. The pregnant teenager has particular nutritional and emotional needs. She is at special risk for sexually transmitted diseases; it has been shown that she benefits particularly from education in areas of childbearing and contraception. The pregnant woman over age 35 is at increased risk for a chromosomally abnormal child,[24] and she must be so advised. Patients should be asked about family histories of Down syndrome, neural tube defects, hemophilia, hemoglobinopathies, and other birth defects, as well as mental retardation. Consultation for genetic counseling and genetic testing, if desired, may be appropriate. The age of the father may be important, as there may be genetic risks to the fetus when the father is older than 55 years.[25] Certain diseases may be race related. Black patients should be screened for sickle cell disease, those of Jewish and French Canadian heritage should be screened for Tay-Sachs disease, and those of Mediterranean descent should be screened for β-thalassemia.

Low socioeconomic status should be identified and appropriate referral to federal programs, such as that for women, infants, and children (WIC), can have real benefits. If a patient has a history of previous neonatal death or stillbirth, records should be carefully reviewed so that the correct diagnosis is made and recurrence risk appropriately assessed. A history of drug abuse or recent blood transfusion should be elicited.

Occupational hazards should be identified. Patients whose occupations require heavy physical exercise or excess stress should be informed that they may need to decrease such activity.

Tobacco, alcohol, and recreational drug use can all adversely affect pregnancy and are a critical part of the history. Specific questions concerning smoking, alcohol, and drugs (prescriptive, over the counter, and illicit) should be asked.[27] Regular screening for alcohol and substance use should be carried out using such tools as the T-ACE questionnaire (Table 1-1).[28] Women

---

Table 1-1   Alcohol Abuse Screening: the T-ACE Questionnaire[a]

T	How many drinks does it take to make you feel "high" (can you hold)? (*tolerance;* a positive response consists of two or more drinks)
A	Have people *annoyed* you by criticizing your drinking?
C	Have you ever felt you ought to *cut down* on your drinking?
E	Have you ever had a drink first thing in the morning to steady your nerves or to get rid of a hangover (*eye-opener*)?

Scoring: The tolerance question has substantially more weight (2 points) than the three other questions (1 point each).

[a] These questions were found to be significant identifiers of risk drinking in pregnancy (i.e., alcohol intake potentially sufficient to damage the embryo/fetus).

From Sokol RJ, Martier SS, Ager JW: The T-ACE questions: practical prenatal detection of risk-drinking. Am J Obstet Gynecol 160:863, 1989, with permission.

should be urged to stop smoking prior to pregnancy and to drink not at all or minimally once they are pregnant. Drug addiction confers a particularly high risk, and addicted mothers require specialized care throughout pregnancy.

Violence against women is increasingly recognized as a problem that should be addressed, with reports suggesting that abuse occurs during 3 to 8 percent of pregnancies. Questions addressing personal safety and violence should be included during the prenatal period.

Medical Risk

Family history of diabetes, hypertension, tuberculosis, seizures, hematologic disorders, multiple pregnancies, mental retardation, congenital abnormalities, and reproductive wastage should be elicited. A better history may be obtained if patients are asked to fill out a pre-interview questionnaire or history form. Any significant maternal cardiovascular, renal, or metabolic disease should be defined. Infectious diseases such as urinary tract disease, syphilis, tuberculosis, or herpes genitalis should be identified. Surgical history with special attention to any abdominal or pelvic operations should be noted. A history of previous cesarean birth should include indication, type of uterine incision, and any complications. Allergies, particularly drug allergies, should be prominent on the problem list.

Obstetric Risk

Previous obstetric and reproductive history are essential to care in subsequent pregnancy, and the outcome for each prior pregnancy should be recorded in detail. Previous miscarriages not only confer risk and anxiety for another pregnancy loss but can increase the risk of genetic disease as well as preterm delivery.[30]

Previous preterm delivery is strongly associated with recurrence; it is important to delineate the events surrounding the preterm birth. Did the membranes rupture before labor? Were there painful uterine contractions? Was there bleeding? Were there fetal abnormalities? What was the neonatal outcome? Diethylstilbestrol (DES) exposure, incompetent cervix, and uterine anomalies are all conditions that may be known from a previous pregnancy. Previous fetal macrosomia makes glucose screening essential.

After all the specific questions, it is recommended to ask the patient a few simple questions: What important items haven't I asked? What else about you and your pregnancy do I need to know? What problems and questions do you have? Leaving time for open-ended questions is the best way to complete the initial visit.

Pregnancy Tests

The scientific basis for pregnancy tests is measurement of human chorionic gonadotropin (hCG). hCG secretion is related to the mass of hCG-secreting trophoblastic tissues. Between 3 and 9 weeks' gestation, rapidly rising hCG coincides with proliferation of immature trophoblastic villi and development of an extensive syncytial layer. Between 10 and 18 weeks' gestation, declining hCG is associated with a relative reduction in syncytiotrophoblasts and cytotrophoblasts. From 20 weeks until term, a gradual increase in hCG corresponds with a gradual increase in placental weight and villus volume.

Several hCG assays are available and the choice depends on the sensitivity required. hCG is first detectable in maternal blood 8 to 11 days after conception, but only through very sensitive research assays (sensitivity 0.1 to 0.3 mIU/ml). Most clinically available pregnancy tests have a sensitivity of 25 mIU/ml.

An hCG level of less than 5 mIU/ml can be confidently considered as negative. Levels exceeding 25 mIU/ml can be confidently stated as positive. In the range of 5 to 25 mIU/ml, false-positive results may occur, especially in perimenopausal and postmenopausal women. This is the result of endogenous pituitary hCG secretion that occurs in synchrony with LH. However, nonpregnancy levels of hCG still fall well under the sensitivity of the most sensitive clinical assays used in pregnancy monitoring. If uncertainty exists, repeating the test in 2 days normally confirms a trend upward, thus documenting a pregnancy. Deviation from the patterns of rising hCG suggests either ectopic gestation or spontaneous abortion. If hCG fails to rise 66 percent in 2 days, algorithms to differentiate between these two conditions become necessary, as described in Chapter 15.

Physical and Laboratory Evaluation

Physical evaluation should include a general physical examination as well as a pelvic examination. Baseline height and weight as well as prepregnancy weight are recorded. Special attention should be given to the initial vital signs, cardiac examination, and reflexes, since many healthy young women have not had a physical examination immediately before becoming pregnant. Any physical finding that might have an impact on

Table 1-2 Recommendations for All Women for Prenatal Care

	Preconception or First Visit	Weeks								
		6–8ᵃ	14–16	24–28	32	36	38	39	40	41
History										
Medical, including genetic	X									
Psychosocial	X									
Update medical and psychosocial		X	X	X	X	X	X	X	X	X
Physical examination										
General	X									
Blood pressure	X	X	X	X	X	X	X	X	X	X
Height	X	X	X	X	X	X	X	X	X	X
Weight	X	X	X	X	X	X	X	X	X	X
Height and weight profile	X									
Pelvic examination and pelvimetry	X	X								
Breast examination	X	X								
Fundal height			X	X	X	X	X	X	X	X
Fetal position and heart rate			X	X	X	X	X	X	X	X
Cervical examination	X									

Laboratory tests				
Hemoglobin or hematocrit	X		X	X
Rh factor, blood type	X			
Antibody screen	X		X	
Pap smear	X			
Diabetic screen			X	
MSAFP, triple screen[b]		X		
Urine				
Dipstick	X			
Protein	X			
Sugar	X			
Culture			X	
Infections				
Rubella titer	X			
Syphilis test	X			
Gonococcal culture	X		X	X
Hepatitis B	X		X	
HIV (offered)	X			
Toxoplasmosis	X			
Illicit drug screen (offered)	X			
Genetic screen	X			

[a] If preconception care has preceded.
[b] MSAFP, maternal serum α-fetoprotein.

pregnancy (e.g., DES changes in the cervix) or that might be affected by pregnancy (e.g., mitral valve prolapse) should be defined. It is particularly important to perform and record a complete physical examination at this initial visit, since less emphasis will be placed on nonobstetric portions of the examination as pregnancy progresses.

The pelvic examination should focus on the uterine size. Before 12 to 14 weeks, size can give a fairly accurate estimate of gestational age. Papanicolaou smear and culture for gonorrhea and chlamydia are done. The cervix should be carefully palpated, and any deviation from normal should be noted. Clinical pelvimetry should be performed and the clinical impression of adequacy noted. The pelvic examination is limited by examiner and patient variation as well as by obesity. If there is difficulty in examining the uterus, an ultrasound study is indicated.

Basic laboratory studies are routinely performed (Table 1-2).

Specific conditions will require further evaluation. A history of thyroid disease will lead to thyroid function testing. Anticonvulsant therapy requires blood level studies to determine adequacy of medication. Identification of problems on screening (e.g., anemia, abnormal glucose screen) will mandate further testing. Screening for varicella has been suggested for women with no known history of chicken pox.

The American College of Obstetricians and Gynecologists (ACOG) has recommended routine screening of all pregnant women for hepatitis B.[33] HIV screening in high-risk populations should also be offered, since maternal therapy with AZT can reduce vertical transmission (see Ch. 22).

Repeat Prenatal Visits

A plan of visits is outlined to the patient. This has been traditionally every 4 weeks for the first 28 weeks of pregnancy, every 2 to 3 weeks until 36 weeks, and weekly thereafter. If the pregnancy progresses normally[34,35] this number of visits can be decreased; especially in parous, healthy women. If there are any complications, the intervals can be decreased appropriately. For example, patients with hypertensive disease may require weekly visits to monitor blood pressure.

If the patient is Rh negative and unsensitized, she should receive Rh immune globulin prophylaxis at 28 weeks. A glucose screening test for diabetes is also appropriately performed at this time (see Ch. 21), and routine fetal movement counting can begin using an organized system. At 36 weeks a repeat hematocrit, especially in those women with anemia or at risk for peripartum hemorrhage (multipara, repeat cesarean), may be performed. Also, appropriate cultures for sexually transmitted disease (gonorrhea, chlamydia) should be obtained as indicated in the third trimester.

At 41 weeks from the last menstrual period, the patient should be entered into a screening program for fetal well-being, which may include electronic monitoring tests or ultrasound evaluation (see Ch. 18).

Intercurrent Problems

It is the practice in prenatal care to evaluate the pregnant patient for the development of certain complications. If a patient shows a tendency to blood pressure elevation at 28 weeks, for example, she should be seen again in a week, not a month. Development of hypertension must be recognized and evaluation and hospitalization appropriately instituted.

Weight gain in pregnancy has been shown to be an important correlate of fetal weight gain and is therefore closely monitored. Too little weight gain should lead to an evaluation of nutritional factors and an assessment of associated fetal growth. Excess weight gain is one of the first signs of fluid retention, but it may also reflect increased dietary intake or decreased activity. Dependent edema is physiologic in pregnancy, but generalized or facial edema can be a first sign of disease.

Proteinuria reflects urinary tract disease, generally either infection or glomerular dysfunction, possibly the result of preeclampsia. Urinary tract infection should be looked for, and the degree of protein quantitated in a 24-hour urine collection.

Growth retardation and macrosomia can often be suspected clinically on the basis of an abnormality in fundal growth.

Nutrition

One of the earliest purposes of prenatal care was to counsel and ensure that women received adequate nutrition for pregnancy. The health care provider may be influential in correcting inappropriate dietary habits. Strict vegetarians may need supplemental vitamin B_{12}. Occasionally, consultation with a registered dietitian may be necessary when there is poor compliance or a special medical need, such as diabetes mellitus.

The U.S. Department of Agriculture has published the new food guide pyramid.[38] Americans are encouraged to eat 6 to 11 servings per day of bread, cereal, rice, and pasta; 3 to 5 servings per day of vegetables; 2 to 4 servings per day of fruit; 2 to 3 servings per day of milk, yogurt and cheese; and 2 to 3 servings per day of meat, poultry, fish, beans, eggs, and nuts. Fats, oils, and sweets should be used sparingly. Pregnant women need three servings per day of dairy products, a serving being a cup of milk or yogurt, 1 1/2 oz of natural cheese, or 2 oz processed cheese.

Recommended dietary allowances (RDAs) for most substances increase during pregnancy. According to the 1989 RDAs, only the recommendations for iron, folic acid, and vitamin D double during gestation.[39] The RDAs for calcium and phosphorus increase by one-half; the RDA for pyridoxine and thiamine increase by about one-third. The RDAs for protein, zinc, and riboflavin increase by about one-fourth. The RDAs for all other nutrients except vitamin A increase by less than 20 percent and vitamin A increases not at all. All of these nutrients, with the exception of iron, are supplied by a well-balanced diet.

The National Academy of Sciences currently recommends that 30 mg of ferrous iron supplements be given to pregnant women daily, since the iron content of the habitual American diet and the iron stores of many women are not sufficient to provide the increased iron required during pregnancy. For those at high nutritional risk, such as adolescents, those with multiple gestation, heavy cigarette smokers, and drug and alcohol abusers, a vitamin/mineral supplement should be given. Increased iron is needed both for the fetal needs and the increased maternal blood volume. Iron-containing foods should also be encouraged, such as liver, red meats, eggs, dried beans, leafy green vegetables, whole-grain enriched bread and cereal, and dried fruits. The 30-mg iron supplement is contained in approximately 150 mg of ferrous sulfate, 300 mg of ferrous gluconate, or 100 mg of ferrous fumarate. Taking iron between meals will facilitate its absorption.

Weight Gain

The total weight gain recommended in pregnancy is 25 to 35 lb for normal women.[41] Underweight women may gain up to 40 lb, and overweight women should limit weight gain to 15 to 25 lb.

If the patient does not show a 10-lb weight gain by midpregnancy, her nutritional status should be reviewed. Inadequate weight gain is associated with an increased risk of a low-birth-weight infant. Inadequate weight gain seems to have its greatest effect in women who are of low or normal weight before pregnancy. Patients should be cautioned against weight loss during pregnancy. Total weight gain in the obese can be modified downward to 15 lb, but less weight gain is associated with an increased risk of intrauterine growth retardation.

When excess weight gain is noted, an assessment for fluid retention is also performed. In the assessment of edema, some dependent edema in the legs is normal as pregnancy advances because of venous compression by the weight of the uterus. Elevation of the feet and bedrest on the left side will help correct this problem. Turning the patient from her back to her left side increases venous return from the legs as the pressure on the vena cava is relieved. This maneuver increases the effective circulating blood volume, cardiac output, and thus the blood flow to the kidney. A diuresis will follow, as well as increased blood flow to the uterus.

Activity and Employment

Most patients are able to maintain their normal activity levels in pregnancy. Mothers tolerate pregnancy with considerable physical activity, such as looking after small children, but heavy lifting and excessive physical activity should be avoided. Recreational exercises should be encouraged, such as those available in prenatal exercise classes. The patient should be counseled to discontinue activity if she experiences discomfort.

Healthy pregnant women may work until delivery. Strenuous physical exercise, standing for prolonged periods, and work on industrial machines may be associated with increased risk of poor pregnancy outcome, and these should be modified as necessary.[42,43]

Travel

The patient should be advised against prolonged sitting during car or airplane travel because of the risk of venous stasis and possible thromboembolism. The usual recommendation is stopping at least every 2 hours for 10 minutes to allow the patient to walk around and increase venous return from the legs.

The patient should be instructed to wear her seatbelt during car travel, but under the abdomen as pregnancy advances. It may also be helpful to take pillows along in a car to increase comfort.

If the patient is traveling a significant distance, it might be helpful for her to carry a copy of her medical record with her in case an emergency arises in a strange city.

Nausea and Vomiting in Pregnancy

Nonpharmacologic measures are usually recommended initially to treat nausea and vomiting in early pregnancy. Frequent small feedings in order to keep some food in the stomach at all times is helpful. A protein snack at night is advised, and the patient is instructed to keep crackers at her bedside so that she can have these before arising in the morning. Drug therapy for nausea in pregnancy is covered in Chapter 2.

Heartburn

Heartburn is a common complaint in pregnancy because of relaxation of the esophageal sphincter. The patient should be advised to save part of her meal for later if she is experiencing postprandial heartburn and also not to eat immediately before lying down. Liquid antacids coat the esophageal lining more effectively than do tablets.

Hemorrhoids

Hemorrhoids are varicose veins of the rectum. Since straining during bowel movements contributes to their aggravation, avoidance of constipation is preventive, and prolonged sitting should also be avoided. Hemorrhoids will often regress after delivery.

Constipation

Constipation is physiologic during pregnancy with decreased bowel transit time, and the stool may be hardened. Dietary modification with increased bulk, such as with fresh fruit and vegetables, and plenty of water can usually help this problem. Constipation is aggravated by the addition of iron supplementation; if dietary measures are inadequate, patients may require stool softeners. Additional dietary fibers such as Metamucil (psyllium hydrophilic muciloid) or surface-active agents such as Colace (docusate) are recommended. Laxatives are rarely necessary.

Urinary Frequency

Often during the first 3 months of pregnancy, the growing uterus places increased pressure on the bladder. Urinary frequency usually will improve as the uterus rises out of the pelvis by the second trimester. However, urinary frequency may return as the head presses against the bladder. If the patient experiences pain with urination, it is appropriate to check for infection.

Round Ligament Pain

Frequently, patients will notice sharp groin pains due to spasm of the round ligaments associated with movement. This is more frequently felt on the right side due to the usual dextrorotation of the uterus. The pain may be helped by local heat or acetaminophen. Modification of activity with gradual rising and sitting down, and avoidance of sudden movement will decrease problems with this type of pain.

Syncope

Compression of the veins in the legs from the advancing size of the uterus places patients at risk of venous pooling associated with prolonged standing. Measures to avoid this possibility include wearing support stockings and exercising the calves to increase venous return. In later pregnancy, patients may have problems with supine hypotension, a distinct problem when undergoing a medical evaluation or an ultrasound examination. A left lateral tilt position with wedging below the right hip will help keep the weight of the pregnancy off the inferior vena cava.

Backache

Backache can be prevented to a large degree by avoidance of excessive weight gain. Exercises to strengthen back muscles can also be helpful. Posture is important, and sensible shoes, not high heels, should be worn.

Sexual Activity

No restriction need be placed on sexual intercourse. For women at risk for preterm labor or with a history of previous pregnancy loss avoidance of sexual activity may be recommended.

Breast-Feeding

During prenatal visits, the patient should be encouraged to breast-feed her infant. Human milk is the most appropriate nutrient for human infants and also provides significant immunologic protection against infection. Infants who are breast-fed have a lower incidence of infection and require fewer hospitalizations than do infants who are fed formula exclusively. The reasons a woman decides to bottle-feed should be explored, as they may be based on a misconception.

Working outside the home need not be a contraindication to breast-feeding. Many women with careers are now finding time to breast-feed their infants. Nursing for only a few weeks or months is better than not nursing at all. Women should be aware that alternative ways of breast-feeding can be used to correspond with their work schedules. They can decrease the frequency of lactation to a few times a day in most cases and still continue to nurse. Other women may pump their breasts at work, leaving milk for the child's caregiver during the day and thus providing breast milk to the infant even more frequently. The milk may be refrigerated and is safe to use for 24 hours. For a longer duration, the milk should be frozen. Because freezing and thawing destroy the cellular content, fresh milk is preferred.

There is no need for specific nipple preparation during pregnancy. Soap and drying agents should not be used on the nipples, which should be washed only with water.

Preparation for Childbirth

The introduction of childbirth education and consumerism has had significant impact on the practice of obstetrics. The success of obstetric practice in preventing disasters has allowed interest to focus on the quality of the child and of the perinatal experience. Prepared childbirth can have a beneficial effect on performance in labor and delivery.[47]

Assessment of Gestational Age

The establishment of an estimated date of delivery and confirmation of that date by accumulation of supportive information remains one of the most important tasks of good prenatal care.

Human pregnancy has a duration of 280 days, measured from the first day of the last menstrual period (LMP) until delivery. The standard deviation is 14 days. Clinicians measure menstrual weeks (not conceptional weeks) with an assumption of ovulation based on day 14 of a 28-day cycle. This gives pregnancy the 40-week gestational period in common clinical use. Confusion exists among patients who try to measure pregnancy in terms of 9 months or who try to measure in conceptional weeks. It is helpful to explain to patients that pregnancy will be described in terms of weeks, rather than months. The common use of a term such as "4 months pregnant" has no meaning (one does not know whether this is 16 or 20 weeks) and has no place on a contemporary prenatal record.

Clinical Dating

The most reliable clinical estimator of gestational age is an accurate LMP. Using Naegele's rule, the estimated date of delivery is calculated by subtracting 3 months and adding 1 week from the first day of the LMP. A careful history must be taken from the patient verifying that the date given is the first day of the period as well as whether the period was normal, heavy, or light. The date of the previous menstrual period will help ascertain the length of the cycle. History should also be taken about previous use of oral contraceptives, which might influence ovulation.

The size of the uterus on early pelvic examination, or by direct measurement of the abdomen from the pubic symphysis to the top of the uterine fundus (over the curve), provides useful information. Fundal height measurement in centimeters using the over-the-curve technique approximates the gestational age from 16 to 38 weeks within 3 cm.

In the first pregnancy, quickening, the first perception of fetal movement by the mother, is usually noted at about 19 weeks; in subsequent pregnancies, probably because of the experience of the observer, it tends to occur about 2 weeks earlier.[48]

Audible fetal heart tones, in addition to being absolute evidence of pregnancy, are another marker of gestational age. Using an unamplified Hillis-DeLee fetoscope, they are generally audible at 19 to 20 weeks.[48] Observer experience, acuity, and the time spent listening can all affect this number.

Use of the electronic Doppler device permits detection of the fetal heart by 11 to 12 weeks. If fetal heart tones are not heard at the expected time, an ultrasound is appropriate.

Ultrasound

Ultrasound plays a major role in assessment of size and duration of pregnancy. A National Institutes of Health consensus conference in 1984 concluded that, in a low-risk pregnancy followed from the first trimester, routine ultrasound examination was not justified for determining gestational age. However, a long list of indications justify an ultrasound examination.[50]

A randomized trial has shown that the risk of being called overdue was reduced from 8 to 2 percent for patients who received early ultrasound.[51] Also, twins were detected more often and perinatal mortality was reduced in the ultrasound group. The RADIUS (Routine Antenatal Diagnostic Imaging with Ultrasound) study reported no improvement in perinatal outcome with use of routine ultrasound in normal, low-risk women.[52,53] However, 61 percent of women were excluded for many reasons, such as an uncertain menstrual history, and only 35 percent of anomalies were detected in the ultrasound-screened group. The authors' practice is to perform ultrasound at 16 to 20 weeks for a baseline gestational age measurement and as a screening for fetal abnormality or multiple gestation. If ultrasound is not done routinely, the caregiver must be vigilant in detecting indications for a scan.

Ultrasound is an accurate means of estimating gestational age in early pregnancy.[55] The crown–rump length, biparietal diameter, and femur length of pregnancy correlate closely with age before 24 weeks. As pregnancy progresses, fetal size varies considerably, and measurement of the fetus is a poor tool for estimation of gestational age in the third trimester (see Ch. 4).

Assessment of Fetal Maturity Before Repeat Cesarean Delivery or Elective Induction of Labor

The ACOG Committee on Obstetrics: Maternal Fetal Medicine[56] states that, in a gestation in which 39 weeks have elapsed since the last menstrual period in a patient with normal menstrual cycles and no immediate antecedent use of oral contraceptives, fetal maturity can be assumed if one of the following clinical criteria for estimating gestational age is supported by at least one of the following laboratory determinations:

Clinical Criteria

1. Fetal heart tones have been documented for at least 20 weeks by nonelectronic fetoscope or at least 30 weeks by Doppler.
2. Uterine size has been established by pelvic examination prior to 16 weeks of gestation.

Laboratory Determinations

1. Thirty-six weeks have elapsed since a positive serum or urine hCG pregnancy test; *or*
2. Ultrasound
   a. Measurement based on the crown–rump

length obtained between 6 and 12 weeks of gestation *or*

b. Other ultrasound confirmation of gestational age obtained before 24 weeks of gestation

Key Points

- Preconceptional evaluation should include rubella testing and hepatitis testing, in addition to medical and family history.
- Preconceptional supplementation with folic acid can reduce the incidence of neural tube defects and other defects. All women of childbearing age should consume 0.4 mg of folic acid daily. Women who have had a child previously affected by a neural tube defect should take 4 mg daily from 4 weeks before conception through the first 3 months of pregnancy.
- The triple screen (α-fetoprotein, hCG, and estriol) can detect women younger than 35 years of age at increased risk for pregnancies with chromosomal abnormalities.
- The number of prenatal visits can be decreased with safety in healthy parous women.
- The total weight gain recommended for healthy women is 25 to 35 pounds. Underweight women may gain up to 40 pounds, and overweight women should limit weight gain to 15 to 25 pounds.
- Bedrest on the left side increases venous return from the legs, as pressure on the vena cava is relieved. This maneuver increases the effective circulating blood volume, cardiac output, and, thus, the blood flow to the kidney. A diuresis follows, as well as increased blood flow to the uterus.
- The pregnant woman should be advised against prolonged sitting during car or airplane travel because of the risk of venous stasis and possible thromboembolism.
- Breast-feeding is best.
- Ultrasound evaluation between 16 and 20 weeks allows accurate assessment of gestational age and screening for fetal abnormality and multiple gestation.

Chapter 2

Drugs in Pregnancy and Lactation

Jennifer R. Niebyl

Virtually all drugs cross the placenta to some degree, with the exception of large organic ions such as heparin and insulin. Approximately 25 percent of birth defects are known to be genetic in origin; drug exposure accounts for only 2 to 3 percent. Approximately 65 percent of defects are of unknown etiology but may be from combinations of genetic and environmental factors.

The incidence of major malformations in the general population is 2 to 3 percent.[1] A major malformation is one that is incompatible with survival, one requiring major surgery for correction, or one producing major dysfunction. If minor malformations are also included, the rate is 7 to 10 percent. The risk of malformation after exposure to a drug must be compared with this background rate.

There is a marked species specificity in drug teratogenesis.[2] For example, thalidomide was not found to be teratogenic in rats and mice but is a potent human teratogen. Conversely, in certain strains of mice, corticosteroids produce a high percentage of offspring with cleft lip, although no studies have shown these drugs to be teratogenic in humans. The Food and Drug Administration (FDA) lists five categories of labeling for drug use in pregnancy:

A. Controlled studies in women fail to demonstrate a risk to the fetus in the first trimester, and the possibility of fetal harm appears remote.
B. Animal studies do not indicate a risk to the fetus; there are no controlled human studies, or animal studies do show an adverse effect on the fetus, but well-controlled studies in pregnant women have failed to demonstrate a risk to the fetus.
C. Studies have shown the drug to have animal teratogenic or embryocidal effects, but no controlled

studies are available in women, or no studies are available in either animals or women.

D. Positive evidence of human fetal risk exists, but benefits in certain situations (e.g., life-threatening situations or serious diseases for which safer drugs cannot be used or are ineffective) may make use of the drug acceptable despite its risks.

X. Studies in animals or humans have demonstrated fetal abnormalities, or evidence demonstrates fetal risk based on human experience, or both, and the risk clearly outweighs any possible benefit.

The classic teratogenic period is from day 31 after the last menstrual period in a 28-day cycle to 71 days from the last period (Fig. 2-1). During this critical period, organs are forming, and teratogens may cause malformations that are usually overt at birth. The timing of exposure is important. Administration of drugs early in the period of organogenesis will affect the organs developing at that time, such as the heart or neural tube. Closer to the end of the classic teratogenic period, the ear and palate are forming and may be affected by

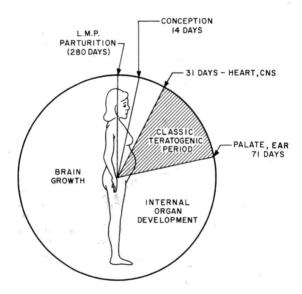

Fig. 2-1 Gestational clock showing the classic teratogenic period. (From Blake DA, Niebyl JR: Requirements and limitations in reproductive and teratogenic risk assessment. *In* Niebyl JR [ed]: Drug Use in Pregnancy [2nd ed]. Philadelphia, Lea & Febiger, 1988, p 1, with permission.)

a teratogen. Before day 31, exposure to a teratogen produces an all-or-none effect. With exposure around conception, the conceptus usually either does not survive or survives without anomalies.

Patients should be educated about avenues other than the use of drugs to cope with tension, aches and pains, and viral illnesses during pregnancy. The risk–benefit ratio should justify the use of a particular drug, and the minimum effective dose should be employed. As long-term effects of drug exposure in utero may not be revealed for many years, caution with regard to the use of any drug in pregnancy is warranted.

Effects of Specific Drugs

Estrogens and Progestins

Recent studies have not confirmed any teratogenic risk for oral contraceptives or progestins. A meta-analysis of first-trimester sex hormone exposure revealed no association between exposure and fetal genital malformations.[6] However, because of the previous conflicting literature, it is wise to do a sensitive pregnancy test before giving progestins to an amenorrheic patient.

Androgenic Steroids

Androgens may masculinize a developing female fetus. Synthetic testosterone derivatives may cause clitoromegaly and labial fusion if given before 13 weeks of pregnancy.[7] Danazol (Danocrine) has been reported to produce mild clitoral enlargement and labial fusion when given inadvertently for the first 10 to 12 weeks after conception.[8]

Anticonvulsants

Infants of epileptic women taking anticonvulsants during pregnancy have approximately double the general population risk of malformations,[14] especially cleft lip with or without cleft palate and congenital heart disease. Valproic acid (Depakene) carries approximately a 1 percent risk of neural tube defects and possibly other anomalies.[15] A combination of more than three drugs or a high daily dose increases the chance of malformations.[17]

Fewer than 10 percent of offspring show the fetal hydantoin syndrome,[20] which consists of microcephaly, growth deficiency, developmental delays, mental retardation, and dysmorphic craniofacial features, and hypoplasia of the nails and distal phalanges. Carbamazepine (Tegretol) is also associated with an increased risk of a dysmorphic syndrome.[22] Children exposed in utero to phenytoin scored 10 points lower on IQ tests than children exposed to carbamazepine or nonexposed controls.[23]

Some women may have taken anticonvulsant drugs for a long period without reevaluation of the need for continuation of the drugs. For patients with idiopathic epilepsy who have been seizure free for 2 years and who have a normal electroencephalogram, it may be safe to attempt a trial of withdrawal of the drug before pregnancy.[27]

Most authorities agree that the benefits of anticonvulsant therapy during pregnancy outweigh the risks of discontinuation of the drug if the patient is first seen during pregnancy. The blood level of drug should be monitored to ensure a therapeutic level but minimize the dosage. Anticonvulsant therapy can affect vitamin K–dependent clotting factors in the newborn. Vitamin K supplementation at 10 mg daily for these mothers has been recommended for the last month of pregnancy.[28,29]

Isotretinoin and Other Vitamin A Derivatives

Isotretinoin (Accutane) is a significant human teratogen, (FDA category X), with appropriate warnings that a negative pregnancy test is required before therapy. The risk of structural anomalies in patients studied prospectively is 25 percent and an additional 25 percent have mental retardation alone.[32] The malformed infants have a characteristic pattern of anomalies including microtia/anotia (small/absent ears), micrognathia, cleft palate, heart defects, thymic defects, retinal or optic nerve anomalies, and central nervous system malformations including hydrocephalus.[31] Microtia is rare as an isolated anomaly yet appears commonly as part of the retinoic acid embryopathy.

Unlike vitamin A, isotretinoin is not stored in tissue. Therefore, a pregnancy after discontinuation of isotretinoin is not a risk as the drug is no longer detectable in serum 5 days after its ingestion.

Topical tretinoin (Retin-A) has not been associated with any teratogenic risk.[34]

Etretinate is used for psoriasis may well have a teratogenic risk similar to that of isotretinoin. Case reports of malformation, especially of the central nervous system,[35] have appeared, but the absolute risk is unknown. The half-life of several months makes levels cumulative, and the drug carries a warning to avoid pregnancy within 6 months of use.

The levels of vitamin A in prenatal vitamins (5,000 IU/day orally) have not been associated with any documented risk. Birth defects have been reported after exposure to levels of greater than 10,000 IU of vitamin A daily.

Psychoactive Drugs

There is no clear risk documented for most psychoactive drugs with respect to overt birth defects. However, effects of chronic use of these agents on the developing brain in humans are difficult to study, and so a conservative attitude is appropriate. Lack of overt defects does not exclude the possibility of behavioral teratogenesis.

Tranquilizers

Conflicting reports of the possible teratogenicity of the various tranquilizers, including meprobamate (Miltown) and chlordiazepoxide (Librium), have appeared, but in prospective studies no risk of anomalies has been confirmed.[36,37] In most clinical situations, the risk–benefit ratio does not justify the use of benzodiazepines in pregnancy. Perinatal use of diazepam (Valium) has been associated with hypotonia, hypothermia, and respiratory depression.

Lithium (Eskalith, Lithobid)

The risk of lithium exposure is less than previously estimated. A prospective study of 148 women exposed to lithium in the first trimester showed one fetus in the lithium-exposed group had Ebstein anomaly, and one infant in the control group had a ventricular septal defect. Lithium is not a major human teratogen but Ebstein's anomaly may be higher than in non-exposed controls.

Lithium is excreted more rapidly during pregnancy; thus, serum lithium levels should be monitored.

Two cases of polyhydramnios associated with maternal lithium treatment have been reported.[44,45] Because nephrogenic diabetes insipidus has been reported in adults taking lithium, the presumed mechanism of this polyhydramnios is fetal diabetes insipidus. Perinatal effects of lithium have been noted, including hypotonia, lethargy, and poor feeding in the infant.

It is usually recommended that drug therapy be changed in pregnant women on lithium to avoid fetal drug exposure. Tapering over 10 days will delay the risk of relapse.[46] However, discontinuing lithium is associated with a 70 percent chance of relapse of the affective disorder in 1 year as opposed to 20 percent in those who remain on lithium. Discontinuation of lithium may pose an unacceptable risk to women who have had significant affective instability. These women should be offered appropriate prenatal diagnosis with ultrasound, including fetal echocardiography.

Antidepressants

Amitriptyline (Elavil) is apparently safe for pregnancy. In the Michigan Medicaid study, 467 newborns were exposed during the first trimester, with no increased risk of birth defects.[48] In two studies of fluoxetine (Prozac), no increased risk of major malformations was found in 237 infants exposed in utero.

Anticoagulants

Warfarin (Coumadin) has been associated with chondrodysplasia punctata. The syndrome, occurring in about 5 percent of exposed pregnancies, includes nasal hypoplasia, bone stippling seen on radiologic examination, ophthalmologic abnormalities, and mental retardation. The ophthalmologic abnormalities and mental retardation may occur even with use only beyond the first trimester.[51]

The alternative drug, heparin, does not cross the placenta, and it should be the drug of choice for patients requiring anticoagulation. Therapy with 20,000 units/day for greater than 20 weeks has been associated with bone demineralization.[53] The risk of spine fractures was 0.7 percent with low-dose heparin and 3 percent with a high-dose regimen.[55] Heparin can also cause thrombocytopenia.

The risks of heparin during pregnancy may not be justified in patients with only a single episode of thrombosis in the past.[56,57] Certainly conservative measures should be recommended, such as elastic stockings and avoidance of prolonged sitting or standing.

In patients with cardiac valve prostheses, full anticoagulation is necessary, as low-dose heparin resulted in three valve thromboses (two fatal) in 35 mothers so treated.[58]

Thyroid and Antithyroid Drugs

Propylthiouracil (PTU) and methimazole (Tapazole) both cross the placenta and may cause mild fetal goiter. The goal of such therapy during pregnancy is to keep the mother slightly hyperthyroid to minimize fetal drug exposure.

The need for thyroxine increases in many women with primary hypothyroidism when they are pregnant, as reflected by an increase in serum thyrotropin (TSH) concentrations.[61] It is prudent to monitor thyroid function and to adjust the thyroid dose to maintain a normal TSH level.

Antineoplastic Drugs and Immunosuppressants

Methotrexate, a folic acid antagonist, is a human teratogen, causing multiple congenital anomalies, including cranial defects and malformed extremities. When low-dose oral methotrexate (7.5 mg/week) was used for rheumatoid disease in the first trimester, five full-term infants were normal, and three patients experienced spontaneous abortions.[73]

Azathioprine (Imuran) has been used by patients with renal transplants or systemic lupus erythematosus, and the frequency of anomalies was not increased.[72,74]

Of 67 infants exposed to cyclosporine (Sandimmune) in utero, there was no increased risk of anomalies.[75,76]

Eight malformed infants have resulted from first-trimester exposure to cyclophosphamide (Cytoxan), but these infants were also exposed to other drugs or radiation.[77]

Chloroquine (Aralen) is safe in doses used for malarial prophylaxis, and there was no increased incidence of birth defects among 169 infants exposed to 300 mg once weekly.[78] However, after exposure to larger anti-inflammatory doses (250 to 500 mg/day), two cases of cochleovestibular paresis were reported.[79]

When cancer chemotherapy is used during embryogenesis, there is an increased rate of spontaneous abortion and major birth defects. Later in pregnancy there is a greater risk of intrauterine growth restriction and stillbirth, and myelosuppression is often present in the infant.[81]

Antiasthmatics

Metaproterenol (Alupent) and Albutenol (Ventolin)

When albutenol and metaproterenol are given as topical aerosols for the treatment of asthma, the total dose absorbed is usually not significant. With oral or intravenous doses, however, the cardiovascular effects of the agents may result in decreased uterine blood flow. No teratogenicity has been reported.[64]

Cromolyn Sodium (Intal)

Cromolyn sodium may be administered in pregnancy, and the systemic absorption is minimal. Teratogenicity has not been reported.

Corticosteroids

When prednisone or prednisolone are maternally administered, the concentration of active compound in the fetus is less than 10 percent of that in the mother as they are inactivated by the placenta. Therefore, these agents are the drugs of choice for treating medical diseases such as asthma. Inhaled corticosteroids are also effective therapy, and very little drug is absorbed. When steroid effects are desired in the fetus, for example, to accelerate lung maturity, betamethasone (Celestone) and dexamethasone (Decadron) are preferred, as these are minimally inactivated by the placenta. In several hundred infants exposed to corticosteroids in the first trimester, no increase in abnormalities was noted.[64,74,75]

Antiemetics

Faced with a self-limited condition occurring at the time of organogenesis, the clinician is well advised to avoid the use of medications whenever possible and to encourage supportive measures initially.

Vitamin B₆

Vitamin B_6 (pyridoxine) 25 mg tid has been reported in two randomized placebo-controlled trials to be effective for treating the nausea and vomiting of pregnancy.[83,84] There was no evidence of teratogenicity.

Doxylamine

Doxylamine (Unisom) is an effective antihistamine for nausea in pregnancy and can be combined with vitamin B_6. Vitamin B_6 (25 mg) and Unisom (25 mg) at bedtime, and one-half of each in the morning and afternoon, is an effective combination.

Other Antiemetics

Although there are no teratogenic effects known for other antiemetics, much less information is available.

Meclizine (Bonine)

In one randomized placebo-controlled study, meclizine gave significantly better results than placebo.[86] Prospective clinical studies have provided no evidence that meclizine is teratogenic in humans.

Dimenhydrinate (Dramamine)

No teratogenicity has been noted with dimenhydrinate, but a 29 percent failure rate and a significant incidence of side effects, especially drowsiness, has been reported.[88]

Diphenhydramine (Benadryl)

In 595 patients treated in the Collaborative Perinatal Project, no teratogenicity was noted with diphenhydramine.[64] Drowsiness can be a problem.

Trimethobenzamide (Tigan)

The data about trimethobenzamide are conflicting. In 193 patients in the Kaiser Health Plan study,[87] there was a suggestion of increased congenital anomalies but no concentration of specific anomalies was observed in these children. In 340 patients in the Collaborative Perinatal Project,[64] no evidence for an association between this drug and malformations was found.

Phenothiazines

Chlorpromazine (Thorazine) has been shown to be effective in hyperemesis gravidarum, with the most important side effect being drowsiness. Teratogenicity does not appear to be a problem.

Ondansetron (Zofran)

Ondansetron is no more effective than promethazine and has not been evaluated for teratogenicity.[90]

Antihistamines and Decongestants

No increased risk of anomalies has been associated with most of the commonly used antihistamines, such as chlorpheniramine (Chlortrimeton). Loratadine (Claritin) has not been studied in human pregnancy. An association between exposure during the last 2 weeks of pregnancy to antihistamines in general and retrolental fibroplasia in premature infants has been reported.[93]

In the Collaborative Perinatal Project[64] an increased

risk of birth defects was noted with phenylpropanolamine (Entex LA) exposure in the first trimester. In one retrospective study, an increased risk of gastroschisis was associated with first-trimester pseudoephedrine (Sudafed) use.[94] Use of these drugs for trivial indications should be discouraged. If decongestion is necessary, topical nasal sprays will result in a lower dose to the fetus than systemic medication.

Patients should be educated that antihistamines and decongestants are only symptomatic therapy for the common cold and have no influence on the course of the disease. Other remedies should be recommended, such as use of a humidifier, rest, and fluids.

Antibiotics and Anti-infective Agents

Penicillins

Penicillin, ampicillin, and amoxicillin (Amoxil) are safe in pregnancy.

Cephalosporins

In a study of 5,000 Michigan Medicaid recipients, there was a suggestion of possible teratogenicity (25 percent increased birth defects) with cefaclor, cephalexin, and cephradine but not other cephalosporins.[97] Because other antibiotics that have been used extensively (e.g., penicillin, ampicillin, amoxicillin, erythromycin) have not been associated with an increased risk of congenital defects, they should be first-line therapy when such treatment is needed in the first trimester.

Sulfonamides

Among 1,455 human infants exposed to sulfonamides during the first trimester, no teratogenic effects were noted.[64] Sulfonamides cause no known damage to the fetus in utero, as the fetus can clear free bilirubin through the placenta. Sulfonamides compete with bilirubin for binding sites on albumin, thus raising the levels of free bilirubin in the serum and increasing the risk of hyperbilirubinemia in the neonate. For that reason, they are not the first choice in the third trimester.

Sulfamethoxazole with Trimethoprim (Bactrim, Septra)

Two small trials failed to show any increased risk of birth defects after first-trimester exposure to trimethoprim.[100,101] However, two studies have suggested an increased risk of cardiovascular defects after exposure in the first trimester,[102] so this is best avoided.

Sulfasalazine (Azulfidine)

Sulfasalazine is used for treatment of ulcerative colitis and Crohn disease due to its relatively poor oral absorption. However, it does cross the placenta, leading to fetal drug concentrations approximately the same as those of the mother, although both are low. No severe neonatal jaundice has been reported following maternal use of sulfasalazine even when the drug was given up to the time of delivery.[103]

Nitrofurantoin (Macrodantin)

No reports have linked the use of nitrofurantoin with congenital defects.

Tetracyclines

The tetracyclines readily cross the placenta and are firmly bound by chelation to calcium in developing bone and tooth structures. This produces brown discoloration of the deciduous teeth, hypoplasia of the enamel, and inhibition of bone growth.[106] The staining of the teeth takes place in the second or third trimester of pregnancy, while bone incorporation can occur earlier. Alternate antibiotics are currently recommended during pregnancy. First-trimester exposure to tetracyclines has not been found to have any teratogenic risk.

Aminoglycosides

Streptomycin and kanamycin have been associated with congenital deafness in approximately 2.3 percent of the offspring of mothers who took these drugs during pregnancy. Neuromuscular blockade may be potentiated by the combined use of aminoglycosides and curariform drugs; therefore, the dosages should be reduced appropriately. Potentiation of magnesium sulfate–induced neuromuscular weakness has also been reported in a neonate exposed to magnesium sulfate and gentamicin (Garamycin).[111]

No known teratogenic effect other than ototoxicity has been associated with the use of aminoglycosides in the first trimester.

Antituberculosis Drugs

There is no evidence of any teratogenic effect of isoniazid, *para*-aminosalicylic acid, rifampin (Rifadin), or ethambutol (Myambutol).

Erythromycin

No teratogenic risk of erythromycin has been reported. The transplacental passage of erythromycin is unpredictable, and so it is not an adequate therapy for syphilis in pregnancy.

Clindamycin (Cleocin)

Of 647 infants exposed to clindamycin in the first trimester, no increased risk of birth defects was noted.[119]

Quinolones

The quinolones (e.g., ciprofloxacin [Cipro], norfloxacin [Noroxin]) have a high affinity for bone tissue and cartilage and may cause arthralgia in children. However, no malformations or musculoskeletal problems were noted in 38 infants exposed in utero in the first trimester.[120]

Metronidazole (Flagyl)

Studies have failed to show any increase in the incidence of congenital defects among the newborns of mothers treated with metronidazole during early or late gestation.

Acyclovir (Zovirax)

The Acyclovir Registry has recorded 601 exposures during pregnancy, including 425 in the first trimester, with no increased risk of abnormalities in the infants.[124] The Centers for Disease Control and Prevention recommends that pregnant women with disseminated infection (e.g., herpes encephalitis, herpes hepatitis or varicella pneumonia) be treated with acyclovir.[125]

Lindane (Kwell)

After application of lindane to the skin, about 10 percent of the dose used can be recovered in the urine. Toxicity in humans after use of topical 1 percent lindane has been observed almost exclusively after misuse and overexposure to the agent. Although no evidence of specific fetal damage is attributable to lindane, the agent is a potent neurotoxin, and its use during pregnancy should be limited. Pregnant women should be cautioned about shampooing their children's hair, as absorption could easily occur across the skin of the

hands of the mother. An alternate drug for lice is usually recommended, such as pyrethrins with piperonyl
butoxide (Rid).

Antifungal Agents

Nystatin (Mycostatin) is poorly absorbed from intact
skin and mucous membranes, and topical use has not
been associated with teratogenesis.[107]

The imidazoles are absorbed in only small amounts
from the vagina. Clotrimazole (Lotrimin) or miconazole (Monistat) in pregnancy is not known to be associated with congenital malformations.

Drugs for Induction of Ovulation

In more than 2,000 exposures, no evidence of teratogenic risk of clomiphene (Clomid) has been noted,[127]
and the percentage of spontaneous abortions is close
to the expected rate. Although infants are often exposed to bromocriptine (Parlodel) in early pregnancy,
no teratogenic effects have been observed in more than
1,400 pregnancies.[128,129]

Mild Analgesics

Aspirin

There is no evidence of any teratogenic effect of aspirin
taken in the first trimester.[64] Aspirin in analgesic doses
does have significant perinatal effects, however, as it
inhibits prostaglandin synthesis. Uterine contractility
is decreased, and patients taking aspirin in analgesic
doses have delayed onset of labor, longer duration of
labor, and an increased risk of a prolonged pregnancy.[130] The ductus arteriosus may be constricted in
utero.

Aspirin also decreases platelet aggregation, which
can increase the risk of bleeding before as well as at
delivery. Platelet dysfunction has been described in
newborns within 5 days of ingestion of aspirin by the
mother.[131]

Acetaminophen (Tylenol, Datril)

Acetaminophen has shown no evidence of teratogenicity. The bleeding time is not prolonged with acetaminophen, in contrast to aspirin,[136] and the drug is not toxic
to the newborn.

Other Nonsteroidal Anti-inflammatory Agents

No evidence of teratogenicity has been reported for other nonsteroidal anti-inflammatory drugs (e.g., ibuprofen [Motrin, Advil], naproxen, [Naprosyn]). Chronic use may lead to oligohydramnios, constriction of the fetal ductus arteriosus, or neonatal pulmonary hypertension.

Propoxyphene (Darvon)

Propoxyphene is an acceptable alternative mild analgesic with no known teratogenicity.[64] It carries potential for narcotic addiction, similar to codeine.

Codeine

In the Collaborative Perinatal Project, no increased relative risk of malformations was observed in 563 codeine users.[64] Codeine can cause addiction and newborn withdrawal symptoms perinatally.

Smoking

Smoking has been associated with small size for gestational age and an increased prematurity rate.[139] The spontaneous abortion rate is up to twice that of nonsmokers. Abortions associated with maternal smoking tend to have a higher percentage of normal karyotypes and occur later than those with chromosomal aberrations[140] (see Ch. 14). The higher perinatal mortality rate associated with smoking is partly attributable to an increased risk of both abruptio placentae and placenta previa as well as premature and prolonged rupture of membranes. The risks of complications and of the associated perinatal loss rise with the number of cigarettes smoked. Discontinuation of smoking during pregnancy can reduce the risk of both pregnancy complications and perinatal mortality.

Alcohol

The fetal alcohol syndrome (FAS) has been reported in the offspring of alcoholic mothers and includes the features of gross physical retardation with onset prenatally and continuing after birth.[142] The diagnosis of FAS requires at least one characteristic from each of the following three categories:

1. Growth retardation before and/or after birth.
2. Facial anomalies.
3. Central nervous system dysfunction.

Among alcoholic mothers, perinatal deaths are about eight times more frequent. Growth restriction, microcephaly, and IQ below 80 are considerably more frequent than among controls.

Heavy drinking remains a major risk to the fetus, and reduction even in midpregnancy can benefit the infant. An occasional drink during pregnancy carries no known risk, but no level of drinking is known to be safe.

Marihuana

No teratogenic effect of marihuana has been documented. One study suggested a mean 73-g decrease in birth weight associated with marihuana use when urine assays were performed rather than on self-reporting.[150]

Cocaine

A serious difficulty in determining the effects of cocaine on the infant is the frequent presence of many confounding variables in the population using cocaine. These mothers often abuse other drugs, smoke, have poor nutrition, fail to seek prenatal care, and live under poor socioeconomic conditions. The neural systems likely to be affected by cocaine are involved in neurologic and behavioral functions that are not easily quantitated by standard infant development tests.

Cocaine-using women have a higher rate of spontaneous abortion than controls.[151] Studies have suggested an increased risk of congenital anomalies after first-trimester cocaine use,[152–154] particularly microcephaly.

Cocaine is a central nervous system stimulant and has marked vasoconstrictive effects. Abruptio placentae has been reported to occur immediately after nasal or intravenous administration.[151] Several studies have also noted increased stillbirths, preterm labor, premature birth, small size for gestational age, dysmorphic features, and neurobehavioral abnormalities in infants after cocaine use.[150–152,155,156]

Cocaine has also been reported to cause fetal disruption,[160] presumably due to interruption of blood flow to various organs. Bowel infarction has been noted with unusual ileal atresia and bowel perforation. Limb infarction has resulted in missing fingers, and central nervous system bleeding in utero may result in porencephalic cysts.

Narcotics

The goal of methadone maintenance is to bring the patient to a level of approximately 20 to 40 mg/day. The dose should be individualized at a level sufficient to minimize the use of supplemental illicit drugs, since they represent a greater risk to the fetus than do the higher doses of methadone required by some patients. Manipulation of the dose in women maintained on methadone should be avoided in the last trimester because of an association with increased fetal complications and in utero deaths attributed to fetal withdrawal in utero.[161]

The infant of the narcotic addict is at increased risk of abortion, prematurity, and growth restriction. Withdrawal should be watched for carefully in the neonatal period.

Caffeine

There is no evidence of teratogenic effects of caffeine in humans. There is still some conflicting evidence concerning the association between heavy ingestion of caffeine and increased pregnancy complications. Some studies suggest that heavy caffeine use is associated with low-birth-weight infants, spontaneous abortions, prematurity, and stillbirths.[162,163] However, these studies were not controlled for the concomitant use of tobacco and alcohol. In another report controlled for smoking, other habits, demographic characteristics, and medical history, no relationship was found between either low birth weight or short gestation and heavy coffee consumption.[164] Among pregnant women who consumed over 300 mg/day of caffeine, one study suggested an increase in term low-birth-weight infants (less than 2,500 g at greater than 36 weeks).[165] A recent prospective cohort study found no evidence that moderate caffeine use increased the risk of spontaneous abortion or growth retardation.[169]

Aspartame (NutraSweet)

The major metabolite of aspartame is phenylalanine,[170] which is concentrated in the fetus by active placental transport. Sustained high blood levels of phenylalanine in the fetus as seen in maternal phenylketonuria (PKU) are associated with mental retardation in the infant. Within the usual range of aspartame ingestion, peak phenylalanine levels do not exceed normal postprandial levels, and even with high doses phenylalanine concentrations are still very far below those associated with mental retardation. These responses have also been studied in women known to be carriers of PKU, and the levels are still normal. Thus it seems unlikely that use of aspartame in pregnancy would cause any fetal toxicity.

Drugs in Breast Milk

The dose to the infant of drugs in breast milk is usually approximately 1 to 2 percent of the maternal dose. This amount is usually so trivial that no adverse effects are noted. In the case of toxic drugs, however, any exposure may be inappropriate. If the mother has unusually high blood concentrations such as with increased dosage or decreased renal function, drugs may appear in higher concentrations in the milk. Also, drugs are eliminated more slowly in the infant with immature enzyme systems. As the benefits of breast-feeding are well known, the risk of drug exposure must be weighed against these benefits.

The American Academy of Pediatrics has reviewed drugs in lactation[173] and categorized the drugs as listed below.

Drugs Commonly Listed as Contraindicated During Breast-Feeding

Cytotoxic Agents

Cyclosporine (Sandimmune), doxorubicin (Adriamycin), and cyclophosphamide (Cytoxan) might cause immune suppression in the infant, although data are limited with respect to these and other cytotoxic agents.

After oral administration to a lactating patient with choriocarcinoma, methotrexate was found in milk in low levels. Most individuals would elect to avoid any exposure of the infant to this drug. However, in environments in which bottle feeding is rarely practiced and presents practical and cultural difficulties, therapy with this drug would not in itself appear to constitute a contraindication to breast-feeding.[174]

Bromocriptine (Parlodel)

This ergot alkaloid derivative has an inhibitory effect on lactation. However, in one report a mother taking 5 mg/day for a pituitary tumor was able to nurse her infant.[176]

Ergotamine (Ergomar)

This medication has been reported to be associated with vomiting, diarrhea, and convulsions in the infant in doses used in migraine medications. However, short-term ergot therapy in the postpartum period for uterine contractility is not a contraindication to lactation.

Lithium (Eskalith, Lithobid)

Lithium reaches one-third to one-half the therapeutic blood concentration in infants, who might develop lithium toxicity, with hypotonia and lethargy.[177,178]

Amphetamines

One report of 103 cases of exposure to amphetamines in breast milk noted no insomnia or stimulation in the infants.[179] However, amphetamines are concentrated in breast milk.

Radioactive Compounds That Require Temporary Cessation of Breast-Feeding

Radiopharmaceuticals require variable intervals of interruption of nursing to ensure that no radioactivity is detectable in the milk. Intervals generally quoted are, for gallium 67, 2 weeks; ^{131}I, 5 days; radioactive sodium, 4 days; and ^{99m}Tc, 24 hours. For reassurance, the milk may be counted for radioactivity before nursing is resumed.[180]

Drugs Whose Effects on Nursing Infants Are Unknown but May Be of Concern

Psychotropic drugs such as antianxiety, antidepressant, and antipsychotic agents may be of concern when given to nursing mothers for long periods. Although there are no data about adverse effects in infants exposed to these drugs via breast milk, they could theoretically alter central nervous system function.[173] Fluoxetine (Prozac) is excreted in breast milk at low levels.[181]

Temporary cessation of breast-feeding after a single dose of metronidazole (Flagyl) may be considered. Its half-life is such that interruption of lactation for 12 to 24 hours after single-dose therapy usually results in negligible exposure to the infant. Even if a woman continued to nurse, the infant would get a trivial dose.

Drugs Usually Compatible With Breast-Feeding

Narcotics, Sedatives, and Anticonvulsants

No evidence of adverse effect is noted with most of the sedatives, narcotic analgesics, and anticonvulsants.

Patients may be reassured that, in normal doses, carbamazepine (Tegretol),[182] phenytoin (Dilantin), magnesium sulfate, codeine, morphine, meperidine (Demerol), and diazepam (Valium) do not cause any obvious adverse effects in infants.[183]

Analgesics

Aspirin is transferred into breast milk in small amounts. The risk is related to high dosages (e.g., greater than 16 300-mg tablets per day), when the infant may get sufficiently high serum levels to affect platelet aggregation or even cause metabolic acidosis. No harmful effects of acetaminophen (Tylenol, Datril) have been noted.

Antihistamines and Phenothiazines

No harmful effects have been noted from antihistamines or phenothiazines, and they have not been found to affect milk supply. Decongestants should be avoided in women who are having trouble with milk supply.

Antihypertensives

Propranolol (Inderal) and atenolol (Tenormin) are excreted in breast milk, at approximately 1 percent of the maternal dose, an amount unlikely to cause any adverse effect.[192–194] Clonidine (Catapres) concentrations in milk are almost twice maternal serum levels.[197] Neurologic and laboratory parameters in the infants of treated mothers are similar to those of controls. ACE inhibitors (e.g., captopril) and calcium channel blockers (e.g., nifedipine) are excreted in breast milk in low concentrations.

Anticoagulants

Most mothers requiring anticoagulation may continue to nurse their infants with no problems. Heparin does not cross into milk and is not active orally.

At a maternal dose of 5 to 12 mg/day, no warfarin was detected in infant breast milk or plasma. This low concentration is probably due to the fact that warfarin is 98 percent protein bound. Thus, with monitoring of neonatal prothrombin times to ensure lack of drug accumulation, warfarin may be safely administered to nursing mothers.

Corticosteroids

Breast-feeding is allowed in mothers taking corticosteroids as the nursing infant ingests only 0.1 percent

of the maternal dose, or less than 10 percent of its endogenous cortisol.[204]

Antibiotics

Penicillin derivatives are safe in nursing mothers. In
susceptible individuals or with prolonged therapy, diarrhea and candidiasis are theoretical concerns.

Dicloxacillin (Pathocil) is 98 percent protein bound.
If this drug is used to treat breast infections, very little
will get into the breast milk, and nursing may be continued.

Cephalosporins appear only in trace amounts in
milk, and the infant is exposed to less than 1 percent
of the maternal dose.

Tooth staining or delayed bone growth from tetracyclines have not been reported after the drug was taken
by a breast-feeding mother, due to the high binding of
the drug to calcium and protein, limiting its absorption
from the milk. The amount of free tetracycline available
is too small to be significant.

Sulfonamides only appear in small amounts in breast
milk and are ordinarily not contraindicated during
nursing. However, the drug is best avoided during the
first 5 days of life or in premature infants when hyperbilirubinemia may be a problem, as the drug may dis-
place bilirubin from binding sites on albumin. When a
mother took sulfasalazine (Azulfidine) 500 mg every 6
hours, the drug was undetectable in all milk samples.

Gentamicin (Garamycin) is transferred into breast
milk, and half of nursing newborn infants have the drug
detectable in their serum. The low levels detected
would not be expected to cause clinical effects.[207]

Nitrofurantoin (Macrodantin) is excreted into breast
milk in very low concentrations. In one study the drug
could not be detected in 20 samples from mothers receiving 100 mg four times a day.[208]

Erythromycin and azithromycin (Zithromax) are excreted into breast milk in small amounts, and no reports of adverse effects on infants have been noted.

Key Points

- Infants of epileptic women taking anticonvulsants
  have double the rate of malformations of unexposed
  infants; the risk of fetal hydantoin syndrome is less
  than 10 percent.
- The risk of malformations after in utero exposure to
  isotretinoin is 25 percent, and an additional 25 percent of infants have mental retardation.

- Heparin is the drug of choice for anticoagulation during pregnancy, although there is some risk of osteoporosis from its use.
- Angiotensin-converting enzyme inhibitors can cause fetal renal failure in the second and third trimesters, leading to oligohydramnios, craniofacial deformities, and hypoplastic lungs.
- Vitamin B_6 25 mg tid is a safe and effective therapy for first-trimester nausea and vomiting; doxylamine (Unisom) is also effective in combination with B_6.
- Most antibiotics are generally safe in pregnancy. Trimethoprim may carry an increased risk in the first trimester, and tetracyclines cause tooth discoloration in the second and third trimesters. Aminoglycosides can cause fetal ototoxicity.
- Aspirin in analgesic doses inhibits platelet function and prolongs bleeding time; alternate analgesics such as acetaminophen are preferred in pregnancy.
- Fetal alcohol syndrome occurs in infants of mothers drinking heavily during pregnancy. A safe level of alcohol intake during pregnancy has not been determined.
- Cocaine has been associated with increased risk of spontaneous abortions, abruptio placentae, and congenital malformations, in particular microcephaly.
- Most drugs are safe during lactation, as subtherapeutic amounts appear in breast milk (approximately 1 to 2 percent of the maternal dose). Lithium is a notable exception.

Chapter 3

Genetic Counseling and Prenatal Diagnosis

Joe Leigh Simpson

Approximately 3 percent of liveborn infants have a major congenital anomaly. Genetic factors are usually responsible. In addition, more than 50 percent of first-trimester spontaneous abortions and at least 5 percent of stillborn infants show chromosomal abnormalities (see Ch. 14).

This chapter first considers the principles of genetic counseling and genetic screening. Thereafter, disorders amenable to genetic screening and prenatal diagnosis are discussed.

Frequency of Genetic Disease

Phenotypic variation—normal or abnormal—may be considered in terms of several etiologic categories: (1) chromosomal abnormalities, numerical or structural; (2) single-gene or mendelian disorders; (3) polygenic and multifactorial disorders, polygenic implying an etiology resulting from cumulative effects of more than one gene and multifactorial implying interaction as well with environmental factors; and (4) teratogenic disorders, caused by exposure to exogenous factors (e.g., drugs) that deleteriously affect an embryo otherwise destined to develop normally.

Chromosomal Abnormalities

The incidence of chromosomal aberrations is 1/160. Table 3-1 shows the incidences of individual abnormalities.[2]

Single-Gene Disorders

Approximately 1 percent of liveborns are phenotypically abnormal due to a single-gene mutation. Several

Table 3-1 Chromosomal Abnormalities
in Liveborn Infants

Type of Abnormality	Incidence[a]
Numerical aberrations	
Sex chromosomes	
47, XYY	1/1,000 MB
47, XXY	1/1,000 MB
Other (males)	1/1,350 MB
47, X	1/10,000 FB
47, XXX	1/1,000 FB
Other (females)	1/2,700 FB
Autosomes	
Trisomies	
13–15 (D group)	1/20,000 LB
16–18 (E group)	1/8,000 LB
21–22 (G group)	1/800 LB
Other	1/50,000 LB
Structural aberrations	
Balanced	
Robertsonian	
t(DqDq)	1/1,500 LB
t(DqGq)	1/5,000 LB
Reciprocal translocations and insertional inversions	1/7,000 LB
Unbalanced	
Robertsonian	1/14,000 LB
Reciprocal translocations and insertional inversions	1/8,000 LB
Inversions	1/50,000 LB
Deletions	1/10,000 LB
Supernumeraries	1/5,000 LB
Other	1/8,000 LB
Total	1/160 LB

[a] LB, live births; MB, male births; FB, female births

Pooled data tabulated by Hook EB, Hamerton JL: The frequency of chromosome abnormalities detected in consecutive newborn studies—differences between studies—results by sex and by severity of phenotypic involvement. p. 63. In Hook EB, Porter IH (eds): Population Cytogenetic Studies in Humans. Academic Press, San Diego 1977, with permission.

thousand single-gene (mendelian) disorders have been recognized, and many more are suspected.[3] However, even the most common mendelian disorders (cystic fibrosis in whites, sickle cell anemia in blacks, β-thalassemia in Greeks and Italians, α-thalassemia in Southeast Asians, Tay-Sachs disease in Ashkenazi Jews) are individually rare. In aggregate, however, mendelian disorders account for 40 percent of the congenital defects seen in liveborn infants.

Polygenic/Multifactorial Disorders

Another 1 percent of neonates are abnormal but possess a normal chromosomal complement and have not undergone mutation at a *single* genetic locus. As will be discussed below, it can be deduced that several different genes are involved (polygenic/multifactorial inheritance).[1] Disorders in this etiologic category include most common malformations limited to a single organ system. These include hydrocephaly, anencephaly, and spina bifida (neural tube defects), facial clefts (cleft lip and palate), cardiac defects, pyloric stenosis, omphalocele, hip dislocation, uterine fusion defects, and clubfoot. After the birth of one child with such anomalies, the recurrence risk in subsequent progeny is usually 1 to 5 percent.[1] This frequency is less than would be expected if only a single gene were responsible but greater than that for the general population. The recurrence risks for malformations are also 1 to 5 percent for offspring of affected parents. That recurrence risks are similar for both siblings and offspring diminishes the likelihood that environmental causes are the exclusive etiologic factor because it is unlikely that households in different generations would be exposed to the same teratogen. Further excluding environmental factors as sole etiologic agents are observations that monozygotic twins are much more often concordant (similarly affected) than are dizygotic twins, despite both types of twins sharing a common intrauterine environment.

The above observations are best explained on the basis of polygenic/multifactorial inheritance. Although more than one gene is involved, only a few genes are necessary to produce the number of genotypes necessary to explain recurrence risks of 1 to 5 percent. That is, large numbers of genes and complex mechanisms need *not* be invoked. Polygenic/multifactorial etiology can thus plausibly be assumed responsible for most liveborns who have an anomaly of a single organ system and who have neither a chromosomal abnormality nor a mendelian mutation.

Teratogenic Disorders

Perhaps 15 to 20 proved teratogens are known. Although many other agents are suspected teratogens, the quantitative combination of known teratogens to the incidence of anomalies seems relatively small (with the possible exception of alcohol).

Genetic History

All obstetrician/gynecologists must attempt to determine whether a couple, or anyone in their family, has a heritable disorder or is at increased risk for abnormal offspring. To address this question, some obstetricians find it helpful to elicit genetic information through the use of questionnaires or checklists that are often constructed in a manner that requires action only for positive responses.

One should inquire into the health status of first-degree relatives (siblings, parents, offspring), second-degree relatives (nephews, nieces, aunts, uncles, grandparents), and third-degree relatives (first cousins, especially maternal). Adverse reproductive outcomes such as repetitive spontaneous abortions, stillbirths, and anomalous liveborn infants should be pursued. Couples having such histories should undergo chromosomal studies in order to exclude balanced translocations. Genetic counseling may prove sufficiently complex to warrant referral to a clinical geneticist, or it may prove simple enough for the well-informed obstetrician to manage. If a birth defect exists in a second-degree relative (uncle, aunt, grandparent, nephew, niece) or third-degree relative (first cousin), the risk for that anomaly will usually not prove substantially increased over that in the general population.

Parental ages should also be recorded. Advanced maternal age (Table 3-2) warrants discussion irrespective of a physician's personal convictions regarding pregnancy termination, as knowledge of an abnormality may affect obstetric management. Ethnic origin should be recorded to exclude disorders noted in Table 3-3. Incidentally, the above applies for both gamete donors and couples achieving pregnancy by natural means.

Genetic Screening

Genetic screening implies routine monitoring for the presence or absence of a given condition in apparently normal individuals. Screening is now offered routinely for (1) all individuals of certain ethnic groups to identify those individuals heterozygous for a given autosomal recessive disorder (Table 3-3), (2) all pregnant women to detect elevated maternal serum α-fetoprotein (MSAP) for diagnosis of fetal neural tube defects

Table 3-2   Maternal Age and Chromosomal
Abnormalities (Live Births)[a]

Maternal Age	Risk for Down Syndrome	Risk for Any Chromosome Abnormalities
20	1/1,667	1/526[b]
21	1/1,667	1/526[b]
22	1/1,429	1/500[b]
23	1/1,429	1/500[b]
24	1/1,250	1/476[b]
25	1/1,250	1/476[b]
26	1/1,176	1/476[b]
27	1/1,111	1/455[b]
28	1/1,053	1/435[b]
29	1/1,000	1/417[b]
30	1/952	1/384[b]
31	1/909	1/385[b]
32	1/769	1/322[b]
33	1/625	1/317[b]
34	1/500	1/260
35	1/385	1/204
36	1/294	1/164
37	1/227	1/130
38	1/175	1/103
39	1/137	1/82
40	1/106	1/65
41	1/82	1/51
42	1/64	1/40
43	1/50	1/32
44	1/38	1/25
45	1/30	1/20
46	1/23	1/15
47	1/18	1/12
48	1/14	1/10
49	1/11	1/7

[a] Because sample size for some intervals is relatively small, confidence limits are sometimes relatively large. Nonetheless, these figures are suitable for genetic counseling.

[b] 47,XXX excluded for ages 20–33 (data not available).

Data from Hook EB: Rates of chromosomal abnormalities of different maternal ages. Obstet Gynecol 58:282, 1981 and Hook EB, Cross PK, Schreinemachers DM et al: Chromosomal abnormality rates at amniocentesis and liveborn infants. JAMA 249:2043, 1983, with permission.

Table 3-3   Genetic Screening in Various Ethnic Groups[a]

Ethnic Group	Disorder	Screening Test	Definitive Test
Ashkenazi Jews	Tay-Sachs disease	Decreased serum hexosamidase-A, possibly molecular analysis	Chorionic villus sampling (CVS) or amniocentesis for assay of hexosamidase-A or possibly direct molecular analysis
Blacks	Sickle cell anemia	Presence of sickle cell hemoglobin, confirmatory hemoglobin electrophoresis	CVS or amniocentesis for genotype determination (direct molecular analysis)
Mediterranean people	β-Thalassemia	Mean corpuscular volume (MCV) <80%, followed by hemoglobin electrophoresis	CVS or amniocentesis for genotype determination (direct molecular analysis or RFLP linkage analysis)
Southeast Asians and Chinese (Vietnamese, Laotian, Cambodian, Filipinos)	α-Thalassemia	MCV <80%, followed by hemoglobin electrophoresis	CVS or amniocentesis for genotype determination (direct molecular studies) (direct or RFLP linkage analysis)
Northern European whites	Cystic fibrosis (CF)	DNA analysis of CF gene for at least ΔF508 mutation and next 20 or more most common mutations	CVS or amniocentesis for genotype determination, definitive diagnosis on fetuses may not be possible

[a] Cystic fibrosis screening is recommended but not yet considered standard.

(NTDs), (3) all pregnant women 35 years of age and above to undergo invasive tests and to detect Down syndrome, and (4) all pregnant women *under* age 35 years to undergo maternal serum screening to detect Down syndrome.

MSAFP Screening for Neural Tube Defects

Relatively few NTDs (5 percent) occur in families who have had previously affected offspring. Thus a method other than a positive family history is needed to identify couples in the general population at risk for a child with an NTD. MSAFP serves this purpose, identifying couples with a negative family history who nonetheless have sufficient risk to justify amniocentesis.

MSAFP is greater than 2.5 multiples of the median (MOM) in 80 to 90 percent of pregnancies in which the fetus has an NTD. Because considerable overlap exists between MSAFP in normal pregnancies and MSAFP in pregnancies characterized by a fetus with an NTD, systematic protocols for evaluating elevated MSAFP values are necessary. Elevated MSAFP occurs for reasons other than an NTD: (1) underestimation of gestational age, inasmuch as MSAFP increases as gestation progresses; (2) multiple gestation (60 percent of twins and almost all triplets produce MSAFP values that would be elevated if judged on the basis of singleton values); (3) fetal demise, presumably due to fetal blood extravasating into the maternal circulation; (4) Rh isoimmunization, cystic hygroma, and other conditions associated with fetal edema; and (5) anomalies other than NTD, usually characterized by edema or skin defects.

The initial MSAFP assay should be performed at 15 to 20 weeks' gestation. Corrections for maternal weight and some other factors are necessary, using various algorithms. Values between 2.0 and 2.5 MOM are usually considered elevated. The precise value above which MSAFP is considered elevated is less important than setting a consistent policy per program. Values above 2.0 MOM are definitely considered elevated in insulin-dependent diabetic women, but in twin gestations MSAFP is judged abnormal only at 4.5 to 5.0 MOM or greater.

Approximately 5 percent of women will have an elevated MSAFP value. If gestational age assessment is determined accurately before MSAFP sampling, the number of women having an abnormal serum value will be lower (3 percent). There is virtue in reassaying MSAFP if the value lies between 2.50 and 2.99 MOM and if gestational age is 18 weeks or less. Ultrasound is ob-

Table 3-4   Likelihood of Having a Fetus with NTD After Various Stages of an MSAFP Screening Program

Time	Risk
Before MSAFP	1/1,000
After one elevated MSAFP	1/50
Before sonogram	1/30
Before amniocentesis	1/15
Amniotic fluid AFP > 5 SD	1/2.2[a]
Acetylcholinesterase present	1/1.1

[a] Approximately equal number of other serious abnormalities or fetal demise.

viously required to exclude erroneous gestational age, multiple gestations, or fetal demise. Amniocentesis for AFP and acetylcholinesterase (AChE) is necessary if no explanation for elevated MSAFP is evident on ultrasound. The presence of AChE indicates an open NTD or other anomalies.

MSAFP screening identifies 90 percent of anencephaly and 80 to 85 percent of spina bifida, albeit at the cost of 1 to 2 percent of all pregnant women undergoing amniocentesis. Approximately 1/15 women having an unexplained elevated serum AFP will prove to have a fetus with an NTD (Table 3-4). Not well appreciated is that sensitivity of detecting an NTD in twin gestations is less than in singleton gestations, being only about 30 percent for spina bifida given a threshold of 4.5 MOM. The poor sensitivity exists because twins are usually discordant for an NTD. Liberal use of comprehensive ultrasound is recommended in twin gestations.

Some physicians recommend comprehensive ultrasound immediately after elevated MSAFP. Thus amniocentesis would not be performed in the absence of ultrasound evidence of an NTD. Although logical, the sensitivity of NTD detection cannot yet be assumed to be as high as with MSAFP followed by amniocentesis.

Maternal Serum Screening for Identifying Younger Women at Increased Risk for a Fetus with Trisomy

In addition to the association between low MSAFP and Down syndrome, an association exists for other analytes. The analyte having the greatest discriminatory value is human chorionic gonadotropin (hCG), which is elevated in Down syndrome pregnancies.[8] In the second trimester either intact hCG or free β-hCG will suffice for assay. The combination of hCG, MSAFP, and maternal age when analyzed with appropriate software allows detection of some 60 percent of cases of Down syndrome with an associated amniocentesis rate of no more than 5 percent.[9] Less certain is the usefulness of unconjugated serum estriol and inhibin, analytes that if present in low values are associated with Down syndrome.

Several years after maternal serum screening for the detection of NTDs was introduced, it became clear that a low MSAFP level was associated with trisomy 21.[7] Maternal serum screening is now offered to women under the age of 35 for detection of Down syndrome. Values may be sufficiently high that women who are not otherwise candidates for invasive procedures like amniocentesis or chorionic villus sampling (CVS) might wish to undergo such. This proposition is attractive because only 25 percent of infants with Down syndrome are born to women ages 35 and above. Thus decreasing the population incidence requires identifying younger women at sufficient risk to justify an invasive procedure.

The sensitivity of detecting Down syndrome is age dependent. Detection rates are 90 percent for women ages 35 and above but less than 25 percent for those in their early third decade. Moreover, utilization of this approach for the detection of Down syndrome in twin gestations is not standard.

Trisomy 18 is associated with low hCG. One can offer an invasive procedure (amniocentesis) whenever the serum values are at or below each of these three thresholds: MSAFP ≤0.6 MOM, hCG ≤0.55 MOM, unconjugated estriol ≤0.5 MOM.[10]

The ACOG recommended women under the age of 35 years be counseled about maternal serum screening to detect Down syndrome.[11] Women ages 35 years and above should continue to be offered invasive procedures. If older women insist on maternal serum screening in lieu of an invasive procedure, they must appreciate that detection is not 100 percent but only 90 percent. Finally, early evidence appears quite strong that first trimester analytes will also detect Down syndrome. Associations exist between Down syndrome and low MSAFP, low PAPP-A, and elevated free β-hCG.[12]

Diagnostic Procedures for Prenatal Genetic Diagnosis

Amniocentesis

Technique

In amniocentesis, amniotic fluid is aspirated, often for the purpose of genetic diagnosis at 15 to 16 weeks' gestation (menstrual weeks). While the procedure has traditionally been performed at 15 to 16 weeks, it can be performed earlier (especially 12 to 14 weeks).[13] A 22-gauge spinal needle with stylet is usually employed. Ultrasound examination is obligatory in order to determine gestational age, placental position, location of amniotic fluid, and number of fetuses. Ultrasound should be performed concurrently with amniocentesis. Rh-immune globulin should be administered to the Rh-negative, Du-negative, unsensitized patient.

In multiple gestations, amniocentesis can usually be performed on all fetuses. Following aspiration of amniotic fluid from the first sac, 2 to 3 ml of indigo carmine, diluted 1:10 in bacteriostatic water, is injected before the needle is withdrawn. A second amniocentesis is then performed at a site determined after visualizing the membranes separating the two sacs. It is important to note the locations of each sac in case selective termination is later required. Aspiration of clear fluid confirms that the second (new) sac was entered. Triplets and other multiple gestations can be managed similarly, sequentially injecting dye into successive sacs. Some obstetricians aspirate the second sac without dye injection or use a single puncture technique; however, I still prefer dye injection for confirmation.

After amniocentesis, the patient may resume all normal activities. Common sense dictates that strenuous exercise such as jogging or "aerobic" exercise be deferred for a day or so. The patient should report persistent uterine cramping, vaginal bleeding, leakage of amniotic fluid, or fever; however, physician intervention is almost never required, unless overt abortion occurs.

If only one fetus in a multiple gestation is abnormal, parents should be prepared to choose between aborting all fetuses or continuing the pregnancy with one or more normal and one abnormal fetuses. Selective termination in the second trimester is possible, but success of this procedure is greater in the first trimester.[14]

Safety of Traditional Amniocentesis

Any procedure that involves entering the pregnant uterus logically carries risk to the fetus. Amniocentesis is no exception. Amniocentesis carries potential danger to both mother and fetus. Maternal risks are quite low, with symptomatic amnionitis occurring only rarely (0.1 percent). Minor maternal complications such as transient vaginal spotting or minimal amniotic fluid leakage occur in 1 percent or fewer of cases, but almost always these are self-limited in nature. Other very rare complications include intra-abdominal viscus injury or hemorrhage.

The risk of pregnancy loss secondary to amniocentesis is 0.5 percent, or perhaps slightly less. At the author's medical center, serious maternal complications and fetal injuries are stated to be "remote" risks. Concurrent ultrasound is now recommended, but its utilization should not be assumed to decrease risks much below 0.5 percent.

Safety of Early Amniocentesis

Amniocentesis at 13 to 14 weeks' gestation should be a relatively safe and efficacious technique. However, reported data cannot yet support the claim that early amniocentesis is equal in safety to traditional amniocentesis. Contentions that procedure-related risks for early amniocentesis are comparable to traditional amniocentesis or even to CVS must be viewed with caution.

Amniocentesis should not be performed earlier than 12 weeks because of the risk (1–2%) of fetal talipes equinovarus.

Chorionic Villus Sampling

CVS allows prenatal diagnosis in the first trimester to permit pregnancy termination early in gestation and also protect patient privacy. Both chorionic villi analysis and amniotic fluid cell analysis offer the same information concerning chromosomal status, enzyme levels, and DNA patterns. The one major difference is that assays requiring amniotic fluid, specifically MSAFP, necessitate amniocentesis.

Technique

CVS can be performed by transcervical, transabdominal, or transvaginal approaches. *Transcervical* CVS is usually performed with a flexible polyethylene catheter that encircles a metal obturator extending just distal to the catheter tip. The outer diameter is usually about 1.5 mm. Introduced through the cervical os (Fig. 3-1), the catheter/obturator is directed toward the trophoblastic tissue surrounding the gestational sac. After withdrawal of the obturator, 10 to 25 mg of villi are aspirated by negative pressure into a 20- or 30-ml syringe containing tissue culture media. The optimal time for transcervical sampling is 10 to 12 completed gestational weeks, but the procedure can be performed later in pregnancy.

In *transabdominal* chorionic villus sampling (Fig. 3-2), concurrent ultrasound is used to direct an 18- or

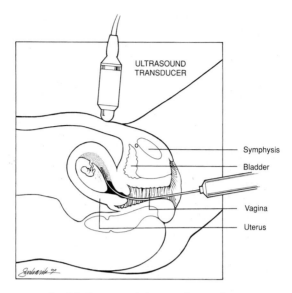

Fig. 3-1 Transcervical chorionic villus sampling.

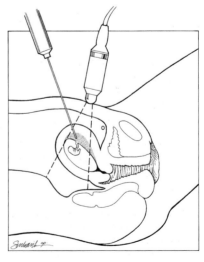

Fig. 3-2 Transabdominal chorionic villus sampling.

20-gauge spinal needle into the long axis of the placenta. After removal of the stylet, villi are aspirated into a 20-ml syringe containing tissue culture media.

Safety of Chorionic Villus Sampling

Pregnancy Losses

The U.S. Cooperative Clinical Comparison of Chorionic Villus Sampling and Amniocentesis study[25] and the Canadian Collaborative CVS-Amniocentesis Trial Group study[26] have reported that pregnancy loss rates after CVS are no different from loss rates after amniocentesis. In the U.S. study,[25] 2,278 women self-selected transcervical CVS; 671 women similarly recruited in the first trimester selected amniocentesis. Randomization did not prove possible. The excess loss rate in the CVS group was 0.8 percent, not statistically significant. In a Canadian randomized study,[26] 1,391 subjects were assigned to transcervical CVS and 1,396 to amniocentesis. The excess loss rate in the former was also 0.8 percent and again not statistically different. Variables shown to influence fetal loss rates adversely in CVS include fundal location of the placenta, number of catheter passages, small sample size, and prior bleeding during the current pregnancy. All except the last are surrogates for technical difficulty. The frequency of intrauterine growth retardation, placental abruption, and premature delivery are no higher in women undergoing CVS than expected in the general population.[27]

Transcervical CVS and transabdominal CVS appear to be equally safe procedures.[28]

Limb Reduction Defects

Controversy about the safety of CVS has more recently shifted focus from concerns about the risk of fetal loss to its being the possible cause for congenital abnormalities. In 1991, Firth and colleagues[37] reported that 5/289 (1.7 percent or 17/1,000) infants exposed to CVS between 56 and 66 days of gestation (i.e., 42 to 50 days after fertilization) had severe limb reduction deformities (LRDs). There quickly followed a number of reports both supporting and refuting such an association.[38–41]

A World Health Organization study group has continued to analyze data collected through an international registry.[48] Pattern analysis of the types of limb defects and overall frequencies of specific LRD were compared with the background population study from British Columbia.[49] Both the types of limb defects and overall incidences were the same in the CVS group and the general population.

At Baylor College of Medicine, we avoid performing CVS under 10 weeks' gestation and further consider it prudent to counsel patients about the LRD controversy. We state that the absolute risk at 10 to 12 weeks is believed to be very low, perhaps 1/3,000 if any increase in risk exists. We also stress that the risk be placed in proper perspective, weighed against the substantial advantages that first-trimester prenatal diagnosis with CVS offers.

Fetal Blood Sampling

The technique most commonly used for fetal blood sampling is ultrasound-directed PUBS. The procedure can be safely undertaken from 18 weeks onward, although successful procedures have been reported as early as 12 weeks.[51] Due to its fixed position, the placental cord root is usually the site of choice whenever it is clearly visible. Alternatively, free loops of cord or the intrahepatic vein are possibilities.[50,51] The spinal needle is inserted into the fetal umbilical cord under direct ultrasound guidance, and a small amount of blood is aspirated.

Fetal blood sampling appears to be relatively safe when performed by experienced physicians, albeit carrying more risk than CVS or amniocentesis. Maternal complications are rare, but include amnionitis and transplacental hemorrhage. Collaborative data from 14 North American centers, sampling 1,600 patients at varying gestational ages and for a variety of indications, revealed an uncorrected fetal loss rate of 1.6 percent.[51] However, no studies directly comparing loss rates in control and treated groups have been published. Assessment is also difficult because loss rates for fetuses subjected to PUBS vary greatly by the indication for the procedure. Loss rates for fetuses with ultrasound-detected anomalies are far greater than for fetuses being evaluated because of maternal blood group sensitization or for suspicion of chromosomal mosaicism.

Indications for Prenatal Genetic Studies

Cytogenetic Disorders

Every chromosomal disorder is potentially detectable in utero. It is not appropriate, however, to perform amniocentesis or CVS in every pregnancy because for many couples the risk of an invasive procedure outweighs diagnostic benefits.

Advanced Maternal Age and Abnormal Maternal Serum Analysis

The most common indication for antenatal cytogenetic studies is advanced maternal age. The incidence of trisomy 21 is 1/800 liveborn births in the United States, but the frequency increases with maternal age (Table 3-2). Trisomy 13, trisomy 18, 47,XXX, and 47,XXY also increase with advanced maternal age.

For approximately 20 years it has been standard medical practice in the United States to offer invasive chromosomal diagnosis to all women who at their expected delivery date will be 35 years or older. The choice of age 35 is largely arbitrary, however, having been chosen during an interval when risk figures were available only in 5-year intervals (i.e., 30 to 34 years, 35 to 39 years, 40 to 44 years). Flexibility is thus appropriate when answering inquiries from women younger than 35 years, for indeed increasing numbers of women age 33 or 34 years seek prenatal diagnosis.

The risk figures shown in Table 3-2 are applicable only for liveborns. The prevalence of abnormalities at the time when CVS or amniocentesis is performed is somewhat higher.[55,56] For example, the risk for a 35-year-old woman is 1/270 for Down syndrome at the time of amniocentesis (midtrimester). (In maternal serum screening for Down syndrome reports state risks at the time of screening, i.e., second trimester.) That the frequency of chromosomal abnormalities is lower in liveborn infants than in first- or second-trimester fetuses is due to the disproportionate likelihood that fetuses lost spontaneously have chromosomal abnormalities. That is, some abnormal fetuses would have died in utero had iatrogenic intervention not occurred in the second trimester. In fact, 5 percent of stillborn infants show chromosomal abnormalities (see Ch. 14).

Maternal serum screening is now recommended for women under age 35 years to detect couples at sufficient risk for a child with fetal trisomy to justify invasive procedures.[11] The logical corollary might be that a normal or slightly elevated MSAFP level decreases the risk of aneuploidy in infants of older women to the extent that amniocentesis could be avoided. British workers in particular recommend against amniocentesis in older women (35 to 37 years) having normal or slightly increased MSAFP values.[57] However, most U.S. authorities do not agree because of the potential legal hazard and because detection rates are not 100 percent but only 90 percent. In many other countries serum screening is offered to women of all ages.[58] If an older woman wishes to undergo maternal serum screening in lieu of an invasive test she should also be informed that sensitivity to detect abnormalities is even less by ultrasound screening.[59]

Previous Child With Chromosomal Abnormality

After the occurrence of one child or abortus with autosomal trisomy, the likelihood that subsequent progeny will also have autosomal trisomy is increased, even if parental chromosomal complements are normal. Recurrence risks are perhaps 1 percent.[60] The risk is not so high as once believed, but antenatal chromosomal studies should be offered for couples having a prior trisomic pregnancy.

Recurrence risk data following the birth of a liveborn infant trisomic for a chromosome other than 21 are limited. Counseling that the risk is 1 percent for either the same or a different chromosomal abnormality seems appropriate.

Parental Chromosomal Rearrangements

An uncommon but important indication for prenatal cytogenetic studies is the presence of a parental chromosomal abnormality. A balanced translocation is the usual indication, but inversions and other chromosomal abnormalities exist. Empirical data invariably reveal that theoretical risks for abnormal (unbalanced) offspring are greater than empirical risks. Empirical risks approximate 12 percent for offspring of either male or female heterozygotes having reciprocal translocations.[61] For Robertsonian (centric fusion) translocations, risks vary according to the chromosomes involved. For t(14q;21q), risks are 10 percent for offspring of heterozygous mothers and 2 percent for offspring of heterozygous fathers (Fig. 3-3).[61] For other nonhomologous Robertsonian translocations, empirical risks for liveborns are less than 1 percent. For homologous translocations (e.g., 21q;21q), all liveborn offspring should have trisomy 21. For other homologous Robertsonian translocations (13q;13q or 22q; 22q), almost all pregnancies result in abortions.

Mendelian Disorders

Increasing numbers of mendelian disorders are now detectable in utero. DNA analysis now permits many diagnoses using any available nucleated cell (chorionic villi, amniotic fluid cells). The nature of the mutant or absent gene product need not necessarily even be

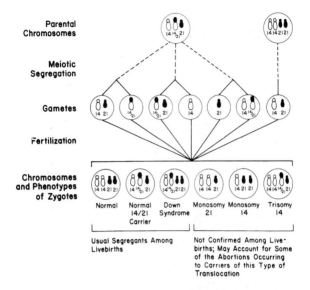

Fig. 3-3 Diagram of possible gametes and progeny of a phenotypically normal individual heterozygous for a Robertsonian translocation between chromosomes 14 and 21 (a form of D/G translocation). Three of the six possible gametes are incompatible with life. The likelihood that an individual with such a translocation would have a child with Down syndrome is theoretically 33 percent. However, the empirical risk is considerably less. (From Gerbie AT, Simpson JL: Antenatal diagnosis of genetic disorders. Postgrad Med 59:129, 1976, with permission.)

known. We can predict confidently that in the foreseeable future all common mendelian disorders will be detectable.

Inborn Errors of Metabolism

If an enzyme is expressed in amniotic fluid cells or chorionic villi, detection of a metabolic error is possible. This requirement is fulfilled by most metabolic disorders, a prominent exception being phenylketonuria (PKU). All metabolic disorders detectable in amniotic fluid have proved detectable as well in chorionic villi. Although cultured cells are usually necessary for diagnosis, occasionally one can arrive at a diagnosis on the basis of a product in amniotic fluid. The most prominent example is 17α-hydroxyprogesterone, an elevated value of which indicates adrenal 21-hydroxylase deficiency (congenital adrenal hyperplasia). This disorder can also be detected by analysis of linked human leukocyte antigen markers in nuclei obtained by CVS or amnio-centesis.[68]

Disorders Detectable by Molecular Methods

The power of molecular prenatal diagnosis is that any available nuclear cell can be utilized for diagnosis. All cells contain the same DNA, and the gene need not be expressed, unlike the situation when a gene product (enzyme protein) must be analyzed. Through molecular techniques developed within the last decade, many previously undetectable disorders have now become diagnosable.

To appreciate these advances, the obstetrician/gynecologist must be aware of the analytical techniques that made possible diagnosis by molecular methods. Pivotal was the discovery of *restriction endonucleases*. These bacterial enzymes recognize specific nucleotide sequences five to seven nucleotides in length and cut DNA only at those sites. Use of restriction enzymes permits DNA to be divided into fragments of reproducible lengths (Fig. 3-4).

In *Southern blotting*, agarose gel electrophoresis is used to separate DNA fragments by size, after exposure to restriction endonucleases. The DNA is then denatured and transferred from the agarose gel to a nitro-cellulose filter, on which specific fragments can be located by hybridization. Labeled strands of known DNA sequences act as probes, hybridizing a specific comple-

RESTRICTION ENDONUCLEASES

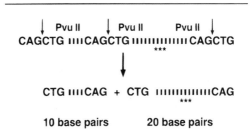

Fig. 3-4 Simplified diagram illustrating the manner in which a restriction endonuclease cuts DNA at a specific nucleotide sequence. PvuII recognizes the sequence CAGCTG and only that sequence. DNA is separated into fragments of different lengths on the basis of distances between restriction enzyme recognition sites. The further the distance between sites, the longer the length of intervening DNA (i.e., 20 versus 30 base pairs). Shorter DNA fragments (e.g., 20 base pairs) show greater mobility and migrate further on agarose gel.

mentary sequence from among the many DNA fragments on the filter. Fragments that contain the sequence that hybridizes with the probe can be detected as bands. Use of size standards facilitates determining whether a particular-sized fragment is or is not present.

A modification of this approach involves use of synthetic oligonucleotides 15 to 18 nucleotides in length, called *allele-specific oligonucleotides* (ASOs). An ASO is designed to hybridize to an unknown sample if and only if the latter is characterized by all 15 to 18 nucleotides. ASOs that recognize normal DNA and any known mutant sequence can be designed and used for "dot blot" DNA analysis or "slot blot" analysis.

Integral to facile diagnosis was development of the *polymerized chain reaction* (PCR) procedure. In PCR, a target sequence can be amplified severalfold (10^5 to 10^6).

If a disorder is known to be characterized by absence of DNA, one can determine whether a probe does or does not hybridize with the relevant sequence of DNA from an individual of unknown genotype. Failure of hybridization indicates that the individual lacks the DNA sequence in question; thus the disorder is assumed present. This approach is currently used to diagnose all forms of α-thalassemia, many cases of Duchenne/Becker muscular dystrophy, some cases of β-thalassemia, and some forms of hemophilia.

A second general approach becomes applicable if the molecular basis involves a point mutation whose nucleotide sequence is known. The most straightforward example is sickle cell anemia, in which the triplet (codon) designating the sixth amino acid has undergone a mutation from adenine to guanine. As a result, codon 6 connotes valine rather than glutamic acid, leading to the abnormal protein (β^s). Fortunately, several restriction enzymes recognize the normal DNA sequence at codons 5, 6, and 7. One could also construct ASOs designed to hybridize only if every single nucleotide is present. Use of a β^s oligonucleotide probe will confirm the specific mutant DNA sequence. Diagnosis with limited amounts of DNA can be achieved by the use of PCR amplification. A hybridized ASO usually appears as a "dot blot" (Fig. 3-5) or "slot blot."

For most mendelian disorders, many different molecular mutations are responsible (heterogeneity). This is the case for cystic fibrosis, hemophilia A and B, adult polycystic kidney disease, PKU, β-thalassemias, and others. Usually one molecular mutation is particularly common, and a limited number considerably less so but in aggregate accounting for a respectable proportion (10 to 15 percent) of mutations; innumerable other

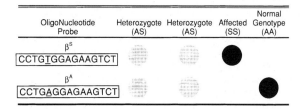

Fig. 3-5 Dot blot analysis. Oligonucleotides are constructed for sequences complementary to normal DNA (β^A) and mutant DNA (β^S). DNA challenged by the oligonucleotide probe will be hybridized if and only if the DNA contains all nucleotides connoted by the probe. Thus, AS individuals will respond to both β^A and β^S probes, whereas AA or SS individuals will respond only to one of the two probes (β^A and β^S, respectively). Homozygous individuals respond with a stronger (darker) signal than heterozygous individuals.

mutations are very rare, some almost unique. A common approach is to amplify the unknown DNA and test with multiple ASOs (multiplex PCR). An important caveat is that a mutation not corresponding to one of the mutations tested will pass unrecognized. Various techniques facilitate identifying all mutations, but all of these procedures are laborious and still incomplete. Despite the molecular revolution, a place often still exists for analysis of the gene product (protein or enzyme).

Diagnosis When the Molecular Basis Is Not Known

The molecular approaches described above are applicable only when the precise molecular basis of a disorder is known. Unfortunately, this requirement is fulfilled less often than one would desire. One reason is that certain genes may not yet be cloned and isolated. Even if the chromosomal location is known, an interval passes before the sequence is determined. A second reason is the considerable heterogeneity noted previously to exist at the molecular level. Mutations at multiple nucleotide sites within the gene can all produce a dysfunctional product. Given that genes are often very large, diagnostic complexities may be daunting. Sequencing the entire gene for every diagnostic situation is not practical, and even then the mutation might not be detected if it were located in a promoter region or involved in translation. If mutations occur in a more limited number of exons (coding sequences) within the gene, the problem is ameliorated but is not obviated.

The problem cited above can be addressed by linkage analysis, taking advantage of the ostensibly innocuous differences in DNA that exist among individuals in the general population. These differences are called *polymorphisms* and are analogous to such well-known polymorphisms as the ABO blood group locus. Clinically insignificant differences in DNA yield differences in DNA fragment lengths following exposure to a given restriction endonuclease. These differences are thus termed *restriction fragment length polymorphisms* (RFLPs). In linkage analysis a diagnosis is made not on the basis of analyzing the mutant gene per se but rather on the basis of presence or absence of a nearby marker. In RFLPs the marker is a DNA variant capable of being recognized following exposure to a given endonuclease. The marker could also be a dinucleotide or trinucleotide polymorphism. Throughout the genome there exist polymorphisms in which the number of nucleotide repeats (e.g., the dinucleotides cytosine and adenine, or CA) vary among individuals at a given locus. For example, some individuals may show 6 CA repeats, others 8, and others 10 at a given locus. The almost innumerable number of such polymorphisms underlies the scientific basis of DNA analysis being used for forensic pathology.

To illustrate the principle of linkage analysis, let us assume that a given RFLP or nucleotide repeat is known to lie close to or preferably within the mutant gene of interest. One next needs to deduce the relationship of the mutant to the status of the marker. Starting with an individual of known genotype, usually an affected fetus or child, one determines on which parental chromosome a given DNA marker is located (*cis–trans* relationship). Is the marker located on the chromosome carrying the mutant gene, and is it located on the chromosome carrying the normal gene?

There are pitfalls in linkage analysis using RFLP or nucleotide repeats. First, the marker may or may not be informative in a given family. If all family members show identical DNA fragment patterns at a given locus, that locus is obviously useless because affected and unaffected individuals cannot be distinguished from each other. If a given marker is uninformative, one searches for another marker that may prove informative. Fortunately, a potentially limitless number of markers exist. Second, the distance between the mutant gene and the marker is crucial because the likelihood of meiotic recombination is inversely related to this distance. Recall that during meiosis I recombination can occur between homologous chromosomes. Genes are linked to one another if, after meiosis I, they remain together more often than expected by chance. Recombination can occur even between closely linked loci; thus prenatal diagnosis based on linkage analysis is never 100 percent accurate. Using polymorphic markers on both sides of the mutant can minimize but not exclude the possibility of a recombinational event.

Neural Tube Defects

Failure of the neural tube to close during embryogenesis leads to anencephaly, spina bifida (myelomeningocele or meningocele), encephalocele, and other less common midline defects (e.g., lipomeningocele). Anencephaly is almost never compatible with long-term survival. Spina bifida is compatible with long-term survival, although it is frequently associated with hemiparesis, urinary incontinence, and hydrocephalus.

Anencephaly and spina bifida represent different manifestations of the same pathogenic process and reflect the same genetic etiology. Couples who have had a child with an NTD have approximately 1 percent risk for any subsequent offspring having spina bifida and 1 percent risk for subsequent offspring having anencephaly (2 percent for any NTD).[71] This holds true irrespective of the type of NTD present in the index case (proband). If a prospective parent has an NTD, the risk is also about 2 percent. Second-degree relatives (nieces, nephews, grandchildren) and third-degree relatives (first cousins) are less likely to be affected. A woman whose sister or brother had a child with an NTD carries a lower (0.5 to 1.0 percent) risk for offspring with an NTD.[40] For reasons that are unclear, risks are slightly lower if the father's sibling had an NTD.

Antenatal diagnosis of an NTD is best accomplished by amniotic fluid α-fetoprotein (AF-AFP) assay. Through AF-AFP analysis, diagnosis of an NTD is possible in all anencephaly cases and in all spina bifida cases except the 5 to 10 percent in which skin covers the lesion. Closed lesions are somewhat more common in encephaloceles. Ultrasonography by experienced physicians should readily exclude anencephaly, and spina bifida theoretically can be detected by serial views of the vertebral column and shape of the cranium, ventricles, cerebellum, and cisterna magna. Unfortunately, few ultrasonographers can state their sensitivity or specificity for detecting NTDs. Until such data are available, AF-AFP analysis should be considered the standard method for detecting an NTD despite frequent hopes and statements to the contrary.

AF-AFP may be spuriously elevated if the amniotic fluid is contaminated with fetal blood. This pitfall can be eliminated if AChE is assayed concurrently. AChE is present in the amniotic fluid of fetuses with open NTDs but is absent in normal amniotic fluid. If AChE is absent but fetal hemoglobin is present, the elevated AFP is probably due to fetal blood. Some confusion may arise if amniocentesis is performed earlier than 13 weeks.

Key Points

- The frequency of major birth defects is 2 to 3 percent. Major etiologic categories include chromosomal abnormalities (1/160 live births), single-gene or mendelian disorders, polygenic/multifactorial disorders, and teratogenic disorders. Of the chromosomal abnormalities, approximately half represent autosomal trisomy and half sex chromosomal abnormalities.

- Principles of genetic counseling include adequate communication, appreciation of psychologic defenses, and philosophy of nondirective counseling.

- Genetic screening in the nonpregnant population for heterozygote detection is appropriate for only selected autosomal recessive disorders: Tay-Sachs disease in Jewish populations, α-thalassemia in Orientals, β-thalassemia in Mediterranean peoples (Greek and Italian), sickle cell in blacks.

- In all pregnancies, genetic screening should be performed for chromosomal abnormalities and NTDs. All women ages 35 years and above at delivery should be offered prenatal cytogenetic diagnosis. For younger women, maternal serum screening should be offered to detect autosomal trisomies. The profile of decreased MSAFP, elevated hCG, and decreased unconjugated serum estriol and possibly other analytes favors Down syndrome. Maternal serum analyte screening in combination with maternal age can detect 60 percent of Down syndrome cases, but the frequency varies according to maternal age (90 percent over age 35 but less than 25 percent in the early third decade). Screening for NTDs involves elevated MSAFP followed by amniotic fluid analysis; approximately 80 to 90 percent of NTDs can be detected at a cost of 5 percent amniocentesis.

- All invasive procedures carry risks. Amniocentesis at 15 weeks and above carries a procedure-related risk of approximately 0.5 percent loss. Amniocentesis before this time has not been subjected to rigorous trials to determine safety. CVS is considered, in experienced hands, equal to amniocentesis in terms of loss rates and diagnostic accuracy. Both transcervical and transabdominal CVS are equal in safety. Availability of both procedures allows the physician to choose the most appropriate technique.

- Controversy exists concerning LRDs associated with CVS. If a risk exists, it appears to be greatest below 10 weeks of gestation, for which reason, in general, the procedure should generally be available at 10 weeks and beyond. A maximum limb reduction risk of 1/3,000 has been reported, and many believe that the risk is not greater than that of the general population. The rate of complications associated with fetal blood sampling is uncertain but appears to be 1 to 2 percent. However, this varies according to the diagnosis being assessed. No studies have directly compared loss rates in control and tested pregnancies.
- Many single-gene disorders are detectable. Some can be detected by enzymatic analysis, whereas others can be recognized best or only through molecular methodologies.
- Two principal types of molecular analysis are employed. Direct analysis is possible if the gene sequence is known. Linkage analysis is necessary if the gene has been localized but not yet sequenced. Linkage analysis takes advantage of markers lying close to the gene in question; accuracy is not 100 percent because recombination can occur between the marker and the mutant gene.

Obstetric Ultrasound: Assessment of Fetal Growth and Anatomy

Frank A. Chervenak and
Steven G. Gabbe

Diagnostic ultrasound is an important tool for antepartum fetal surveillance. This technology has permitted accurate assessment of gestational age and has enabled the obstetrician to follow fetal growth serially and detect fetal growth disorders.

Biophysics of Ultrasound

To use ultrasound most effectively, the obstetrician must understand the basic biophysics of the technique.[1] Sound is a waveform of energy that causes small particles in a medium to oscillate. The frequency of sound refers to the number of peaks or waves that traverse a given point per unit of time and is expressed in hertz. Sound with a frequency of one cycle or one peak per second would have a frequency of 1 Hz. Ultrasound applies to high-frequency sound waves exceeding 20,000 Hz. Diagnostic ultrasound instruments operate in a higher range of frequencies, varying from 2 to 10 million Hz, or 2 to 10 MHz. The duty factor of diagnostic ultrasound, defined as the ratio between the emission of a sound wave and the reception of the sound wave, is 1/1,000 or 0.001. During a 15-minute diagnostic evaluation, the fetus is exposed to only 1 second of ultrasound energy.

Principles of Imaging

A two-dimensional picture is created when the returning ultrasound echoes are displayed on an oscilloscope screen.[1] The ultrasound signal returning to the transducer is converted to an electrical impulse, and the strength of that electrical impulse is directly proportional to the strength of the returning echo. The density of the medium into which the sound wave has been transmitted and through which it is reflected will determine the strength of the signal. The velocity of the reflected sound wave will be faster and its signal on the oscilloscope brighter after reflection off bone than off tissues that are less dense, such as muscle, fat, brain, or water. Air greatly decreases the transmission of sound waves. For this reason, a coupling medium or gel is applied between the surface of the transducer and the skin.

A storage oscilloscope is used to create a compounded image and produce a two-dimensional picture. The standard transducer used in these systems is 3.5 MHz. The higher the frequency of the sound, the better the reproduction and resolution but the shallower the depth of penetration.

Safety of Ultrasound

Studies of clinical outcomes of infants exposed to ultrasound have failed to demonstrate any significant effects.[7,8] In 1993, the American Institute of Ultrasound in Medicine Bioeffects Committee concluded[6]:

> No confirmed biological effects on patients or instrument operators caused by exposure at intensities typical of the present diagnostic ultrasound instruments have ever been reported. Although the possibility exists that such biological effects may be identified in the future, current data indicate that the benefits to patients of the prudent use of diagnostic ultrasound outweigh the risks, if any, that may be present.

In considering the safety of any diagnostic procedure, one must also consider the skill with which the examination is conducted and the way in which the results are interpreted and utilized. False-positive and false-negative diagnoses appear to be the greatest risk for the patient undergoing an obstetric ultrasound examination.

Transvaginal Ultrasound

Transvaginal ultrasound, with its ability to use higher frequency transducers, can result in better visualization of the early pregnancy.[10-14] A gestational sac can be seen with transvaginal ultrasound as early as 4.5 menstrual weeks.[15] Once seen, the gestational sac grows at a fairly constant rate of 1 mm in mean diameter per day.[16] The yolk sac is visualized when the gestational sac is 10 mm or larger. Between the seventh and the thirteenth menstrual weeks the yolk sac gradually in-

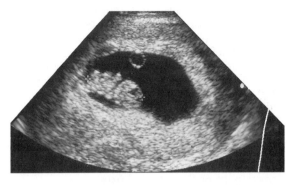

Fig. 4-1 Sonogram demonstrating crown–rump length (between crosses) of 8-week fetus. Yolk sac is in the near field.

creases in diameter from about 3 to 6 mm (Fig. 4-1).[17,18] The amnion develops about the same time as the yolk sac but, because it is thinner, is more difficult to visualize. The amnion grows rapidly during early pregnancy, and fusion with the chorion is usually complete by the sixteenth week.

Cardiac activity is usually the first manifestation of the embryo, at about 6 menstrual weeks. Once the embryo is 5 mm, cardiac activity should be present; its absence is indicative of early demise.[19–21] Embryonic movements can be seen between 7 and 8 menstrual weeks.

Although the gestational sac can be used to date an early pregnancy, the most accurate sonographic measure is the crown–rump length.[23] During the first trimester, this method is accurate to within 4 to 5 days. As this is the single best tool to assess gestational age at any time in pregnancy, it should be considered for patients at risk for growth restriction and other complications of pregnancy.

Between the eighth and twelfth weeks, there is a normal midgut herniation.[24] This should not be confused with an omphalocele, which can be diagnosed with certainty after that time. The liver can be seen at 9 to 10 weeks, the stomach at 10 to 12 weeks, the bladder at 11 to 13 weeks, and the four chambers of the heart at about 12 weeks.[10–14] First-trimester ultrasound should *not* be used as a substitute for a second-trimester evaluation of fetal anatomy.[25]

Although the main value of vaginal ultrasound is in early pregnancy, it may be of clinical use later in gestation. Vaginal ultrasound permits direct visualization of the internal cervical os and allows accurate assessment of the location of the placenta and its distance from the internal os. With vaginal ultrasound, one can identify early signs of preterm labor or incompetent cervix, such as funneling or shortening of the cervical length. Vaginal ultrasound can also improve visualization of intracranial anatomy when the head is engaged and permits enhanced views of cranial structures in coronal and sagittal planes.[29]

Second Trimester

Assessment of Gestational Age

When performed during the first 18 weeks of gestation, ultrasound permits an extremely accurate assessment of gestational age. The fetal crown–rump length, a measurement from the top of the fetal head to its rump, can define gestational ages between 6 and 10 weeks with an error of ±3 to 5 days (Table 4-1). In general, the gestational age of the pregnancy in weeks is equal to 6.5 plus the crown–rump length of the fetus in centimeters. When performing a crown–rump length measurement, care must be taken to avoid confusing the yolk sac with the fetal head. Beyond 12 weeks, the fetus begins to curve and the crown–rump length loses its accuracy.

The biparietal diameter (BPD) is the measurement most often used for establishing fetal gestational age. The transaxial or transverse BPD is best obtained at the level of the thalami and cavum septum pellucidum

Table 4-1   Ultrasonographic Assessment of Fetal Age

Measurement	Gestational Age (Menstrual Weeks)	Range (Days)
Crown–rump length	5–12	± 3
Biparietal diameter	12–20	± 8
	20–24	± 12
	24–32	± 15
	>32	± 21
Femur length	12–20	± 7
	20–36	± 11
	>36	± 16

From Gabbe SG, Iams JD: Intrauterine growth retardation. *In* Iams JD, Zuspan FP (eds): Manual of Obstetrics and Gynecology. St. Louis, CV Mosby Company, 1990, p 169, with permission.

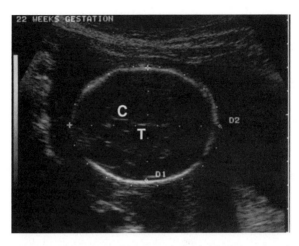

Fig. 4-2 A determination of the BPD at the level of the thalami (T) and cavum septum pellucidum (C). The BPD measurement is made from the outer edge of the skull to the opposite inner edge (D1) and on a line perpendicular to the midline. The occipitofrontal diameter (D2) is also shown. The electronic calipers (dots) have been placed to obtain a measurement of the HC.

(Fig. 4-2). The BPD measurement is made from the outer edge of the skull to the inner edge of the opposite side.

From 12 to 28 weeks' gestation, the relationship between BPD and gestational age is linear.[32] However, growth of the fetal head slows late in gestation, and errors of several weeks may be made in estimating gestational age. In addition, later in gestation, the fetal head becomes more elongated in its anterior–posterior plane. Such dolichocephaly may be assessed by measuring the cephalic index, the ratio of the BPD divided by the occipital–frontal diameter. This ratio should normally be 0.75 to 0.85. If the ratio falls outside this range, the BPD should not be used to estimate gestational age. Femur length may be applied in such cases. At a given gestational age, a group of fetuses will vary in their BPD. This biologic variation is another source of error in estimating gestational age with advancing gestation. Serial determinations of BPD in the second and early third trimesters can reduce the significance of this biologic variation by determining the normal growth rate for a given fetus.

Assessment of Fetal Viability

Real-time ultrasound can be used to confirm the presence of fetal death in utero. The absence of fetal cardiac motion as well as the presence of fetal scalp edema and overlapping of the fetal cranial bones confirms fetal death.

Third Trimester

Evaluation of Fetal Growth

When establishing gestational age and evaluating fetal growth, it is best to evaluate a variety of parameters, including the BPD, the long bones, especially the femur and humerus, and the abdominal circumference (AC) (Fig. 4-3) and transcerebellar diameter. The uniformity of fetal growth that characterizes early gestation is lost after 20 weeks. Therefore, a single ultrasound study performed late in pregnancy cannot accurately establish gestational age (Table 4-1). Fetal AC or perimeter measured at the level of the umbilical vein has been used not only to assess gestational age but to detect the presence of intrauterine growth restriction and macrosomia. Composite tables estimat-

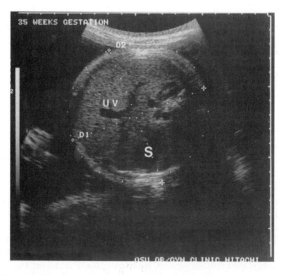

Fig. 4-3 Transverse or axial view of the abdomen demonstrates the fetal stomach (S) and umbilical vein (uv). Note that the abdomen is round and the umbilical vein is well within the substance of the liver. This is the proper level for determination of the fetal AC; electronic calipers (dots) have been placed to make this measurement. The AC may also be calculated using measurements of the anteroposterior (D1) and transverse (D2) abdominal diameters using the following formula: AC = D1 + D2 × 1.57.

ing fetal weight have been constructed by several authors and are usually based on a combination of (1) head size as measured by BPD or head circumference (HC), (2) femur length (FL), and (3) AC. The BPD and fetal AC may be combined to calculate estimates of fetal weight that are likely to be within 10 percent of actual weight.

Abnormal Fetal Growth

Fetal growth restriction is discussed in Chapter 17.

Fetal Macrosomia

Macrosomia has been defined as a birth weight in excess of 4,000 to 4,500 g.[36] Infants with a birth weight above the 90th percentile are also categorized as large for gestational age (LGA). Excessive fetal growth resulting in macrosomia has long been recognized as an important cause of perinatal morbidity and mortality, especially in the pregnancy complicated by diabetes mellitus. At delivery, the macrosomic fetus is more likely to suffer shoulder dystocia, traumatic injury, and asphyxia.

Macrosomia in the infant of the diabetic mother (IDM) is characterized by selected organomegaly, with increases in both fat and muscle mass resulting in a disproportionate increase in the size of the abdomen and shoulders. However, brain growth is not altered, and, therefore, the HC is usually normal. Thus the macrosomia of the IDM is asymmetric. The macrosomic infant of an obese woman without glucose intolerance will demonstrate excessive growth of *both* the AC and HC, or symmetric macrosomia.

Antenatal sonographic detection of the LGA fetus could allow improved selection of the route of delivery to reduce the likelihood of birth trauma. Unfortunately, our clinical ability to evaluate fetal size at term remains poor, with only 35 percent of large infants being identified by excessive symphysis–fundal height measurements.[37]

Several studies have emphasized the limited predictive value of ultrasound to identify the macrosomic fetus. Overall, both the sensitivity and positive predictive value in these reports range between 50 and 60 percent. It must be remembered that formulas for estimation of fetal weight are associated with a 95 percent confidence range of at least 10 to 15 percent.[34] Thus the predicted weight using ultrasonography would have to exceed 4,700 g for all fetuses with weights in excess of 4,000 g to be accurately identified!

In summary, detection of the macrosomic infant using both clinical *and* ultrasonographic techniques remains challenging. In patients at risk for fetal macrosomia—women who have diabetes mellitus, who are obese, or whose pregnancies go beyond 41 weeks—a "growth profile" including ultrasound measurements of estimated fetal weight and HC/AC and FL/AC ratios may improve the identification of excessive fetal growth.[48] In patients at low risk for macrosomia, a fundal height measurement of 4 cm or more than expected for gestational age should signal the need for an ultrasound study.

Assessment of Amniotic Fluid Volume

Ultrasound has proved valuable in the evaluation of amniotic fluid volume. Early application of this technology included measurements of the largest vertical pocket of fluid. Oligohydramnios, a reduction in amniotic fluid volume, was diagnosed when the largest pocket of amniotic fluid measured in two perpendicular planes was less than 1 cm. Hydramnios, or excessive amniotic fluid, was defined as the largest pocket of amniotic fluid exceeding 8 cm in two perpendicular planes.[50] Fetal structural anomalies have been observed in 36 to 63 percent of cases with polyhydramnios.[60,61]

The amniotic fluid index (AFI) has improved the reproducibility and quantitation of amniotic fluid volume. The AFI measurement is performed with the patient in the supine or semi-Fowler position. The maternal abdomen is divided into quadrants (Fig. 4-4). The umbilicus is used as one reference point to divide the uterus into upper and lower halves, and the linea nigra is used as the midline to divide the uterus into right and left halves. The ultrasound transducer head is then placed on the maternal abdomen along the longitudinal axis. The transducer head is maintained perpendicular to the floor, and the vertical diameter of the largest amniotic fluid pocket in each quadrant is identified and measured. These measurements are summed to obtain the AFI in centimeters. If a fetal extremity or portion of the umbilical cord is observed in the quadrant to be measured, the transducer head is moved slightly to exclude these structures. A linear array, sector, or curvilinear transducer may be used to determine the AFI.[55] Care must be taken to avoid excessive pressure on the transducer, as this might decrease the AFI.[56] Only those amniotic fluid pockets completely clear of cord or extremities should be measured. The technique is extremely reproducible. When the AFI is determined in a patient at 20 weeks' gestation

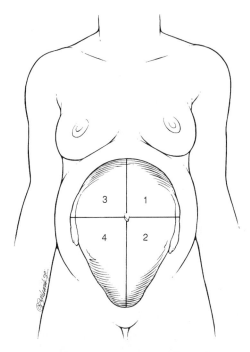

Fig. 4-4 The AFI measurement utilizes ultrasound to assess the depth of fluid pockets in each quadrant of the uterus. Note that the umbilicus divides the uterus into upper and lower halves, and the linea nigra divides the uterus into right and left halves.

or less, the uterus is divided into halves using the linea nigra and the largest pocket identified in each half is added to produce an AFI.

Using this technique, the mean AFI in over 350 pregnancies at 36 to 42 weeks was 12.9 ± 4.6 cm. The normative values for AFI are shown in the appendix to this volume. Patients with an AFI less than 5.0 cm at term were considered to have oligohydramnios, while those with an AFI of 20 cm or greater were considered to have polyhydramnios. When the AFI fell below 5 cm, the frequency of nonreactive nonstress tests, fetal heart rate decelerations, meconium staining, cesarean sections for fetal distress, and low Apgar scores increased.

Sonographic Evaluation of Fetal and Placental Anatomy

Evaluation of fetal and placental anatomy is an integral part of ultrasound examinations during the second and third trimesters. A basic ultrasound examination that documents fetal life, fetal number, fetal presentation, gestational age and growth, amniotic fluid volume, and placental localization without an evaluation of fetal anatomy, therefore, should be considered incomplete. The following description represents the examination of fetal anatomy that should be part of the basic study. A comprehensive sonographic examination of fetal anatomy is often more detailed when it is targeted to look for a certain anomaly.[64-73]

The fetal skull should be elliptical, with the cranium ossified and intact. The ventricular system should be evaluated by assessment of the width of the atrium. The cerebellum should be visualized (Fig. 4-5). An attempt should be made to visualize the face, especially to rule out a facial cleft. The spine is easier to evaluate in its entirety in the second trimester than in the third. A sagittal sonogram should be complemented by a series of transverse sonograms to identify normal anterior and normal posterior ossification elements (Figs. 4-6

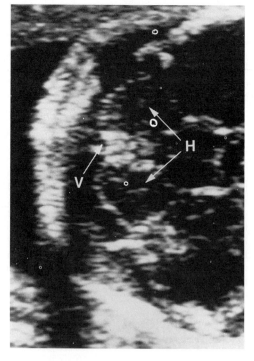

Fig. 4-5 Sonogram demonstrating cerebellar hemispheres (H). V, cerebellar vermis.

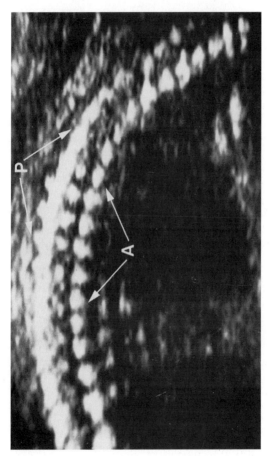

Fig. 4-6 Longitudinal view of the spine demonstrating anterior (A) and posterior (P) ossification elements.

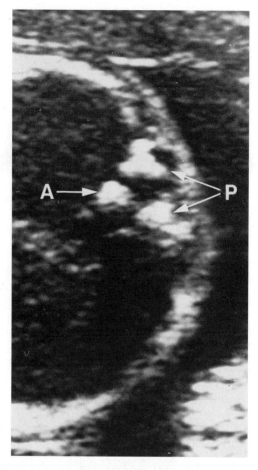

Fig. 4-7 Transverse view of the spine demonstrating anterior (A) and posterior (P) ossification elements.

and 4-7). A four-chambered view of the heart should be obtained. Ventricles and atria of equal and appropriate sizes and an intact ventricular septum should be observed (Fig. 4-8). Real-time ultrasound is invaluable in diagnosing most fetal cardiac anomalies. Examination of the fetal outflow tracts increases the detection of heart anomalies. In cases of a suspected fetal arrhythmia, atrial and ventricular rates can be determined. The fetal bladder (Fig. 4-9), stomach (Fig. 4-10), and kidneys (Fig. 4-11) should be visualized. The abdominal wall should be intact (Fig. 4-12). The long bones of at least the lower extremities should be visualized (Fig.

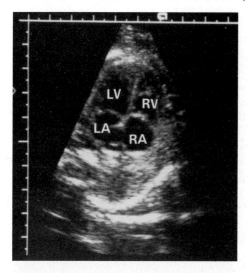

Fig. 4-8 Four-chamber view of the heart. LA, left atrium; LV, left ventricle; RA, right atrium; RV, right ventricle.

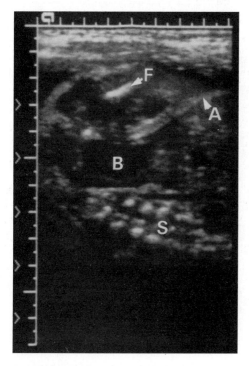

Fig. 4-9 Sonogram demonstrating fetal bladder (B), spine (S), abdominal wall (A), and femur (F).

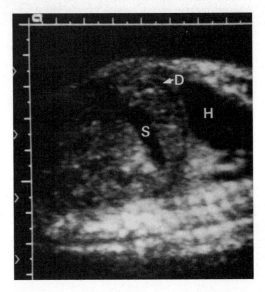

Fig. 4-10 Sonogram demonstrating fetal stomach (S), diaphragm (D), and heart (H).

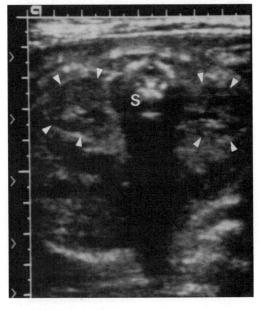

Fig. 4-11 Sonogram demonstrating fetal kidneys (outlined by arrows). S, fetal spine.

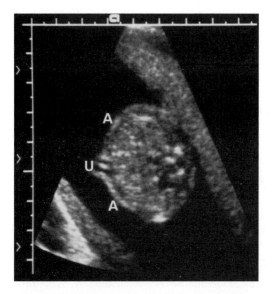

Fig. 4-12 Sonogram demonstrating intact abdominal wall (A) and umbilical cord insertion (U).

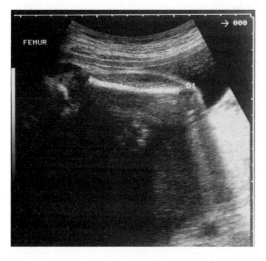

Fig. 4-13 Sonogram demonstrating femur.

4-13). Although fetal gender often may be identified in the second and third trimesters, this should not be considered an integral part of the examination.[64–73]

In addition to the assessment of placental location, ultrasound can provide an evaluation of placental anatomy.[25,26] Placental thickness can be directly related to gestational age, with the thickness of the placenta in millimeters corresponding approximately to the weeks of gestation. For example, at 20 weeks' gestation, the placenta will be approximately 20 mm thick.

Ultrasound Diagnosis of Fetal Anomalies

Antenatal ultrasound scanning at about 18 to 20 weeks of gestation permits the detection of most major fetal structural anomalies.[64,65,71,77–79] It is important to appreciate, however, that even a thorough ultrasound evaluation during the second trimester will not detect all structural malformations. Anomalies such as hydrocephalus, duodenal atresia, microcephaly, achondroplasia, and polycystic kidneys may not manifest until the third trimester, when the degree of anatomic distortion is sufficient to be sonographically detectable.

What fetal malformations should be identified during a basic ultrasound examination? The anomalies believed to be observable in the majority of cases include anencephaly, hydranencephaly, ventriculomegaly of greater than 15 mm, alobar holoprosencephaly, open spina bifida, a large amount of ascites, bilateral hydronephrosis greater than 20 mm, omphalocele, gastroschisis, and hydrothorax with a mediastinal shift. A useful classification of fetal anomalies is based on the nature of the dysmorphology that permits sonographic detection.

Absence of a Normally Present Structure

A dramatic example of the absence of a structure normally detected by ultrasound is anencephaly, the absence of calvaria and forebrain (Fig. 4-14).

The kidneys are normally visualized as bilateral, ovoid, paraspinal masses with echospared renal pelves. When not visualized, the diagnosis of renal agenesis should be suspected. Severe oligohydramnios and the inability to visualize the bladder support the diagnosis of renal agenesis.

Presence of an Additional Structure

Masses that distort normal fetal anatomy can be readily identified with ultrasound.

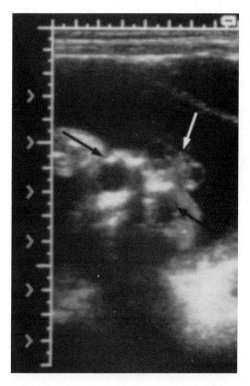

Fig. 4-14 Coronal sonogram of fetal head demonstrating anencephaly. Black arrows point to orbits. White arrow points to area cerebrovasculosa.

Fetal cystic hygromas are fluid-filled masses of the fetal neck that arise from abnormal lymphatic development. They are generally anechoic, with scattered septations and the presence of a midline septum arising from the nuchal ligament[85,86] (Fig. 4-15).

Fetal hydrops or fetal anasarca may be identified by the distortion of the normal fetal surface by skin edema. Ascites, pleural effusions, and pericardial effusions also may be identified[87–89] (Fig. 4-16).

Herniation Through Structural Defects

A common theme in the development of the fetus is the formation by folding and midline fusion of compartments containing vital structures. Incomplete fusion in a variety of locations can lead to defects and herniations of contained structures.[90]

Incomplete closure of the neural tube at the rostral end produces cephaloceles, with herniations of menin-

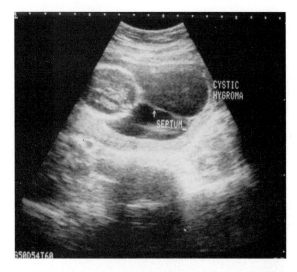

Fig. 4-15 Sonogram demonstrating nuchal cystic hygroma divided by midline septum.

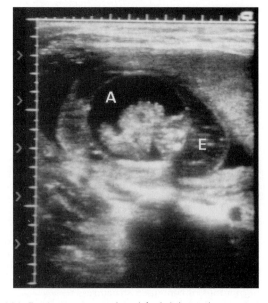

Fig. 4-16 Transverse sonogram through fetal abdomen demonstrating fetal hydrops. E, edema of abdominal wall; A, ascites.

ges and, frequently, of brain substance through a defect in the cranium.[91] Failed fusion at the caudal end produces spina bifida with protruding meningoceles and meningomyeloceles (Fig. 4-17). Sonographic diagnosis of each of these anomalies depends on the demonstration of a defect in the normal structure of the cranium or spine and of a protruding sac, often containing tissue.[92,93]

Most, if not all, cases of spina bifida are complicated by the Arnold-Chiari malformation.[94] The Arnold-Chiari malformation therefore can serve as an important marker for spina bifida. Two characteristic sonographic signs (the "lemon" and the "banana") of the Arnold-Chiari malformation have been described.[95] A scalloping of the frontal bones can give a lemon-like configuration, in axial section, to the skull of an affected fetus during the second trimester. The cerebellar hemispheres are centrally curved in a banana-like sonographic appearance (Fig. 4-18).[95]

Omphaloceles result from failure of the intestines to retract from their temporary location in the umbilical cord and the subsequent herniation of other abdominal contents, including both hollow and solid structures contained within a peritoneal sac. Insertion of the umbilical cord into the sac helps to differentiate an omphalocele from gastroschisis, which has no covering membrane. Distinguishing these two entities may be difficult[96] (Figs. 4-19 and 4-20).

Dilatation Behind an Obstruction

In this class of anomalies, the structural defect itself is rarely seen. Rather, what is observed is the distention of structures behind a defect. Such dilatation is caused by obstruction to the normal flow of cerebrospinal fluid, urine, or swallowed amniotic fluid.

Abnormal Fetal Biometry

Several fetal anomalies are best diagnosed not by observing alterations in shape or consistency, but by determining abnormalities in size. The science of fetal biometry has generated many nomograms defining normal values for parts of the fetal anatomy at various gestational ages[109] (see appendix; Obstetric Ultrasound Measurement Tables).

Ultrasound Detection of Chromosomal Abnormalities

Ultrasound examination can suggest a chromosomal aberration. Sonographic markers for the most serious

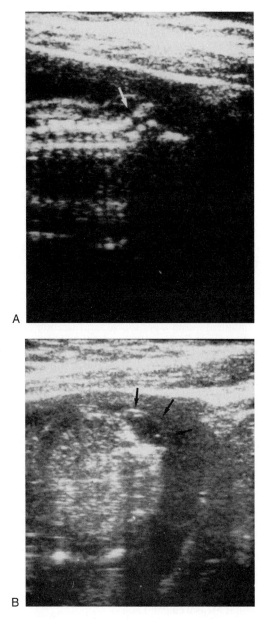

Fig. 4-17 (A) Longitudinal sonogram of fetal spine with arrows pointing to meningomyelocele. (B) Transverse sonogram through fetal spine with arrow pointing to meningomyelocele.

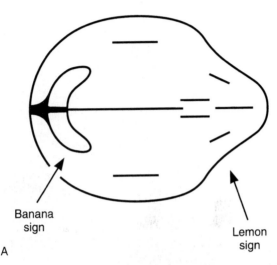

Banana
sign

Lemon
sign

A

Fig. 4-18 (A) Diagrammatic representation of "banana" and "lemon" signs in fetus with spina bifida. *(Figure continues.)*

karyotype abnormalities are often present. Holoprosencephaly, facial clefts, hypotelorism, omphalocele, polydactyly, and heart defects are associated with trisomy 13, while growth restriction, micrognathus, overlapping fingers, omphalocele, horseshoe kidney, and heart defects are associated with trisomy 18. Early-onset severe growth restriction, large head, syndactyly, and heart defects suggest triploidy. Turner syndrome (45,X) is classically associated with nuchal cystic hygroma, but this ultrasound finding can occur in a wide variety of genetic disorders.[64,68]

Major structural malformations, including hydrops, duodenal atresia, and heart defects, are associated with trisomy 21.[126,127] Nuchal skin thickness, defined as 6 mm or more, is a useful screening tool for trisomy 21 and other chromosomal malformations (Fig. 4-21).[123,128,129] Other sonographic signs used to screen for Down syndrome include short femur, short humerus, pyelectasis, mild cerebral ventriculomegaly, clinodactyly with hypoplastic middle phalanx of the fifth digit, widely spaced first and second toes, low set ears, and echogenic bowel.[126,127,130]

Choroid plexus cysts can occur in about 1 percent of fetuses and, while most are closely associated with trisomy 18, can be a marker for other chromosomal

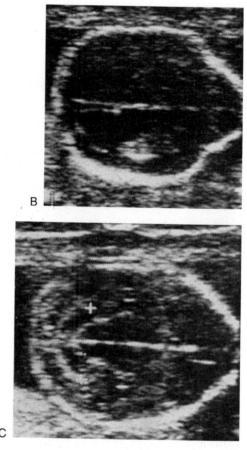

Fig. 4-18 *(Continued)*. (B) Transverse section of fetal head at level of cavum septi pellucidi in an 18-week fetus with open spina bifida showing "lemon" and "banana" sign. (C) Suboccipital bregmatic view of fetal head in an 18-week fetus with open spina bifida, demonstrating "banana" sign (+). (From Nicolaides KM, Campbell S, Gabbe SG, Guidetti R: Ultrasound screening for spina bifida: cranial and cerebellar signs. Lancet 2:72, 1986 © The Lancet Ltd, 1986, with permission.)

abnormalities[131,132] (Fig. 4-22). The need for a karyotype determination when the only structural abnormality seen is a choroid plexus cyst remains controversial.[133,134]

In summary, if a major structural malformation is detected with ultrasound, karyotype determination should be considered.

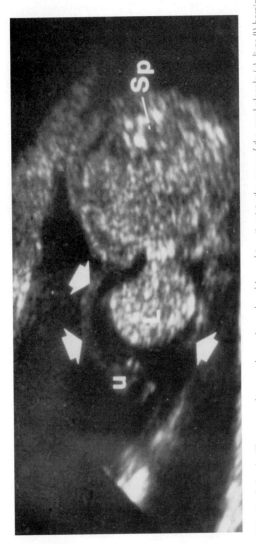

Fig. 4-19 Omphalocele. The surrounding membrane (arrowheads), cord insertion into the apex of the omphalocele (u), liver (L) herniated into the omphalocele sac, and spine (Sp) can be seen.

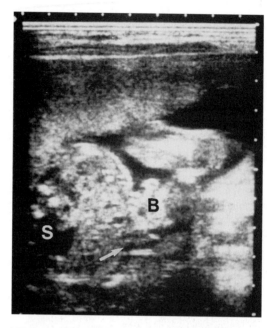

Fig. 4-20 Loops of bowel (B) without a surrounding membrane are characteristic of gastroschisis. The arrow points to the insertion of the umbilical cord. Since the stomach (S) is on the left of the fetus, the site of the bowel herniation is to the right of the umbilical cord.

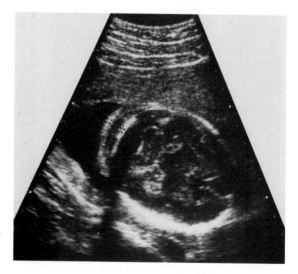

Fig. 4-21 Sonogram demonstrating nuchal skin thickness greater than 6 mm.

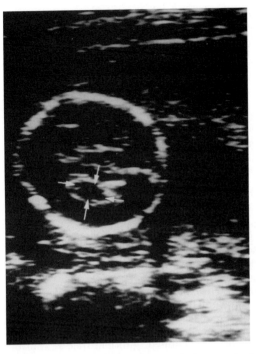

Fig. 4-22 Sonogram demonstrating choroid plexus cyst (outlined by arrows).

Management of a Pregnancy Complicated By an Ultrasonically Diagnosed Fetal Anomaly

If a fetal anomaly is diagnosed by obstetric ultrasound, the fetus should be carefully evaluated for other anomalies before management options can be considered. Echocardiography and karyotype determination should usually be part of this evaluation.

Who Should Have an Obstetric Ultrasound Examination?

Routine performance of obstetric ultrasound examinations—the performance of an ultrasound study on every obstetric patient at approximately 18 weeks' gestation—remains controversial.

A routine obstetric ultrasound examination describes what the American College of Obstetricians and Gynecologists (ACOG) has called a *basic* ultrasound examination, which would include the following information: fetal number, fetal presentation, documentation of fetal life, placental location, assessment of amniotic fluid volume, assessment of gestational age, survey of fetal anatomy for gross malformations, and evaluation for maternal pelvic masses.[68,165] When the findings of a basic ultrasound examination suggest a fetal abnormality or in patients at greater risk of a fetal abnormality, a comprehensive ultrasound examination may be indicated. As noted by ACOG, the comprehensive ultrasound study should be conducted by an individual experienced in these evaluations.

Routine obstetric ultrasound offers at least six advantages: accurate dating of all pregnancies; accurate evaluation of maternal serum levels of α-fetoprotein, human chorionic gonadotropin, and unconjugated estriol (triple screening); early detection of multiple pregnancies; placental localization to rule out placenta previa; detection of structural abnormalities of the fetus; and psychological benefit to the parents.[169,170]

The ideal timing for a routine ultrasound study would appear to be approximately 18 weeks' gestation. At this gestational age, the pregnancy can be accurately dated and fetal anatomy well visualized. Should a fetal abnormality be identified, sufficient time is available to perform a comprehensive ultrasound, obtain a fetal karyotype if necessary, and counsel the patient and her partner.

An ultrasound performed at 18 weeks' gestation will reveal that approximately 10 percent of placentas overlie the cervical os, allowing the obstetrician to exclude placenta previa in the remaining 90 percent of cases. Of patients with a low-lying placenta at 18 weeks, only those women in whom the placenta completely covers the os are at risk for a placenta previa in the third trimester. A repeat ultrasound evaluation should be performed in these cases.[165,176]

One of the most important benefits of routine ultrasound appears to be the identification of major congenital malformations. Major anomalies occur in 2 to 3 percent of all births and account for more than 20 percent of all infant deaths (see Ch. 5). Systematic examination of fetal structure as part of the basic ultrasound study outlined by ACOG can identify a significant proportion of these abnormalities. Data from six European studies demonstrate that routine ultrasound has a sensitivity of 52.9 percent and a positive predictive value of 95.9 percent in identifying major structural anomalies.[177] The specificity and negative predictive value were 99.9 and 99.2 percent, respectively.

In its most recent publications, the ACOG offered the following recommendations concerning routine ultrasound:

> Routine ultrasonography in early pregnancy can help to reduce the incidence of labor induction for suspected postdatism, and decrease the frequency of undiagnosed major fetal anomalies and undiagnosed twins. However, significant effects on infant outcome are not confirmed by randomized, controlled trials. Although obstetric ultrasound studies are performed routinely in many European countries, in the United States the routine use of ultrasonography cannot be supported from a cost-benefit standpoint. Thus ultrasound should be performed for specific indications in low-risk pregnancy.

Conclusions

In summary, studies of routine ultrasound have failed to demonstrate any associated adverse effects on the mother or fetus. Routine ultrasound has a high positive predictive value for conditions known to be associated with poor perinatal outcome, such as twins, placenta previa, and congenital malformations. To date, two large prospective randomized studies have evaluated the benefits of routine ultrasound in obstetric practice.[186–189] One, performed in Finland,[186] demonstrated a reduction in perinatal mortality, resulting from the identification of major fetal anomalies. The second, the RADIUS trial,[187–189] performed in the United States, failed to show an improvement in perinatal outcome. Nevertheless, a large clinical experience from several centers in both the United States and Europe has repeatedly found that routine ultrasound screening at 18 weeks can improve gestational dating in approximately 10 to 25 percent of patients, detect nearly all multiple gestations, exclude placenta previa in most patients and recognize those at greatest risk for this condition, detect one-third to one-half of major fetal malformations, and reduce parental anxiety and increase compliance with the recommendations of health care providers. The cost of routine ultrasound screening must be compared with the costs created by false-positive diagnoses, which may lead to unnecessary patient anxiety and further intervention, and to the cost savings resulting from reduction in the rate of inductions for suspected prolonged pregnancy, a decrease in the rate of preterm delivery for twins, and the identification of a fetus with an anomaly likely to survive but with a poor quality of life. Finally, as with any analytic technique, the value of ultrasound screening is dependent on the skill with which the study is performed and the manner in which the results are interpreted and utilized in clinical care.[170]

Key Points

- Ultrasound energy is produced by a transducer containing crystal structures that convert electrical energy to ultrasound waves and the returning echoes to electrical energy.
- No deleterious effects on the pregnant woman or fetus caused by exposure to ultrasound at the intensities used for imaging have ever been reported.
- Although the gestational sac can be used to date an early pregnancy, measurement of the crown–rump length is the single best method to assess gestational age at any time in pregnancy.
- From 12 to 28 weeks' gestation, the relationship between the biparietal diameter and gestational age is linear.
- Formulas for estimation of fetal weight are associated with a 95 percent confidence range of at least 10 to 15 percent.
- Measurement of the fetal abdominal circumference is probably the most reliable sonographic parameter for the detection of macrosomia.
- At term, an AFI less than 5.0 cm indicates oligohydramnios and greater than 20 cm polyhydramnios.
- The thickness of the placenta in millimeters corresponds to the number of weeks of gestation.
- The "lemon" and "banana" signs are important cranial markers for spina bifida.
- Major structural malformations, including hydrops, duodenal atresia, and cardiac anomalies, are observed in 30 percent of cases of Down syndrome (trisomy 21).

Chapter 5

Antepartum Fetal Evaluation

Maurice L. Druzin and
Steven G. Gabbe

Antepartum fetal deaths now account for nearly 40 to
60 percent of all perinatal mortality in the United
States. The obstetrician must be concerned not only
with prevention of this mortality, but with the detection
of fetal compromise and the timely delivery of such
infants in an effort to maximize their future potential.[2]

The Etiology of Perinatal Mortality

The perinatal mortality rate (PMR) has been defined
by the National Center for Health Statistics (NCHS) as
the number of late fetal deaths (fetal deaths at 28 weeks'
gestation or more) plus early neonatal deaths (deaths
of infants 0 to 6 days of age) per 1,000 live births plus
fetal deaths.[3] According to the NCHS, the neonatal
mortality rate is defined as the number of neonatal
deaths (deaths of infants 0 to 27 days of age) per 1,000
live births; the postneonatal mortality rate, the number
of postneonatal deaths (the number of infants 28 to
365 days of age) per 1,000 live births; and the infant
mortality rate, the number of infant deaths (deaths of
infants under 1 year of age) per 1,000 live births. The
American College of Obstetricians and Gynecologists
(ACOG) has recommended that only deaths of fetuses
and infants weighing 500 g or more at delivery be used
to compare data among states in the United States.[4]
For international comparisons, only deaths of fetuses
and infants weighing 1,000 g or more at delivery should
be included.[4]

Since 1965, the PMR in the United States has fallen
steadily. Using the NCHS definition, the PMR reported
in 1993 was 9.1/1,000. The overall neonatal mortality rate was 5.3/1,000, with fetal deaths at 3.8/1,000
(Fig. 5-1.

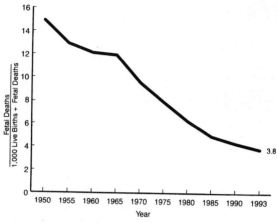

More than 28 weeks gestation.

Fig. 5-1 Late fetal deaths*: 1950–1993. (National Center for Health Statistics.)

While the majority of fetal deaths occur before 32 weeks' gestation, fetuses at 40 to 41 weeks are at a 3-fold greater risk and those at 42 or more weeks are at a 12-fold greater risk for intrauterine death than fetuses at 28 to 31 weeks.

Fetal deaths may be divided into those that occur during the antepartum period and those that occur during labor (intrapartum stillbirths). More than 90 percent of fetal deaths occur before the onset of labor.[9] Antepartum deaths may be divided into four broad categories: (1) chronic asphyxia of diverse origin; (2) congenital malformations; (3) superimposed complications of pregnancy, such as Rh isoimmunization, placental abruption, and fetal infection; and (4) deaths of unexplained cause. If it is to succeed, a program of antenatal surveillance must identify malformed fetuses (see Ch. 4) and recognize those at risk for asphyxia.

Late fetal deaths have fallen markedly since 1935 (Fig. 5-1). At the Royal Victoria Hospital in Montreal, fetal death rate declined by 70 percent, from 11.5/1,000 in the 1960s to 3.2/1,000 during 1990 to 1993.[12] The decline in the fetal death rate may be attributed to the prevention of Rh sensitization, antepartum and intrapartum fetal surveillance, improved detection of intrauterine growth restriction (IUGR) and fetal anomalies with ultrasound, and improved care of maternal diabetes mellitus and preeclampsia. While fetal mortality resulting from IUGR fell 60 percent, from

17.9/1,000 to 7.0/1,000 births, the growth-restricted fetus still had a more than 10-fold greater risk for fetal death than an appropriately grown fetus. Most of these deaths occurred between 28 and 36 weeks' gestation, and the diagnosis of IUGR was rarely identified before death. In addition to IUGR, leading causes of fetal death after 28 weeks' gestation included abruption and unexplained antepartum losses. Unexplained fetal deaths were responsible for more than 25 percent of all stillbirths. Fetal–maternal hemorrhage may occur in 10 to 15 percent of these cases of unexplained fetal deaths. Fetal deaths due to infection, most often associated with premature rupture of the membranes before 28 weeks' gestation, did not decline over the 30 years of the study. After controlling for risk factors such as multiple gestation, hypertension, diabetes mellitus, placenta previa and abruption, previous abortion, and prior fetal death, women 35 years of age or older had a nearly twofold greater risk for fetal death than women under 30.

In summary, approximately 30 percent of antepartum fetal deaths may be attributed to asphyxia, including IUGR and post-term gestations; 30 percent to maternal complications, especially placental abruption, hypertension, and preeclampsia; 15 percent to congenital malformations such as anencephaly and chromosomal abnormalities, including trisomies 21 and 18 and 45,XO; and 5 percent to infection. At least 20 percent of stillbirths will have no obvious etiology.

A decade of experience with antepartum fetal heart rate monitoring revealed that the perinatal mortality rate was significantly lower in the tested high-risk population (evaluated with contraction stress tests and nonstress tests) as compared to the nontested patients. Most stillbirths within 7 days of testing were due to congenital anomalies and placental abruption. In obstetric populations in which high-risk patients are monitored, the majority of stillbirths now occur in what had previously been considered normal pregnancies.

The first box, p 98, lists the information one might predict from an antepartum fetal test, while the second box below lists those aspects of obstetric management that might be influenced by antepartum testing, p 98.

Testing can be initiated at early gestational ages, 25 to 26 weeks, to identify the fetus at risk. Maternal and fetal interventions can then be considered. Obviously, prolongation of intrauterine life is the primary goal, and better understanding of the pathophysiology of the premature fetus and the use of combinations of tests will allow this to be accomplished.

In selecting the population of patients for antepar-

Aspects of Fetal Condition That Might Be Predicted by Antepartum Testing

Perinatal death
Intrauterine growth restriction (IUGR)
Nonreassuring fetal status, intrapartum
Neonatal asphyxia
Postnatal motor and intellectual impairment
Premature delivery
Congenital abnormalities
Need for specific therapy

Adapted from Chard T, Klopper A: Placental Function Tests. New York, Springer-Verlag, 1982, p 1, with permission.

tum fetal evaluation, one would certainly include those pregnancies known to be at high risk of uteroplacental insufficiency (Table 5-1). Routine antepartum fetal evaluation would be necessary to detect most infants dying in utero as the result of hypoxia and asphyxia.[17] It would seem reasonable, therefore, to consider extending some form of antepartum fetal surveillance to all obstetric patients. As described below, assessment of

Obstetric Management That Might Be Influenced by Antepartum Testing

Preterm delivery
Route of delivery
Bedrest
Observation
Drug therapy
Operative intervention in labor
Neonatal intensive care
Termination of pregnancy for a congenital anomaly

Adapted from Chard T, Klopper A: Placental Function Tests. New York, Springer-Verlag, 1982, p 1, with permission.

Table 5-1   Indications for Antepartum Fetal
Monitoring

1. Patients at high risk of uteroplacental insufficiency
   Prolonged pregnancy
   Diabetes mellitus
   Hypertension
   Previous stillbirth
   Suspected IUGR
   Advanced maternal age
2. When other tests suggest fetal compromise
   Suspected IUGR
   Decreased fetal movement
3. Routine antepartum surveillance

fetal activity by the mother may be an ideal technique
for this purpose.

Statistical Assessment of Antepartum Testing

To determine the clinical application of antepartum
diagnostic testing, the predictive value of the tests must
be considered. The sensitivity of the test is the probability that the test will be positive, or abnormal, when the
disease is present. The specificity of the test is the probability that the test result will be negative when the disease is not present. Note that the sensitivity and specificity refer not to the actual numbers of patients with
a positive or abnormal result, but to the proportion or
probability of these test results. The predictive value of
an abnormal test would be that fraction of patients with
an abnormal test result who have the abnormal condition, while the predictive value of a normal test would
be the fraction of patients with a normal test result who
are normal.

The prevalence of the abnormal condition has great
impact on the predictive value of antepartum fetal tests.
When the prevalence of the disease is low, as it is for
intrauterine fetal deaths, even tests with a high sensitivity and specificity are associated with many false predic-
tions.

For most antepartum diagnostic tests, a cutoff point
used to define an abnormal result must be arbitrarily
established.[31] The cutoff point is selected to maximize
the separation between the normal and diseased populations.

Biophysical Techniques of Fetal Evaluation

Fetal State

When interpreting tests that monitor fetal biophysical characteristics, one must appreciate that, during the third trimester, the normal fetus may exhibit marked changes in its neurologic state.[32,33] The near-term fetus spends approximately 25 percent of its time in a quiet sleep state (state 1F) and 60 to 70 percent in an active sleep state (state 2F). Active sleep is associated with rapid eye movements (REM), regular breathing movements, and intermittent abrupt movements of the head, limbs, and trunk. The fetal heart rate in active sleep exhibits increased variability and frequent accelerations with movement. During quiet, or non-REM, sleep, the fetal heart rate slows and heart rate variability is reduced. The fetus may make infrequent breathing movements. Near term, periods of quiet sleep may last 20 minutes, and those of active sleep approximately 40 minutes.[33]

When evaluating fetal condition using the nonstress test or the biophysical profile, one must ask whether a fetus that is not making breathing movements or shows no accelerations of its baseline heart rate is in a quiet sleep state or is neurologically compromised. In such circumstances, prolonging the period of evaluation will usually allow a change in fetal state, and more normal parameters of fetal well-being will appear.

Maternal Assessment of Fetal Activity

Maternal assessment of fetal activity may be ideal for routine antepartum fetal surveillance. During the third trimester the human fetus spends 10 percent of its time making gross fetal body movements, and 30 such movements are made each hour.[34] Periods of active fetal body movement last approximately 40 minutes, while quiet periods last about 20 minutes. The longest period without fetal movements in a normal fetus is approximately 75 minutes. The mother is able to appreciate about 70 to 80 percent of gross fetal movements. Fetal movement appears to peak between 9:00 P.M. and 1:00 A.M., a time when maternal glucose levels are falling.[34] Of note, the normal fetus does not decrease its activity in the week before delivery.[36,37]

Maternal evaluation of fetal activity may reduce fetal deaths due to asphyxia. A small fall in fetal Po_2 is associated with a cessation of limb movements in the fetal lamb.

Several methods have been used to monitor fetal activity in clinical practice. In general, the presence of fetal movements is a reassuring sign of fetal health. However, the absence of fetal activity requires further assessment before one can conclude that fetal compromise exists. Pearson and Weaver[41] advocated the use of the Cardiff Count-to-Ten chart. They found that only 2.5 percent of 1,654 daily movement counts recorded by 61 women who subsequently delivered healthy infants fell below 10 movements per 12 hours. Therefore, they accepted 10 movements as the minimum amount of fetal activity the patient should perceive in a 12-hour period. The patient is asked to start counting the movements in the morning and to record the time of day at which the tenth movement has been perceived. Should the patient not have 10 movements during 12 hours, or should it take longer each day to reach 10 movements, the patient is told to contact her obstetrician.

Moore and Piacquadio[52] demonstrated an impressive reduction in fetal deaths resulting from a formal program of fetal movement counting. Patients used the Count-to-Ten approach but were told to monitor fetal activity in the evening, a time of increased fetal movement. Most women observed 10 movements in an average of 21 minutes, and compliance was greater than 90 percent. Patients who did not perceive 10 movements in 2 hours, a level of fetal activity slightly more than five standard deviations below the mean, were told to report immediately for further evaluation.

Whatever technique is used must be carefully explained to the patient. While there will be a wide but normal range in fetal activity, with fetal movement counting, each mother and her fetus serve as their own controls.[6] Fetal and placental factors that influence maternal assessment of fetal activity include an anterior placental location, short duration of fetal movements, increased amniotic fluid volume, and fetal anomalies.[45] Approximately 80 percent of all mothers will be able to comply with a program of counting fetal activity.[6,48] Maternal factors that decrease the appreciation of fetal movement include increased maternal activity, obesity, and medications such as narcotics or barbiturates.

In conclusion, there appears to be a clearly established relationship between decreased fetal activity and fetal death. Therefore, it would seem prudent to request that *all* pregnant patients, regardless of their risk status, monitor fetal activity starting at 28 weeks' gestation. The Count-to-Ten approach developed by Moore and Piacquadio[53] seems ideal.

Contraction Stress Test

The contraction stress test (CST) or oxytocin challenge test was the first biophysical technique widely applied for antepartum fetal surveillance. Analyses of intrapartum fetal heart rate monitoring had demonstrated that a fetus with inadequate placental respiratory reserve would demonstrate late decelerations in response to hypoxia (see Ch. 7). The CST extended these observations to the antepartum period. The response of the fetus at risk for uteroplacental insufficiency to uterine contractions formed the basis for this test.

Performing the CST

The CST may be conducted in the labor and delivery suite or in an adjacent area, although the likelihood of fetal distress requiring immediate delivery in response to uterine contractions or hyperstimulation is extremely small. The patient is placed in the semi-Fowler position at a 30- to 45-degree angle with a slight left tilt to avoid the supine hypotensive syndrome. The fetal heart rate is recorded using a Doppler ultrasound transducer, while uterine contractions are monitored with the tocodynamometer. Maternal blood pressure is determined every 5 to 10 minutes to detect maternal hypotension.[54] Baseline fetal heart rate and uterine tone are first recorded for a period of approximately 10 to 20 minutes. In some cases, adequate uterine activity will occur spontaneously, and additional uterine stimulation will not be necessary. An adequate CST requires uterine contractions of moderate intensity lasting approximately 40 to 60 seconds with a frequency of three in 10 minutes. These criteria were selected to approximate the stress experienced by the fetus during the first stage of labor. If uterine activity is absent or inadequate, nipple stimulation is used to initiate contractions or intravenous oxytocin is begun. Oxytocin is administered by an infusion pump at 0.5 mU/min. The infusion rate is doubled every 20 minutes until adequate uterine contractions have been achieved.[55] One does not usually need to exceed 10 mU/min to produce adequate uterine activity. After the CST has been completed, the patient should be observed until uterine activity has returned to its baseline level. With nipple stimulation, the test may take approximately 30 minutes. If oxytocin is needed, 90 minutes may be required to perform the CST.

Contraindications to the test include those patients at high risk for premature labor, such as patients with premature rupture of the membranes, multiple gestation, and cervical incompetence, although the CST has not been associated with an increased incidence of premature labor.[56] The CST should also be avoided in conditions in which uterine contractions may be dangerous, such as placenta previa and a previous classic cesarean section or uterine surgery.

Interpreting the CST

The interpretation of the CST is outlined in Table 5-2. A negative test is one in which there are three uterine contractions in 10 minutes with no late decelerations (Figs. 5-2 and 5-3). The term *equivocal* may be used rather than *suspicious* for a CST with an occasional late deceleration.

Variable decelerations that occur during the CST may indicate cord compression often associated with oligohydramnios. In such cases, ultrasonography should be performed to assess amniotic fluid volume.

A negative CST has been consistently associated with good fetal outcome. A negative result therefore permits the obstetrician to prolong a high-risk pregnancy safely. Only one preventable fetal death was reported in 1,337 high-risk patients within 7 days after a negative CST. Fetal deaths after a negative CST can be attributed to cord accidents, malformations, placental abruption, and acute deterioration of glucose control in patients with diabetes mellitus. Thus the CST, like most methods of antepartum fetal surveillance, cannot predict acute fetal compromise. If the CST is negative, a repeat study is usually scheduled in 1 week. Changes in the patient's clinical condition may warrant more frequent studies.

A positive CST has been associated with an increased incidence of intrauterine death, late decelerations in labor, low 5-minute Apgar scores, IUGR, and meconium-stained amniotic fluid (Fig. 5-4).[66] The likelihood of perinatal death after a positive CST has ranged from 7 to 15 percent. There has been a significant incidence of false-positive CSTs that, depending on the endpoint used, averages approximately 30 percent.[54] The positive CST is more likely to be associated with fetal compromise if the baseline heart rate lacks accelerations or "reactivity" and the latency period between the onset of the uterine contractions and the onset of the late deceleration is less than 45 seconds.[68,69]

The high incidence of false-positive CSTs is one of the greatest limitations of this test, as such results could lead to unnecessary premature intervention. False-positive CSTs may be due to misinterpretation of the tracing; supine hypotension, which decreases uterine per-

Table 5-2 Interpretation of the Contraction Stress Test

Interpretation	Description	Incidence (%)
Negative	No late decelerations appearing anywhere on the tracing with adequate uterine contractions (three in 10 minutes)	80
Positive	Late decelerations that are consistent and persistent, present with the majority (>50 percent) of contractions without excessive uterine activity; if persistent late decelerations seen before the frequency of contractions is adequate, test interpreted as positive	3–5
Suspicious	Inconsistent late decelerations	5
Hyperstimulation	Uterine contractions closer than every 2 minutes or lasting >90 seconds, or five uterine contractions in 10 minutes; if no late decelerations seen, test interpreted as negative	5
Unsatisfactory	Quality of the tracing inadequate for interpretation or adequate uterine activity cannot be achieved	5

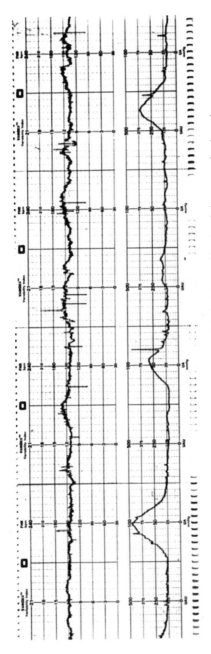

Fig. 5-2 A reactive and negative CST. With this result, the CST would ordinarily be repeated in 1 week.

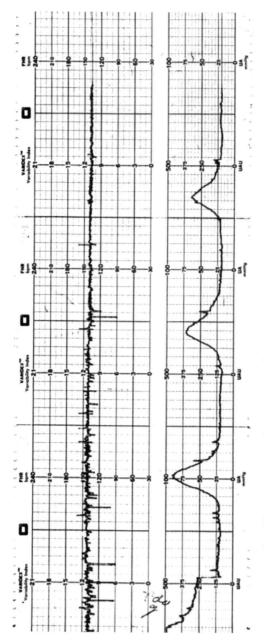

Fig. 5-3 A nonreactive and negative CST. After this result, the test would ordinarily be repeated in 24 hours.

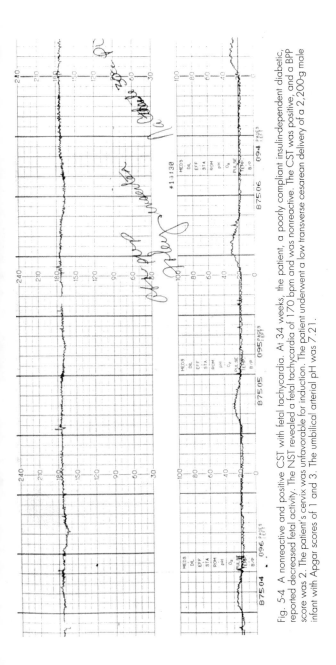

Fig. 5-4 A nonreactive and positive CST with fetal tachycardia. At 34 weeks, the patient, a poorly compliant insulin-dependent diabetic, reported decreased fetal activity. The NST revealed a fetal tachycardia of 170 bpm and was nonreactive. The CST was positive, and a BPP score was 2. The patient's cervix was unfavorable for induction. The patient underwent a low transverse cesarean delivery of a 2,200-g male infant with Apgar scores of 1 and 3. The umbilical arterial pH was 7.21.

fusion; uterine hyperstimulation, which is not appreciated using the tocodynamometer; or an improvement in fetal condition after the CST has been performed. The high false-positive rate also indicates that a patient with a positive CST need not necessarily require an elective cesarean delivery. If a trial of labor is to be undertaken after a positive CST, the cervix should be favorable for induction so that direct fetal heart rate monitoring and careful assessment of uterine contractility with an intrauterine pressure catheter can be performed. False-positive results are not increased when the CST is used early in the third trimester.[70]

A suspicious or equivocal CST should be repeated in 24 hours. Most of these tests will become negative. Like the suspicious CST, a test that is unsatisfactory or shows hyperstimulation should be repeated in 24 hours.

The Nipple Stimulation CST

Many centers utilize nipple stimulation to produce the uterine contractions needed for the CST. With nipple stimulation, the CST can generally be completed in less time, and an intravenous infusion is not required. Therefore, this approach would appear to be an ideal first step in performing a CST.

The patient may first apply a warm moist towel to each breast for 5 minutes. If uterine activity is not adequate, the patient is asked to massage one nipple for 10 minutes. With intermittent nipple stimulation, the patient gently strokes the nipple of one breast with the palmar surface of her fingers through her clothes for 2 minutes and then stops for 5 minutes. This cycle is repeated only as necessary to achieve adequate uterine activity. Intermittent rather than continuous nipple stimulation is important in avoiding hyperstimulation. Defined as contractions lasting more than 90 seconds or five or more contractions in 10 minutes, hyperstimulation has been reported in approximately 2 percent of tests when intermittent nipple stimulation is employed.[79,80]

The Nonstress Test

Accelerations of the fetal heart rate in response to fetal activity, uterine contractions, or stimulation reflect fetal well-being and are the basis for the nonstress test (NST), the most widely applied technique for antepartum fetal evaluation.

In late gestation, the healthy fetus exhibits an average of 34 accelerations above the baseline fetal heart rate each hour.[82] These accelerations require intact neurologic coupling between the fetal central nervous system (CNS) and the fetal heart.[82] Fetal hypoxia will disrupt this pathway. Fetal heart rate accelerations may be absent during periods of quiet fetal sleep. The longest time between successive accelerations in the healthy term fetus is approximately 40 minutes. However, the fetus may fail to exhibit heart rate accelerations for up to 80 minutes and still be normal.

While an absence of fetal heart rate accelerations is most often due to a quiet fetal sleep state, CNS depressants such as narcotics and phenobarbital as well as β-blockers can reduce heart rate reactivity.[83,84] Fetal heart rate accelerations are also decreased in smokers.[85]

The NST is usually performed in an outpatient setting. In most cases, only 10 to 15 minutes are required to complete the test. It has virtually no contraindications, and few equivocal test results are observed. The patient may be seated in a reclining chair, with care being taken to ensure that she is tilted to the left to avoid the supine hypotensive syndrome.[55,86] The patient's blood pressure should be recorded before the test is begun and then repeated at 5- to 10-minute intervals. Fetal heart rate is monitored using the Doppler ultrasound transducer, and the tocodynamometer is applied to detect uterine contractions or fetal movement. Fetal activity may be recorded by the patient using an event marker or noted by the staff performing the test. The most widely applied definition of a reactive test requires that at least two accelerations of the fetal heart rate of 15 bpm amplitude and 15 seconds' duration be observed in 20 minutes of monitoring (Fig. 5-5).[86] Since almost all accelerations are accompanied by fetal movement, fetal movement need not be recorded with the accelerations for the test to be considered reactive. However, fetal movements do provide another index of fetal well-being.

If the criteria for reactivity are not met, the test is considered nonreactive (Fig. 5-6). The most common cause for a nonreactive test will be a period of fetal inactivity or quiet sleep. The test may be extended for an additional 20 minutes with the expectation that fetal state will change and reactivity will appear. If the test has been extended for 40 minutes, and reactivity has not been seen, a CST or fetal biophysical profile (BPP) should be performed. Of those fetuses that exhibit a nonreactive NST, approximately 25 percent will have a positive CST on further evaluation.[86,90,91] Reactivity that occurs during preparations for the CST has proved to be a reliable index of fetal well-being.

On initial testing, 85 percent of NSTs will be reactive

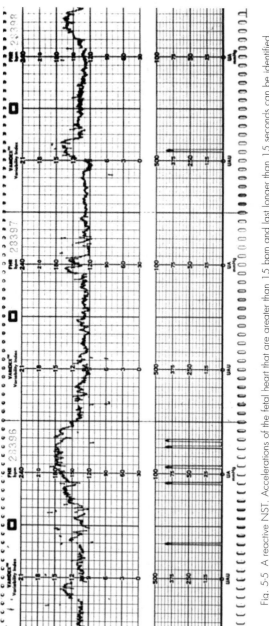

Fig. 5-5 A reactive NST. Accelerations of the fetal heart that are greater than 15 bpm and last longer than 15 seconds can be identified. When the patient appreciates a fetal movement, she presses an event marker on the monitor, creating the arrows on the lower portion of the tracing.

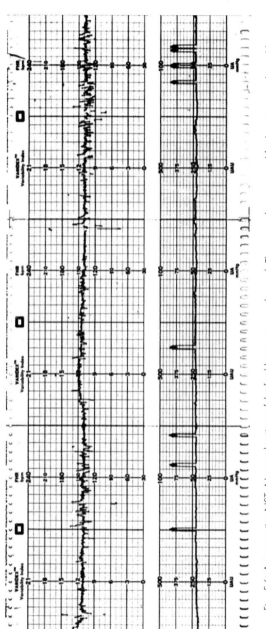

Fig. 5-6 A nonreactive NST. No accelerations of the fetal heart rate are observed. The patient has perceived fetal activity as indicated by the arrows in the lower portion of the tracing.

and 15 percent will be nonreactive.[86] Fewer than 1 percent of NSTs will prove unsatisfactory because of inadequately recorded fetal heart rate data. On rare occasions, a sinusoidal heart rate pattern may be observed as described in Chapter 7. This undulating heart rate pattern with virtually absent variability has been associated with fetal anemia, fetal asphyxia, congenital malformations, and medications such as narcotics.

The NST is most predictive when normal or reactive. A reactive NST has been associated with a perinatal mortality of approximately 5/1,000.[86,93] At least one-half of the deaths of babies dying within 1 week of a reactive test may be attributed to placental abruption or cord accidents. The perinatal mortality rate associated with a nonreactive NST, 30 to 40/1,000, is significantly higher, for this group includes those fetuses who are truly asphyxiated. A nonreactive NST has a considerable false-positive rate. Most fetuses exhibiting a nonreactive NST will not be compromised but will simply fail to exhibit heart rate reactivity during the 40-minute period of testing. Malformed fetuses also exhibit a significantly higher incidence of nonreactive NSTs.[94] Overall, the false-positive rate associated with the nonreactive NST is approximately 75 to 90 percent.[86] However, if the NST is extended for 80 minutes and a persistent absence of reactivity is observed, the fetus is likely to be severely compromised.

The likelihood of a nonreactive test is substantially increased early in the third trimester.[95] Between 24 and 28 weeks' gestation, approximately 50 percent of NSTs are nonreactive.[96] Fifteen percent of NSTs remain nonreactive between 28 and 32 weeks. After 32 weeks, the incidences of reactive and nonreactive tests are comparable to those seen at term. When accelerations of the baseline heart rate are seen during monitoring in the late second and early third trimester, the NST has been associated with fetal well-being.

Vibroacoustic stimulation (VAS) may be utilized to change fetal state from quiet to active sleep and shorten the length of the NST. Most clinicians use an electronic artificial larynx. The incidence of nonreactive NSTs is halved with VAS.[107,108] A reactive NST after VAS stimulation appears to be as reliable an index of fetal well-being as spontaneous reactivity. However, those fetuses that remain nonreactive even after VAS may be at increased risk for poor perinatal outcome.[109] The incidence of reactive NSTs after VAS is significantly increased after 26 weeks' gestation.

In most centers, if the baseline fetal heart rate pattern is nonreactive after 10 to 20 minutes, a stimulus of 3 seconds or less is applied near the fetal head. If the NST remains nonreactive, the stimulus is repeated at 1-minute intervals up to three times. If there continues to be no response to VAS, further evaluation should be carried out with a CST or BPP. VAS may be helpful in shortening the time required to perform an NST and may be especially useful in centers where large numbers of NSTs are done. Studies have confirmed the safety of VAS use during pregnancy and report no long-term evidence of hearing loss in children followed in the neonatal period and up to 4 years of age.

Significant fetal heart rate bradycardias, defined as a fetal heart rate of 90 bpm or a fall in the fetal heart rate of 40 bpm below the baseline for 1 minute or longer, have been observed in 1 to 2 percent of all NSTs.[116–120] Such bradycardias are associated with increased perinatal morbidity and mortality, particularly antepartum fetal death, cord compression, IUGR, and fetal malformations.[121] Clinical management decisions should be based on the finding of bradycardia, *not* on the presence or absence of reactivity. Bradycardia has a higher positive predictive value for fetal compromise (fetal death or fetal intolerance of labor) than does the nonreactive NST. In this setting, antepartum fetal death is most likely due to a cord accident.[116,119,120]

If a bradycardia is observed, an ultrasound examination should be performed to assess amniotic fluid volume and to detect the presence of anomalies. When expectant management has been followed, such bradycardias have been associated with a perinatal mortality rate of 25 percent. Several reports have therefore recommended that delivery be undertaken if the fetus is mature. When the fetus is premature, one might elect to administer corticosteroids to accelerate fetal lung maturation before delivery. Continuous fetal heart rate monitoring is necessary if expectant management is followed.

In most cases, mild variable decelerations are not associated with poor perinatal outcome. When mild variable decelerations are observed, even if the NST is reactive, an ultrasound examination should be done to rule out oligohydramnios. A low amniotic fluid index and mild variable decelerations increase the likelihood of a cord accident.

In selected high-risk pregnancies, the false-negative rate associated with a weekly NST may be unacceptably high.[123,124] It appears that the frequency of the NST should be increased to twice weekly in pregnancies complicated by diabetes mellitus, prolonged gestation, and IUGR.[125]

Which antepartum heart rate test is best? The NST has proved to be an ideal screening test and remains the primary method for antepartum fetal evaluation at most centers. It can be quickly performed in an outpatient setting and is easily interpreted. In contrast, the CST is usually performed near the labor and delivery suite, may require an intravenous infusion of oxytocin, and may be more difficult to interpret. In initial studies, a reactive NST appeared to be as predictive of good outcome as a negative CST. Nevertheless, as more data have been gathered, it appears that the ability of the CST to stress the fetus provides an earlier warning of fetal compromise. In most centers, the NST is used as the primary method for fetal evaluation, with more frequent testing in higher risk pregnancies. The CST is generally utilized to evaluate the fetus with a nonreactive NST. The type of test and its application should be "condition" or diagnosis specific, in which a similar basic screening approach is used, adding different types of evaluation and increased frequency of testing as appropriate for the clinical situation.

The healthy fetus should exhibit a reactive baseline heart rate with no late decelerations when a CST is performed. However, as the fetus deteriorates, one will first observe late decelerations and, finally, the most ominous fetal heart rate pattern, the nonreactive NST and positive CST[64,69,130] (Fig. 5-4). The unusual combination of a reactive NST and a positive CST has been associated with a higher incidence of IUGR and late decelerations in labor than that seen with a negative CST.[131] The likelihood of fetal death is increased in patients demonstrating a nonreactive NST followed by a negative CST.[65,132,133] Consequently, repeating the NST in 24 hours appears the prudent course in such cases.

Fetal Biophysical Profile

With real-time ultrasonography, fetal breathing movement (FBM) is evidenced by downward movement of the diaphragm and abdominal contents and by an inward collapsing of the chest. FBMs, when present, demonstrate intact neurologic control. While the absence of FBMs may reflect fetal asphyxia, this finding may also indicate that the fetus is in a period of quiet sleep.[32,33]

The evaluation of FBM has been used to distinguish the truly positive CST from a false-positive CST. Those fetuses that displayed FBM but had a positive CST were unlikely to exhibit fetal distress in labor. However, when a fetus failed to show FBM and demonstrated late decelerations during the CST, the likelihood of fetal compromise was great. A pattern emerged from these studies that, as long as one antepartum biophysical test was normal, the likelihood that the fetus would have a normal outcome was high.[139,140] As the number of abnormal tests increased, however, the likelihood that fetal asphyxia was present increased as well.

The fetal BPP score combines the NST with four parameters that can be assessed using real-time ultrasonography: FBM, fetal movement, fetal tone, and amniotic fluid volume. FBMs, fetal movement, and fetal tone are mediated by complex neurologic pathways and should reflect the function of the fetal CNS at the time of the examination. A nonreactive NST and absent FBM are the earliest signs of fetal compromise. Amniotic fluid volume should provide information about the presence of chronic fetal asphyxia. In most cases, the ultrasound-derived BPP parameters and NST can be completed within a relatively short time, each requiring approximately 10 minutes. Use of VAS for an equivocal BPP does not increase the false-negative rate and may reduce the likelihood of unnecessary obstetric intervention.[151] The ultrasound examination performed for the BPP has the added advantage of detecting previously unrecognized major fetal anomalies.

In calculating the BPP score, the presence of a normal parameter, such as a reactive NST, is awarded 2 points, while the absence of that parameter is scored as 0. The highest score a fetus can receive is 10, while the lowest score is 0. The BPP may be used as early as 26 to 28 weeks' gestation. Twice-weekly testing is recommended in pregnancies complicated by IUGR, diabetes mellitus, prolonged gestation, and hypertension with proteinuria. The scoring criteria and the clinical actions recommended in response to these scores are presented in Tables 5-3 and 5-4. Of all patients tested, almost 97 percent had a score of 8, which means that only 3 percent require further evaluation for scores of 6 or less. A significant inverse linear relationship has been observed between the last BPP score and both perinatal morbidity and mortality.[143] The false-positive rate, depending on the endpoint used, ranges from 75 percent for a score of 6 to less than 20 percent for a score of 0. In eight investigations using the BPP for fetal evaluation, the corrected perinatal mortality rate, excluding lethal anomalies, was 0.77/1,000.

Several drawbacks of the BPP should be considered. Unlike the NST and CST, unless the BPP is videotaped it cannot be reviewed. If the fetus is in a quiet sleep state, the BPP can require a long period of observation. The present scoring system does not consider the impact of hydramnios.

Table 5-3   Technique of Biophysical Profile Scoring

Biophysical Variable	Normal (Score = 2)	Abnormal (Score = 0)
Fetal breathing movements	At least one episode of > 30 seconds' duration in 30 minutes' observation	Absent or no episode of ≥30 seconds' duration in 30 minutes
Gross body movement	At least three discrete body/limb movements in 30 minutes (episodes of active continuous movement considered a single movement)	Up to two episodes of body/limb movements in 30 minutes
Fetal tone	At least one episode of active extension with return to flexion of fetal limb(s) or trunk; opening and closing of hand considered normal tone	Either slow extension with return to partial flexion or movement of limb in full extension or absent fetal movement
Reactive fetal heart rate	At least two episodes of acceleration of ≥15 bpm and 15 seconds' duration associated with fetal movement in 30 minutes	Fewer than two accelerations or acceleration <15 bpm in 30 minutes
Qualitative amniotic fluid volume	At least one pocket of amniotic fluid measuring 2 cm in two perpendicular planes	Either no amniotic fluid pockets or a pocket <2 cm in two perpendicular planes

Adapted from Manning FA: Biophysical profile scoring. *In* Nijhuis J (ed): Fetal Behaviour. New York, Oxford University Press, 1992, p 241, with permission.

Table 5-4 Management Based on Biophysical Profile

Score	Interpretation	Management
10	Normal infant; low risk of chronic asphyxia	Repeat testing at weekly intervals; repeat twice weekly in diabetic patients and patients at ≥42 weeks' gestation
8	Normal infant; low risk of chronic asphyxia	Repeat testing at weekly intervals; repeat testing twice weekly in diabetics and patients at ≥42 weeks' gestation; oligohydramnios is an indication for delivery
6	Suspect chronic asphyxia	If ≥36 weeks' gestation and conditions are favorable, deliver; if at <36 weeks and L/S <2.0, repeat test in 4–6 hours; deliver if oligohydramnios is present
4	Suspect chronic asphyxia	If ≥36 weeks' gestation, deliver; if <32 weeks, repeat score
0–2	Strongly suspect chronic asphyxia	Extend testing time to 120 minutes; if persistent score ≥4, deliver, regardless of gestation age

Adapted from Manning FA, Harman CR, Morrison I et al: Fetal assessment based on fetal biophysical profile scoring. Am J Obstet Gynecol 162:703,1990; and Manning FA: Biophysical profile scoring. *In* Nijhuis J (ed): Fetal Behaviour. New York, Oxford University Press, 1992, p 241, with permission.

Doppler Velocimetry

The principle of Doppler ultrasound has been utilized to measure blood flow in the uterine and fetal vessels. The Doppler effect is the key principle upon which flow studies are based.[152] A moving column of red blood cells will scatter and reflect a beam of ultrasound with a frequency shift proportional to the velocity of the blood flow. In other words, the frequency of the reflected sound is proportional to the speed of the moving red blood cells. Determining blood flow velocity will provide an indirect assessment of changes in blood flow. Calculation of flow velocity is derived from the equation

$$f_d = 2 f_0 \frac{V\cos\theta}{2} ,$$

where f_d is the change in ultrasound frequency or Doppler shift; f_0 is the transmitted frequency of the incident ultrasound; V is the velocity of the reflector or red blood cells; θ is the angle between the beam and the direction of movement of the reflector or red blood cells; and c is the velocity of sound in the medium (Fig. 5-7). The

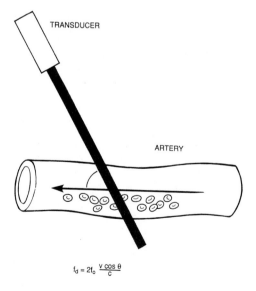

$$f_d = 2f_0 \frac{V\cos\theta}{c}$$

Fig. 5-7 Application of the Doppler principle to determine blood flow velocity. The frequency (f_0) of the ultrasound beam directed at a moving column of red blood cells with velocity V will be increased to f_d in proportion to V and the cosine of the angle of intersection of the vessel by the beam (θ).

velocity of sound in tissues is constant, and the frequency of the incident ultrasound is fixed by the transducer. Therefore, if the angle between the blood vessel studied and the ultrasound beam remains constant, the Doppler shift frequency, f_d, will be directly proportional to the flow velocity, V. The frequency of ultrasound used in Doppler velocimetry studies is 3 to 5 MHz.

Duplex systems to assess blood flow combine real-time imaging with pulsed-wave Doppler. The vessel to be insonated can be identified, and the ultrasound beam placed across that vessel using range gating.

However, for both technical and practical reasons, continuous-wave Doppler systems have been more widely applied.[152,153] These units are less expensive and employ considerably less power than the pulsed Doppler systems. Continuous-wave systems do not allow one to image the vessel to be insonated. Rather, one must depend on the identification of characteristic waveforms produced by maternal and fetal vessels.

Continuous-wave Doppler systems generate flow velocity waveforms that are directly proportional to changes in flow velocity within the vessel. The upswing of the frequency shift reflects stroke volume or cardiac contractility, while the downswing reflects vessel compliance and indicates peripheral resistance.

A variety of indices have been developed to quantify the flow velocity waveforms produced.[153,154] Most commonly used is the peak systolic (S)/diastolic (D) or S/D ratio, also know as the A/B ratio (Figs. 5-8 and 5-9). The greater the diastolic flow, the lower the ratio. As peripheral resistance increases, diastolic flow falls, and the S/D ratio increases.

The normal umbilical artery demonstrates a peak in systole with a large amount of end-diastolic flow, reflecting decreased placental resistance.[153] There is a progressive reduction in pulsatility and increase in diastolic flow throughout gestation. Abnormal umbilical artery flow shows decreased end-diastolic flow or, in extreme situations, absent or reversed end-diastolic flow (Fig. 5-10).[153,157]

While the umbilical artery S/D ratio can provide an approximation of umbilical artery flow, it best reflects changes in placental vascular resistance. How the fetus has responded to this placental abnormality and whether it is hypoxemic cannot be judged by flow velocity waveform indices. Umbilical artery waveforms are characterized by a progressive decline in S/D ratio from early pregnancy until term. This change reflects growth of small muscular arteries in the tertiary stem villi of the placenta. By 30 weeks' gestation, the S/D ratio in the umbilical artery should be below 3 (Fig. 5-11).[158]

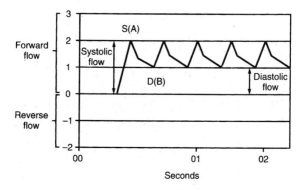

Fig. 5-8 Diagram of a normal umbilical artery flow velocity waveform. Note the forward flow during both systole and diastole, the latter indicating low resistance in the placental bed. (Adapted from Warsof SL, Levy, DL: Doppler blood flow and fetal growth retardation. *In* Gross TL, Sokol JR [eds]: Intrauterine Growth Retardation: A Practical Approach. Chicago, Year Book, 1989, p 163, with permission.)

The broadest application of Doppler flow has been the study of the pregnancy at risk for or demonstrating IUGR. This subject is discussed in Chapter 18. An elevation in the S/D ratio in the umbilical artery may precede the onset of growth restriction. When IUGR has been identified, an abnormal umbilical S/D ratio may be more predictive of neonatal morbidity than the

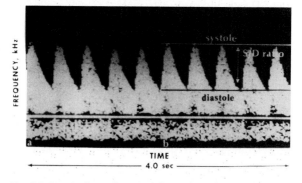

Fig. 5-9 Doppler flow velocity waveforms of the normal umbilical artery. Note that umbilical arterial flow velocities are recorded above the baseline, while nonpulsatile umbilical vein flow in the opposite direction is found below the baseline (A). Measurement of the S/D ratio is also illustrated (B). (From Bruner JP, Gabbe SG, Levy DW et al: Doppler ultrasonography of the umbilical cord in normal pregnancy. J South Med Assoc 86:52, 1993, with permission.)

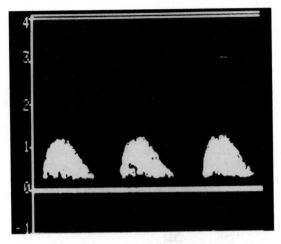

Fig. 5-10 This Doppler flow study reveals absent end-diastolic flow.

NST.[160] The absence of end-diastolic flow in the pregnancy complicated by growth restriction has been associated with nonreassuring intrapartum fetal heart rate patterns and an increased perinatal mortality rate.

The absence or reversal of umbilical end-diastolic frequencies has been considered an extremely ominous finding, and recommendations for immediate delivery

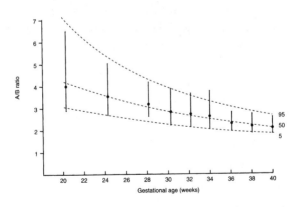

Fig. 5-11 Normal reference values for the S/D or A/B ratio in the umbilical artery throughout gestation. The 95th, 50th, and 5th percentiles are shown at each gestational age. Note that the ratio falls below 3 after 30 weeks' gestation. (From Thompson RS, Trudinger BJ, Cook CM et al: Umbilical artery velocity waveforms: normal reference values for A/B ratio and Pourcelot ratio. Br J Obstet Gynaecol 95:589, 1988, with permission.)

to avoid fetal death or irreversible compromise have been made by many.[166–168] It has also been suggested that reverse flow is more predictive of poor perinatal outcome than absent diastolic flow because it implies virtual cessation of effective uteroplacental circulation.[169] Absent or reversed end-diastolic flow has a sensitivity of 67 percent (20/30) in predicting perinatal death. The relatively high frequency of congenital malformations, including chromosomal abnormalities, in patients with markedly abnormal Doppler studies should lead to further evaluation of the fetus.

Doppler velocimetry is most reliable in conditions predisposing to IUGR, such as chronic hypertension, pregnancy-induced hypertension, collagen vascular disorders, and other diseases in which vasospasm plays a major role. This technique is also valuable in the follow-up of pregnancies with a diagnosis of IUGR or growth discordancy, such as in discordant twins (see Ch. 16). In other common obstetric conditions requiring fetal surveillance, such as prolonged pregnancy and diabetes mellitus, Doppler velocimetry offers no advantage over conventional techniques. Use of umbilical artery Doppler velocity for screening in low-risk pregnancies has not been shown to be either predictive of poor perinatal outcome or cost effective.[172]

The Assessment of Fetal Pulmonary Maturation

Assessment of Fetal Pulmonary Maturity

Available methods for evaluating fetal pulmonary maturity can be divided into four categories: (1) quantitation of pulmonary surfactant, such as the L/S ratio; (2) measurement of surfactant function, including the foam stability index; (3) evaluation of amniotic fluid turbidity; and (4) association with placental grade and cephalometry using ultrasonography.

Quantitation of Pulmonary Surfactant

Lecithin/Sphingomyelin Ratio

The amniotic fluid concentration of lecithin increases markedly at approximately 35 weeks' gestation, while sphingomyelin levels remain stable or decrease. Amniotic fluid sphingomyelin exceeds lecithin until 31 to 32 weeks, when the lecithin/sphingomyelin (L/S) ratio reaches 1. Lecithin then rises rapidly, and an L/S ratio of 2.0 is observed at approximately 35 weeks. A ratio of 2.0 or greater has been reliably associated with pulmonary maturity, predicting the absence of RDS in 98 percent of neonates. The L/S ratio, like most indices of fetal pulmonary maturation, rarely errs when predicting fetal pulmonary maturity but is frequently incorrect when predicting subsequent RDS.[181] Many neonates with an immature L/S ratio will not develop RDS.

Several variables must be considered in interpreting the predictive accuracy of the L/S ratio. A prolonged interval between the determination of an immature L/S ratio and delivery will necessarily increase the number of falsely immature results. It is probably best to discard amniotic fluid samples heavily contaminated by blood or meconium, because the effects of these compounds on the determination of the L/S ratio are quite unpredictable.[182,183] The presence of PG in a bloody or meconium-stained amniotic fluid sample remains a reliable indicator of pulmonary maturity.[184] Finally, it is essential that the obstetrician know the analytical technique used and the predictive value of a mature L/S ratio in his or her laboratory.

Many perinatal processes alter the final interpretation of the L/S ratio. Surfactant deficiency, immaturity, and intrapartum complications are the prime factors in determining the pathogenesis of RDS.[187] Birth asphyxia may lead to RDS in many infants despite an L/S ratio greater than 2.0.

Slide Agglutination Test for PG

PG, which does not appear until 35 weeks' gestation and increases rapidly between 37 and 40 weeks, is a marker of completed pulmonary maturation. A rapid immunologic semiquantitative agglutination test (Amniostat-FLM) can be used to determine the presence of PG.[195] The test takes 20 to 30 minutes to perform, while an L/S ratio may require 1 to 3 hours. No cases of RDS were observed when the Amniostat-FLM assay demonstrated PG. This technique can be applied to samples contaminated by blood and meconium.

Microviscosimeter

The relative lipid content of amniotic fluid may be evaluated by fluorescence depolarization analysis.[196] A lipid-soluble dye is incubated for 30 minutes with the amniotic fluid specimen, and the amount of dye absorbed into the phospholipid membrane structures within the fluid is determined by measuring the fluorescence of polarized light with the microviscosimeter (Felma, Elscint). The fluorescence polarization, or P value, falls as the L/S ratio rises. Few falsely mature results have been reported with P values ranging from less than 0.310 to 0.336. Specimens contaminated with blood cannot be used for this analysis.

TDx Test (Surfactant/Albumin Ratio)

The TDx analyzer, an automated fluorescence polarimeter, has been utilized to assess surfactant content in amniotic fluid.[197-199] The test requires 1 ml of amniotic fluid and can be run in less than 1 hour. The surfactant/albumin ratio is determined with amniotic fluid albumin used as an internal reference. A ratio of 50 to 70 mg surfactant per gram of albumin has been considered mature. The TDx test correlates well with the L/S ratio and has few falsely mature results, making it an excellent screening test. Approximately 50 percent of infants with an immature TDx result will develop RDS.

Measurement of Surfactant Function—Foam Stability Index

The foam stability test is based on the manual foam stability index (FSI), a variation of the shake test. The kit currently available contains test wells with a predispensed volume of ethanol to which amniotic fluid is added. The amniotic fluid–ethanol mixture is shaken, and the FSI value is read as the highest value well in which a ring of stable foam persists.[202] This test appears to be a reliable predictor of fetal lung maturity.[203] Subsequent RDS is very unlikely with an FSI value of 47 or higher. The assay appears to be extremely sensitive, with a high proportion of immature results being associated with RDS, as well as moderately specific, with a high proportion of mature results predicting the absence of RDS. Contamination of the amniotic fluid specimen by blood or meconium invalidates the FSI results.

Visual Evaluation of Amniotic Fluid Turbidity

During the first and second trimesters, amniotic fluid is yellow and clear. It becomes colorless in the third trimester. By 33 to 34 weeks' gestation, cloudiness and flocculation are noted and, as term approaches, vernix appears. Amniotic fluid with obvious vernix or fluid so turbid it does not permit the reading of newsprint through it will usually have a mature L/S ratio.[208]

Placental Grading and Cephalometry

With the exception of amniotic fluid specimens obtained from the vaginal pool, the evaluation of fetal pulmonary maturation requires that a sample of amniotic fluid be obtained by amniocentesis. In the past, third-trimester amniocentesis was associated with significant fetal and maternal risks. Fetal complications have included fetal bleeding from laceration of the placenta or umbilical cord, fetomaternal bleeding, premature labor and premature rupture of the membranes, placental abruption, and fetal injury. Maternal complications, although rare, have included hemorrhage, in some cases from perforation of the uterine vessels, abdominal wall hematomas, Rh sensitization, and infection. Ultrasound guidance for third-trimester amniocentesis has significantly decreased the risks of the procedure.

A bloody tap warrants careful observation. When a bloody tap occurs, the patient should have continuous electronic fetal heart rate monitoring until an Apt or Kleihauer-Betke test confirms that the blood is of maternal origin and the fetus has demonstrated no evidence of compromise. Should a nonreassuring fetal heart rate pattern be observed, cesarean delivery is performed. When fetal blood is recovered, the fetus is delivered if its pulmonary status is mature even if it has not exhibited fetal distress. For those fetuses with pulmonary immaturity, treatment with corticosteroids should be considered, with delivery thereafter.

Placental morphology on ultrasound has been correlated with fetal pulmonary maturation. Four stages of placental maturation have been described based on the appearance of the basal and chorionic plates of the placenta and the placental substance. With progression from the least mature placenta, grade 0, to the most mature placenta, grade 3, one observes increasing deposition of calcium within the placental septa. An excellent correlation has been observed between the presence of a grade 3 placenta at term and a mature L/S ratio in an uncomplicated pregnancy.

There is also a correlation between the BPD and fetal pulmonary maturation. A BPD of at least 9.2 cm will reliably predict the absence of RDS in uncomplicated pregnancies.[226] This approach should not be used for patients with diabetes mellitus.

In summary, ultrasound parameters that correlate with fetal pulmonary maturation may be helpful when the risk of amniocentesis is increased, as with an anterior placenta. However, the most appropriate use of ultrasound in predicting fetal lung maturity is early documentation of gestational age so that elective delivery later in pregnancy can be safely undertaken.

Determination of Fetal Pulmonary Maturation in Clinical Practice

A large number of techniques are now available to assess fetal pulmonary maturation. Several rapid screening tests, including the TDx test, FSI, and Amniostat-FLM, appear to be highly reliable when mature. In an uncomplicated pregnancy, when a screening test such as the TDx demonstrates fetal pulmonary maturation, one can safely proceed with delivery. This approach is also extremely cost effective.[228,229] However, when the screening test is immature, the L/S ratio and PG assay should be used. Similarly, in complicated pregnancies such as those with diabetes mellitus, IUGR, and Rh isoimmunization, the L/S ratio and PG should be determined to assess fetal pulmonary maturation. As noted above, in an uncomplicated pregnancy at term, when an amniocentesis would be difficult because of placental or fetal location, placental grade and fetal BPD may be used as an indirect measure of fetal pulmonary maturation.

Summary

How can one most efficiently use all the techniques available for antepartum fetal surveillance? Obstetricians should take a "diagnosis-specific" approach to testing. They must consider the pathophysiology of the disease process that will be evaluated and then select the best method or methods of testing for that problem. In a pregnancy complicated by diabetes mellitus, careful monitoring of maternal glucose levels should accompany antepartum heart rate testing. In a pregnancy complicated by suspected growth restriction, one would want to make serial evaluations of amniotic fluid volume with ultrasound to detect oligohydramnios.

In a prolonged pregnancy, one would use a parallel testing scheme. In this situation, the obstetrician is concerned not with fetal maturity, but rather with fetal well-being. Several tests are performed at the same time, such as antepartum fetal heart rate testing and the BPP. It is acceptable in this high-risk situation to intervene when a single test is abnormal. One is willing to accept a false-positive test result to avoid the intrauterine death of a mature and otherwise healthy fetus.

In most other high-risk pregnancies, such as those complicated by diabetes mellitus or hypertension, it is preferable to allow the fetus to remain in utero as long as possible. In these situations, a branched testing scheme is used. To decrease the likelihood of unnecessary premature intervention, the obstetrician uses a series of tests and, under most circumstances, would only deliver a premature infant when all parameters suggest fetal compromise. In this situation, one must consider the likelihood of neonatal RDS as predicted by the evaluation of amniotic fluid indices and review these risks with colleagues in neonatology.

Maternal assessment of fetal activity would appear to be an ideal first-line screening test for both high-risk and low-risk patients. The use of this approach may decrease the number of unexpected intrauterine deaths in so-called normal pregnancies. Although a negative CST has been associated with fewer intrauterine deaths than a reactive NST, the NST appears to have significant advantages in screening high-risk patients. It can be easily and rapidly performed in an outpatient setting. The nipple stimulation CST provides an excellent alternative for those who favor primary use of the CST, particularly in the prolonged pregnancy and those cases complicated by diabetes mellitus and IUGR. Most clinicians, however, use the BPP or CST to assess fetal condition further in patients

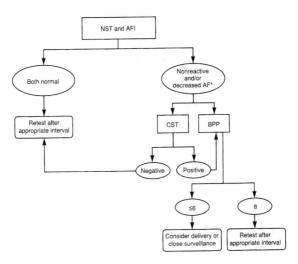

Fig. 5-12 Flow chart for antepartum fetal surveillance in which the NST and AFI are used as the primary methods for fetal evaluation. A nonreactive NST and decreased AFI are further evaluated using either the CST or the BPP. Further details regarding the use of the BPP are provided in Table 5-4. *If the fetus is mature and amniotic fluid volume is reduced, delivery should be considered before further testing is undertaken. (Adapted from Finberg HJ, Kurtz AB, Johnson RL et al: The biophysical profile: a literature review and reassessment of its usefulness in the evaluation of fetal well-being. J Ultrasound Med 9:583, 1990, with permission.)

exhibiting a persistently nonreactive NST. This sequential approach may be particularly valuable in avoiding unnecessary premature intervention.

Figure 5-12 presents a practical testing scheme that has been utilized successfully by several centers.[104,134,230,231] The NST, an indicator of present fetal condition, may be combined with the amniotic fluid index (AFI) (Ch. 4), a marker of long-term status, in a modified BPP. VAS may be used to shorten the time required to achieve a reactive NST. While most patients are evaluated weekly, patients with diabetes mellitus, IUGR, or a prolonged gestation are tested twice weekly. If the NST is nonreactive despite VAS or extended monitoring, or if the AFI is abnormal, either a CST or full BPP is performed.

Key Points

- The prevalence of an abnormal condition (i.e., fetal death) has great impact on the predictive value of antepartum fetal tests.
- The near-term fetus spends approximately 25 percent of its time in a quiet sleep state (state 1F) and 60 to 70 percent in an active sleep state (state 2F).
- Approximately 5 percent of women monitoring fetal movement will report decreased fetal activity.
- The incidence of perinatal death within 1 week of a negative CST is less than 1/1,000.
- The observation that accelerations of the fetal heart rate in response to fetal activity, uterine contractions, or stimulation reflect fetal well-being is the basis for the NST.
- The frequency of the NST should be increased to twice weekly in pregnancies complicated by diabetes mellitus, prolonged gestation, and IUGR.
- Use of VAS for an equivocal BPP does not increase the false-negative rate and may reduce the likelihood of unnecessary obstetric intervention.
- The absence of end-diastolic flow in the umbilical artery flow velocity waveform has been associated with an increased perinatal mortality rate.
- Most amniotic fluid indices of fetal pulmonary maturation rarely err when predicting maturity, but are frequently incorrect when predicting subsequent RDS.
- The NST, an indicator of present fetal condition, and the amniotic fluid index, a marker of long-term fetal status, have been combined in the modified BPP.

SECTION 2
Intrapartum Care

Chapter 6

Labor and Delivery

William F. O'Brien and
Robert C. Cefalo

Management of Labor and Delivery

Definitions

Labor is defined as progressive dilatation of the uterine cervix in association with repetitive uterine contractions. This definition serves to exclude instances in which cervical dilatation occurs without uterine contractions, such as an incompetent cervix. Also excluded are uterine contractions that occur without true progressive dilatation, as is common in the latter stage of pregnancy.

Normal Mechanisms of Labor

Stages and Phases of Labor

Normal labor is a continuous process, and is divided into three stages. The first stage of labor is the interval between the onset of labor and full cervical dilatation. The second stage is the interval between full cervical dilatation and the delivery of the infant. The third stage of labor encompasses the period between the delivery of the infant and delivery of the placenta.

The first stage of labor has been subdivided by Friedman[1] into three phases. The latent phase is defined as the period between the onset of labor and a point at which a change in the slope of cervical dilatation is noted. The phase of maximal dilatation is that period of labor when the rate of cervical dilatation is maximal. A short deceleration phase follows the acceleration phase and ends at full cervical dilatation. The descent phase usually coincides with the second stage of labor.

The Mechanisms of Labor

The mechanisms of labor are the changes in the position of the fetal head during passage through the birth canal. The cardinal movements of labor are (1) engagement, (2) descent, (3) flexion, (4) internal rotation, (5) extension, (6) external rotation, and (7) expulsion.

Engagement

In the normal flexed position, the largest transverse diameter of the fetal head is the biparietal diameter (Fig. 6-1). Engagement is the descent of the biparietal diameter of the fetal head to a level below the plane of the pelvic inlet. Clinically, if the lowest portion of the occiput is at or below the level of the maternal ischial spines, engagement has usually taken place. Engagement is considered an important clinical parameter, as it demonstrates that, at least at the level of the pelvic inlet, the maternal bony pelvis is sufficiently large to allow the descent of the fetal head. Engagement often occurs before the onset of true labor, especially in nulliparas.

Descent

The greatest rate of descent in the deceleration phase of the first stage of labor and during the second stage of labor.

Flexion

Complete flexion with the placement of the fetal chin on the thorax usually occurs only during the course of labor.

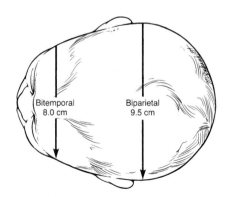

Bitemporal
8.0 cm

Biparietal
9.5 cm

Fig. 6-1 Average transverse diameters of the term fetal skull.

Internal Rotation

During internal rotation, the fetal occiput gradually rotates from its original position (usually transverse with regard to the birth canal) toward the symphysis pubis or, less commonly, toward the hollow of the sacrum. This facilitates the presentation of the smallest possible diameters of the fetal head to the birth canal. As the coccygeus and ileococcygeus muscles form a V-shaped hammock diverging anteriorly, the occiput of the fetus rotates toward the symphysis pubis.

Extension

Descent brings the base of the occiput into contact with the inferior margin of the symphysis pubis. The fetal head is delivered by extension from the flexed to the extended position.

External Rotation

After delivery of the head, the fetus resumes its previous position.

Expulsion

After external rotation of the fetal head, further descent brings the anterior shoulder to the level of the symphysis pubis. After the shoulders, the rest of the body is usually quickly delivered.

Management of Normal Labor and Delivery

The fetal heart rate should be recorded at least every 30 minutes during the first stage of labor. The heart rate should be auscultated immediately after uterine contractions. During the second stage of labor, the fetal heart rate should be auscultated at least every 15 minutes, and preferably after each uterine contraction.

Aspiration pneumonitis, a major cause of anesthetic-associated maternal mortality, is related to the acidity of gastric contents. The use of a clear antacid such as 0.3-M sodium citrate during the course of labor has been recommended by many authors.

Management of Labor in High-Risk Patients

Continuous electronic fetal monitoring is recommended for patients identified as high risk. Internal uterine pressure monitoring provides important information regarding the quality and quantity of contractions. An assessment of fetal scalp capillary pH can be performed in situations of potential fetal distress and may clarify suspicious or confusing fetal heart rate patterns. In patients at high risk, if no specific problems have been identified during the course of labor, management should proceed in a manner similar to that recommended for low-risk patients.

Assisted Spontaneous Delivery

The goals of assisted spontaneous delivery are the reduction of maternal trauma, prevention of fetal injury, and initial support of the newborn.

Episiotomy

A midline, or median, episiotomy is made vertically toward the anus, and a mediolateral episiotomy is made at a 45-degree angle from the inferior portion of the hymenal ring. Although there is general agreement that episiotomy is indicated in cases of arrested or protracted descent or accompanying forceps or vacuum delivery, the role of prophylactic episiotomy is widely debated. Cited advantages include the substitution of a straight surgical incision for ragged spontaneous lacerations and reduction in the duration of the second stage. Although elective episiotomy has been advocated principally as a method to reduce the likelihood of subsequent pelvic relaxation,[7] this association has never been proven.[8]

Disadvantages of episiotomy include increased blood loss, and an increase in third- and fourth-degree lacerations, which sometimes leads to long-term morbidity. Although a mediolateral episiotomy may serve to reduce the likelihood of third-degree lacerations, this procedure is considerably more painful than a median episiotomy, causes increased blood loss, and is more difficult to repair. Routine episiotomy is no longer recommended.

Delivery of the Head

The goal of assisted delivery of the head is the prevention of rapid delivery. If extension does not occur with ease, assistance in the form of a modified Ritgen maneuver may be provided. The hand, protected by a sterile towel, is placed on the perineum and the fetal chin palpated. The chin is then gently pressed upward, effecting extension of the fetal head.

After expulsion of the head, external rotation is allowed. If the cord is palpable around the neck, it should be looped over the head or, if not reducible, doubly clamped and cut. Mucus should be aspirated from the fetal mouth, oropharynx, and nares. Although aspiration is usually performed with a bulb syringe, in the presence of meconium thorough aspiration with a DeLee suction catheter reduces the risk of meconium aspiration syndrome.

Delivery of the Shoulders and Body

Once the fetal airway has been cleared, the physician places his or her hands along the parietal bones of the fetus, and the mother is asked to bear down gently. The fetus is directed posteriorly until the anterior shoulder has passed beneath the symphysis.

After delivery of the anterior shoulder, the mother should be asked to pant. The fetus is slowly directed anteriorly until the posterior shoulder passes the perineum.

After delivery of the shoulders, the fetus should be grasped with the palm of one hand above the shoulders and the other hand along the spine. The infant should be cradled as delivery is completed.

Cord Clamping

The umbilical vein permits passage of blood for up to 3 minutes after birth. Gravitational effects are important in cord blood flow. The physician can therefore influence the degree of postnatal placental transfusion both by the interval between delivery and cord clamping and by altering the height at which the infant is held after delivery.

Pelvimetry and Labor

Clinical Pelvimetry

The diagonal conjugate is the distance from the inferior border of the symphysis pubis to the sacral promontory. It is an easily obtainable index of the anteroposterior (AP) diameter of the pelvic inlet. The measurement is made by positioning the tip of the middle finger at the sacral promontory and noting the point on the hand that contacts the symphysis pubis. The diagonal conjugate is generally 1.5 to 2.0 cm longer than the obstetric conjugate.

The second clinical measurement is the bisischial diameter. With the patient in the lithotomy position, the ischial tuberosities are palpated and the distance between them measured. A value of greater than 8 cm is considered adequate. A small measurement may imply a generally small pelvis or convergence of the pelvic sidewalls.

Other characteristics of the pelvis are described qualitatively (small, average, large). These include the angulation of the pubic rami beneath the pubic arch, the apparent size of the ischial spines, the size of the sacrospinous notch, and the degree of curvature of the sacrum and coccyx.

X-Ray Pelvimetry

X-ray pelvimetry still plays a role in the management of patients with breech presentation. The most commonly used measurements are the AP and transverse diameters and their totals at the pelvic inlet and at the pelvic midplane. More recently, Morgan and Thurman[13] have utilized the fetal–pelvic index, combining ultrasound measurements of the fetus with x-ray pelvimetry.

Risks of X-Ray Pelvimetry

The primary concern governing the use of x-ray pelvimetry is exposure of the fetus to ionizing radiation. The likelihood of childhood malignancy is approximately 1 cancer per 5,000 infants exposed. This risk is small in comparison to the hazard of perinatal mortality associated with cephalopelvic disproportion.

Most authorities agree that the hazards of breech presentation are sufficient to warrant x-ray pelvimetry for cases in which vaginal delivery is contemplated. Most modern authors have recommended that women with pelvic diameters of less than average size are best managed by cesarean delivery.[9,20]

Obstetric Palpation — Leopold Maneuvers

Leopold divided abdominal palpation into four separate maneuvers that can identify fetal landmarks and reveal fetal–maternal relationships.

Leopold's 4 maneuvers:

1. *What is at the fundus?* The examiner places his or her hands at the fundus of the uterus. Palpation ascertains the presence or absence of a fetal pole (vertical vs. transverse lie) and the nature of the fetal pole. The fetal breech is larger, less well defined, and less ballottable than the cranium.
2. *Where are the spine and small parts?* The lateral walls

of the uterus are examined. In vertical lies, the sides will usually be occupied by the fetal back and small parts (extremities).

3. *What is presenting in the pelvis?* The fingertips are placed above the symphysis and brought toward the midline. When the fetus is encountered, the characteristics and degree of descent of the fetal pole are noted.

4. *Where is the cephalic prominence?* In cephalic presentations, a point of the fetal head may be noted as a protuberance that arrests the hand outlining the fetus.

Disorders of Labor

Abnormal Patterns

Abnormal patterns of labor are defined by deviation from the norms for the phases of labor. For all phases except the latent phase, the abnormality may be either protraction or arrest (an arrested latent phase implies that labor has not truly begun).

Prolonged Latent Phase

The latent phase of labor is defined as the period of time starting with the onset of regular uterine contractions and terminated by the onset of the active phase. This phase is considered prolonged if it exceeds approximately 20 hours in nulliparas or 14 hours in multiparas. Most patients will simply be those who have entered labor without substantial cervical effacement. For these women the process that normally occurs over weeks must be compressed into hours.

Most authorities agree that the management of prolonged latent phase consists of therapeutic rest with a rather large dose of morphine (15 to 20 mg). After several hours of rest (usually sleep), approximately 85 percent of patients so treated will progress to the active phase. Approximately 10 percent will cease to have contractions, and the diagnosis of false labor may be made. For the approximately 5 percent of patients in whom therapeutic rest fails and in patients for whom expeditious delivery is indicated, oxytocin infusion may be used.

Two other methods of management must be condemned. Amniotomy holds little benefit for the patient with prolonged latent phase and may serve only to increase the risk of intrauterine infection or cord prolapse. Finally, cesarean delivery for this indication alone benefits neither the fetus nor the mother.

Disorders of the Active Phase

Inefficient uterine activity is also divided into hypertonic and hypotonic dysfunction. In either circumstance, the contraction pattern fails to result in cervical effacement and dilatation.

Hypotonic dysfunction may be seen at any point during labor. Uterine contractions are infrequent, of low amplitude, and accompanied by low or normal baseline pressures. Maternal discomfort is minimal. Hypertonic dysfunction is primarily a condition of nulliparas and is usually associated with early labor. Frequent contractions of low amplitude are often associated with an elevated baseline pressure. Maternal discomfort is significant and backache frequent.

Primary Dysfunctional Labor

Primary dysfunctional labor is defined as active-phase dilatation that occurs at a rate less than 1.2 cm/hr in nulliparas and 1.5 cm/hr in multiparas. An example of this disorder is shown in Figure 6-2.

Optimal management of primary dysfunctional labor is a major distinction between the American and Irish schools of labor management. At the National Maternity Hospital in Dublin, prompt amniotomy and oxytocin infusion[28] have been associated with lower cesarean section rates (see "Active Management of Labor" p 140). Primary dysfunctional labor is a frequent prede-

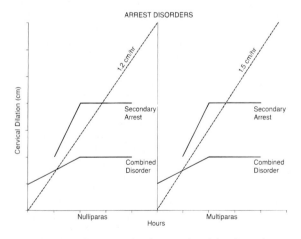

Fig. 6-2 Active-phase arrest disorders. Combined disorder implies an arrest in a gravida previously exhibiting primary dysfunctional labor.

cessor of secondary arrest of labor and requires careful maternal and fetal surveillance. Primary dysfunctional labor alone is not an indication for cesarean delivery.

Secondary Arrest of Cervical Dilatation and Combined Disorders of Active Phase

Secondary arrest is defined as cessation of a previously normal dilatation for a period of 2 hours. A combined disorder of active-phase dilatation is defined as arrest of dilatation occurring when the patient has previously exhibited primary dysfunctional labor (Fig. 6-2).

A generally accepted management program consists of a careful examination, including assessment of fetal and pelvic size, followed by amniotomy and initiation of intrauterine monitoring. If hypotonic uterine dysfunction exists oxytocin infusion may be used with a high degree of success and safety. Most authorities cite continued arrest over 2 to 4 hours as an indication for cesarean delivery. It must be noted, however, that even in the group in which progress is noted, there is an increased frequency of second-stage abnormalities and operative deliveries.

Abnormalities of the Second Stage

Protraction of descent is defined as descent occurring at less than 1 cm/hr in nulliparas and 2 cm/hr in multiparas.[31]

Reviews of electronic fetal heart rate tracings obtained during this stage have documented a high incidence of variable decelerations and prolonged decelerations.[33] The gradual fall in fetal scalp capillary pH that occurs throughout labor is accelerated during the second stage.[34] Until recently, these factors led to a policy of intervention whenever the second stage exceeded 2 hours. When electronic fetal monitoring is reassuring, operative intervention may be avoided provided that descent is progressive.[35]

Arrest of descent requires prompt reevaluation of uterine contractility, maternal and fetal well being, and cephalopelvic relationships. Obvious problems such as hypotonic dysfunction, overdistended bladder, or conduction anesthesia with ineffectual bearing down should be treated appropriately with a high expectation of success. In the absence of such factors, however, careful judgment is required. For patients in whom low forceps delivery is possible, this is the procedure of choice. When a low forceps delivery is not possible, the choice among mid-forceps delivery, vacuum extraction, oxytocin infusion, or cesarean delivery is difficult, and consultation is often helpful.

Stimulation of Uterine Activity

Measurements of Uterine Activity

External tocodynamometry measures the change in shape of the abdominal wall as a function of uterine contractions. This method permits graphic display of uterine activity in relationship to fetal heart rate patterns.

The most precise method for determination of uterine activity is the direct method, with insertion of a fluid-filled catheter directly into the uterine cavity through the cervix after rupture of the membranes.

The most commonly used units of uterine activity are the Montevideo Unit (average intensity frequency/10 min) and the Uterine Activity Unit (1 mm Hg/min).[37] When an abnormality in the progression of labor is noted and uterine activity is not optimal (i.e., contractions of less than 50 mm Hg every 3 minutes, or below 250 Montevideo Units),[39] administration of an oxytocic agent is recommended.

Oxytocic Agents

Sensitivity of the uterus to oxytocin increases between the 20th and 40th weeks of pregnancy. Very high infusion rates of oxytocin have been associated with hypertension, and bolus injections may cause hypotension. When it is administered intravenously as dilute solutions with strict control of the infusion rate, few cardiovascular side effects are noted.

The recommended rate of administration for oxytocin is usually that which simulates normal labor. This rate may vary from 0.5 mIU/min to greater than 30 mIU/min. When used in patients demonstrating a protraction disorder, oxytocin infusion rates greater than 6 mIU/min are rarely required.[43] Approximately 30 to 40 minutes are needed for the full effect of an increase in dosage to be evident in the contraction pattern.

Active Management of Labor

Considerable interest has been directed toward the disparity in the incidences of cesarean delivery between the United States and Ireland. O'Driscoll et al.[45] have maintained that the low rate of cesarean delivery at the National Maternity Hospital in Dublin is due to a philosophy of labor management known as active management. The basic principles of active management include

1. Strict criteria for admission to the labor suite
2. Early amniotomy
3. Hourly cervical examinations
4. Oxytocin administration for dilatation rates less than 1 cm/hr
5. High concentrations of oxytocin in patients requiring augmentation
6. Expected durations of less than 12 hours for the first stage of labor and 2 hours for the second stage

Adherence to these principles at the National Maternity Hospital in Dublin has been associated with a primary cesarean delivery rate of 5 to 6 percent. Direct comparison of cesarean delivery rates between countries is difficult. It would seem, however, that active management offers the potential for the safe reduction in the rate of caesarean delivery due to dystocia.

Forceps Delivery and Vacuum Extraction

Types of Forceps and Specialized Functions

Each half-forceps consists of the blade proper (which is applied to the fetal head), a shank, and a handle. The halves are joined by a lock usually located at the junction of the shanks and the handles. The overall architecture of a forceps is determined by two curves, the cephalic curve, which allows for the area of the fetal head, and the pelvic curve, compensating for the curvature of the birth canal.

The blades may be either solid or fenestrated, and the shanks may be either separated or overlapping. Instruments are illustrated in Figures 6-3 and 6-4. Three commonly used instruments are the Simpson forceps (fenestrated blade, separated shanks), the Elliot forceps (fenestrated blade, overlapping shanks), and the Tucker-McLane forceps (solid blade, overlapping shanks). "Specialized" forceps have been designed to facilitate delivery in cases requiring rotation of the fetal head (Kielland) or for breech delivery (Piper).

Classification of Forceps Delivery

Forceps deliveries are classified according to the station of the fetal head at the time of application:

1. *Outlet forceps:* Application of forceps when the

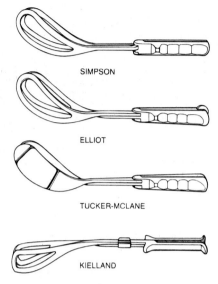

Fig. 6-3 Lateral views of some obstetric forceps. The pelvic curve, a prominent feature of classic instruments, is lacking in the Kielland forceps.

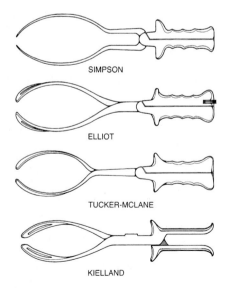

Fig. 6-4 AP view of some forceps. Note the difference between the separated shanks of the Simpson forceps and the overlapping shanks of the Elliot forceps.

scalp is visible at the introitus without separating the labia, the fetal skull has reached the pelvic floor, the fetal head is at or on the perineum, and the angle between the AP line and the sagittal suture does not exceed 45 degrees

2. *Low forceps:* Application when the leading point of the skull is at station +2 or more, subclassified as to whether the angle between the sagittal suture and AP exceeds 45 degrees

3. *Mid-forceps:* Application of forceps when the head is engaged but the presenting part is above station +2

Indications and Contraindications

The major controversy surrounds the mid-forceps delivery. As a group, infants delivered by this method demonstrate an increased incidence of perinatal mortality, perinatal morbidity, and long-term neurologic defects.[50,51] Opponents of the continued use of this technique argue that mid-forceps delivery should be abandoned in a manner similar to high forceps.[52,53] Proponents of the continued usage of mid-forceps believe that the great majority of infants with poor outcome after mid-forceps delivery result from deliveries that are considered difficult.[54]

Outlet forceps may be used to shorten the second stage of labor when it is in the best interests of the mother or fetus. More difficult forceps delivery (low or mid-forceps) may be considered when the second stage is prolonged, for fetal distress, or for maternal indications such as cardiac disease. Mid-forceps deliveries should be reserved for competent operators following careful consideration of the potential fetal risks.

Prerequisites for Forceps Delivery

All forceps deliveries require that several criteria be met before the application of the forceps. These include

1. The membranes must be ruptured.
2. The cervix must be fully dilated.
3. The operator must be fully acquainted with the use of the instrument.
4. The position and station of the fetal head must be known with certainty.
5. Adequate maternal anesthesia for proper application of the forceps must be present.
6. The maternal pelvis must be adequate in size for atraumatic delivery.
7. The characteristics of the maternal pelvis must be

appropriate for the type of delivery being considered.

8. The fetal head must be engaged.

The Use of Vacuum Extraction

Suction induces a caput succedaneum (chignon) within the cup to which tractional force is applied during uterine contractions. Randomized studies comparing forceps with vacuum have not shown a significant difference in success rate or complications.

The indications and contraindications to vacuum extraction are essentially the same as those for forceps delivery. An advantage of vacuum extraction, however, is that delivery may be accomplished with minimal maternal analgesia.

The Third Stage of Labor

The interval between delivery of the infant and delivery of the placenta is less than 15 minutes in approximately 95 percent of all deliveries. If the placenta has not delivered within 30 minutes or if excessive bleeding occurs, manual removal is indicated.

Separation of the placenta is a consequence of continued uterine contractions following expulsion of the fetus. Continued powerful and prolonged contractions serve to control blood loss from the spiral arteries through compression and transport the placenta from the fundus into the lower uterine segment.

Separation of the placenta can usually be detected by the occurrence of the classic signs of placental detachment. These include (1) a gush of blood from the vagina, (2) descent of the umbilical cord, (3) a change in shape of the uterine fundus from discoid to globular, and (4) an increase in the height of the fundus as the lower uterine segment is distended by the placenta.

Fundal compression or traction on the umbilical cord can increase the incidence of complications such as hemorrhage or uterine inversion. Proper management requires only gentle palpation of the uterine fundus for uterine contractions and observation for excessive blood loss. After delivery of the placenta, oxytocin administration can reduce blood loss. The physician should conduct a careful and thorough examination of the cervix, vagina, and perineum. The uterine fundus should be examined transabdominally to ensure that it is firm and that the uterine size is appropriate.

In the absence of anesthesia, intravaginal exploration for obstetric trauma can be quite uncomfortable, and the mother should be notified in advance of the procedures to be performed. Three or four fingers of one hand placed against the posterior vaginal wall and depressed will provide excellent visualization of the vagina and cervix in most cases. Using a sponge forceps, the obstetrician should grasp the anterior lip of the cervix and visualize the entire rim of the cervix either simultaneously or sequentially. After cervical inspection, visualization of both vaginal sidewalls for evidence of lacerations or hematoma formation should be accomplished.

Perineal inspection involves examination of the AP fourchette, vaginal vestibule, hymenal ring, perineal body, external rectal sphincter, and rectal mucosa.

After delivery, the placenta, cord, and membranes should be examined. The classic hallmark of placental abruption is a depressed area on the maternal side of the placenta with an attached blood clot. These findings, however, may not be present if the event is recent or sufficiently remote from delivery to allow organization of the clot.

The cord itself should be inspected for the correct number of vessels and true knots. A single umbilical artery is associated with other anomalies in about 20 percent of infants. Opaque membranes usually indicate chorioamnionitis, which may or may not be associated with other findings of intrauterine infection.

The placenta and membranes should be examined for signs of tearing or missing pieces. A vessel coursing along the membranes should arouse suspicion of an accessory lobe. Intrauterine exploration is required when there is suspicion of retained tissue and in cases of premature delivery.

Induction of Labor

Before the decision to induce labor, the physician should document whether the induction is elective or indicated and that the patient has been informed and accepts the indications, the methods, and potential complications, including the possibility of cesarean delivery.

The maternal pelvis should be assessed clinically as to its adequacy for vaginal delivery. Bishop[64] evaluated multiparous patients for elective induction of labor and developed a score for different variables found from the vaginal exam. Table 6-1 represents a modification of Bishop's method for predicting the ease of induction in which a score of 0, 1, 2, or 3 is given for dilatation, effacement, consistency, and position of the cervix and for station of the vertex. A total score of 9 or above

Table 6-1   Bishop Prelabor Scoring System

Factor	Score			
	0	1	2	3
Dilation (cm)	Closed	1–2	3–4	5 or more
Effacement (%)	0–30	40–50	60–70	80 or more
Station	−3	−2	−1.0	+1, +2
Consistency	Firm	Medium	Soft	
Position of cervix	Posterior	Mid-position	Anterior	

indicates that induction of labor should be successful. It should be recognized that the induction process attempts to accomplish in hours what may take several days of spontaneous prelabor.

Methodology

Surgical

Stripping of Membranes

Digitally separating the chorioamniotic membrane from the wall of the cervix and lower uterine segment releases prostaglandins produced locally from the membranes and adjacent decidua.[67,68] In addition, the method may excite an autonomic neural reflex or cause the release of maternal oxytocin from the posterior pituitary, which may initiate labor.[69] The vertex should be well applied to the cervix. The effects of membrane stripping are not predictable and the efficacy of this method has not been proven.

Amniotomy

In patients with a high Bishop score, artificial rupture of the membranes has been reported to be highly successful in inducing labor in multiparous patients. The amniotic fluid should be released without dislodging the vertex.

Advantages of amniotomy are (1) high success rate, (2) observation of the amniotic fluid for blood or meconium, and (3) ready access for an intrauterine pressure catheter, a direct fetal scalp electrode, and fetal scalp blood sampling. Risks include (1) umbilical cord prolapse, (2) adverse change in fetal position, (3) prolonged rupture of membranes and increased risk of ascending uterine or fetal infection, (4) fetal injury, and (5) rupture of vasa previa and subsequent fetal hemorrhage.

After amniotomy, the fetal heart rate should be carefully monitored. Decelerations or bradycardia of the fetal heart rate are rare without overt or occult umbilical cord prolapse.

If uterine contractions do not ensue after 2 to 4 hours, then intravenous oxytocin should be initiated.

Medical: Oxytocin

The safest method of induction is with a properly regulated continuous intravenous infusion of oxytocin. The prepared solution of oxytocin is piggybacked into the primary line through a sidearm near the intravenous insertion site in the patient's arm so that it can be discontinued and the intravenous line left open.

The rate of administration is usually recommended as that which produces contractions every 2 to 3 minutes, lasting 60 to 90 seconds with 50 to 60 mm Hg intrauterine pressure and a resting uterine tone of 10 to 15 mm Hg. Dosage may vary from 0.5 to 40 mU/min of oxytocin and induction protocols vary. As labor progresses, the frequency and intensity of contractions may increase. The infusion rate of oxytocin can then be reduced to prevent hyperstimulation.

Monitoring of uterine contractions and fetal heart rate is recommended throughout the induction and is best accomplished with continuous electronic monitoring. Constant surveillance of uterine activity is recommended to avoid uterine hyperstimulation.

Prostaglandins

Prostaglandin E_1 and E_2 derivatives have been successfully used to ripen the cervix before amniotomy or oxytocin infusion. Prepidil gel contains dinoprostone as the naturally occurring form of prostaglandin E_2. The dosage recommended is 0.5 mg in the cervical canal every 6 hours. Cervidil vaginal inserts contain 10 mg of dinoprostone released at 0.3 mg/h and can be easily removed if hyperstimulation occurs. Misoprostol, a synthetic PGE_1 analog, has also been used for cervical ripening. It is associated with a higher risk of hyperstimulation than oxytocin.

Complications

Hypercontractility

The most frequently encountered complication of intravenously administered oxytocin is uterine hyperstimulation which may produce fetal distress, abruptio placentae, or uterine rupture. The use of electronic monitoring has increased the early detection of these potentially lethal maternal or fetal complications.

Water Intoxication

Oxytocin is related structurally and functionally to vasopressin, or antidiuretic hormone (ADH), and shares its effect. The use of regulatory infusion pumps and electrolyte-containing solutions can help to prevent water intoxication, which can lead to hyponatremia, confusion, convulsions, coma, congestive heart failure, and death. The ADH effect is rarely seen when the dosage of oxytocin remains below 20 mU/min.

Uterine Rupture

Uterine rupture may occur with the use of oxytocin. This obstetric disaster is more common in grand multiparous patients, in women who have undergone prior uterine surgery, with fetal malpresentations, and with a markedly overdistended uterus.

Elective Induction

Elective induction of labor refers to the initiation of labor without a medical indication. It may be considered when control over the timing of labor may be beneficial, such as in patients who live a great distance from the hospital or have a history of rapid labors. A major problem associated with elective induction is increased cesarean delivery due to failed induction. Fetal maturity must be assured.

Glossary

Asynclitism   When the biparietal diameter of the fetal head is parallel to the planes of the pelvis, the head is in synclitism. The sagittal suture is midway between the front and back of the pelvis. When either the anterior or posterior parietal bone precedes the sagittal suture, asynclitism is present.

Dilatation   Also referred to as dilation. The degree of opening, expressed in centimeters of diameter, of the internal os of the cervix.

Effacement A process that occurs in the latter part of pregnancy and labor by which the cervix is drawn intra-abdominally by the uterine corpus. This process is demonstrable by a shortening and thinning of the remaining intravaginal portion of the cervix. Effacement is expressed as the percentage by which the length of the cervix has been reduced and ranges from 0 (no reduction in length) to 100 percent (no cervix palpable below the fetal presenting part). It is sometimes described in centimeters of cervical length.

Engagement Engagement occurs when the largest transverse diameter of the presenting part has descended past the plane of the pelvic inlet.

Labor Repetitive uterine contractions associated with progressive cervical dilatation.

Lie Relationship between the long axis of the fetus and that of the mother.

Position Relationship between the fetus (occiput in cephalic presentations) and the planes of the birth canal.

Presentation The fetal part that lies closest to the pelvic inlet. The two main presentations are cephalic (vertex), and breech.

Station A measure of the degree of descent of the presenting part of the fetus through the birth canal. Divided into seven stations (-3 to $+3$), with the midpoint (zero station) at the plane of the maternal ischial spines.

Key Points

- The hazards of breech delivery are sufficient to warrant radiographic pelvimetry for cases in which vaginal delivery is contemplated.
- The duration of the latent phase of labor has no direct impact on perinatal mortality.
- The classification of abnormalities of the active phase of labor is based on the cervicographic analysis of labor.
- In some settings, application of the principles of active management of labor has led to a reduction in the rate of cesarean delivery, with no change in perinatal mortality.
- Prior to forceps delivery, fetal position and the characteristics of the maternal pelvis must be known with certainty.
- Examination of the placenta, umbilical cord, and membranes is an important part of delivery management.
- Induction of labor may be indicated when the benefit

of delivery to the mother or fetus outweighs the potential problems if the pregnancy continues.

- The induction process attempts to accomplish in hours what may take several days of spontaneous pre-labor.
- Variability in patient sensitivity and response to oxytocin is the rule rather than the exception.

Chapter 7

Intrapartum Fetal Evaluation

Rosemary E. Reiss,
Steven G. Gabbe, and
Roy H. Petrie

In most prospective randomized studies, the incidence of neurologic damage and perinatal death associated with the use of electronic fetal heart rate monitoring is not significantly lower than that documented with older methods of fetal surveillance, including intermittent fetal heart rate auscultation by stethoscope or Doppler. In several trials, electronic fetal heart rate monitoring was associated with an increased incidence of cesarean delivery. Consequently, the routine use of electronic fetal monitoring for intrapartum fetal evaluation has been disparaged by some.

Despite this controversy, there has been little interest among obstetricians in reverting to the more traditional fetal monitoring techniques, especially in patients judged to be at high risk. The reasons for this include (1) the undisputed reliability and assurance (greater than 98 percent) that a good fetal/neonatal outcome is associated with normal continuous fetal heart rate data and/or acid–base measurement, which safely allows continuation of labor; (2) the unacceptably great expense involved in providing the one-on-one nursing that is mandatory to perform adequate intermittent fetal heart rate auscultation; and (3) the knowledge that, although nonreassuring continuous fetal heart rate data may not be uniformly associated with poor perinatal outcome, they do provide a warning of potential problems and a gauge of fetal response to actions undertaken to improve fetal condition.

With the introduction of continuous fetal heart rate monitoring, the term *fetal distress* came into wide use to describe situations of abnormal fetal heart rate patterns. However, growing experience with fetal assessment techniques has also brought awareness that these tests have many false-positive results and that abnormalities do not necessarily indicate the fetus is jeopardized. The American College of Obstetricians and Gynecologists (ACOG) issued a Committee Opinion[1] in 1994 recommending that the term *nonreassuring fetal status* replace *fetal distress*. In this chapter, both terms are used, but fetal distress is used to indicate fetal hypoxia and acidosis.

Intermittent Fetal Heart Rate Monitoring

Low-Risk Patients

The current ACOG recommendations[21] suggest auscultation after contractions every 30 minutes during the first stage of labor and at least every 15 minutes in second stage for low-risk patients. If the patient is in the hospital during early latent-phase labor, intermittent fetal heart rate monitoring during ambulation is frequently performed at intervals of 45 to 60 minutes until contractions become regular at 3- to 4-minute intervals.

High-Risk Patients

In higher risk patients, the fetal heart rate is intermittently obtained and recorded every 15 minutes during the first stage of labor and every 5 minutes during the second stage of labor. The heart rate is preferably obtained during and 30 seconds following a uterine contraction. Continuous internal fetal heart rate monitoring with appropriate fetal blood acid–base determination should be used to clarify an abnormality of the auscultated fetal heart rate.

Continuous Fetal Heart Rate Monitoring

To evaluate the effects of intrapartum events on the fetus, continuous monitoring is often desirable.

To record the fetal heart rate continuously and instantaneously, a signal must be obtained each time the heart beats, and some mechanical or electronic device must measure the interval between two successive heart beats, calculate the fetal heart rate, and plot each successive rate that is calculated. In clinical practice, the utilization of either an ultrasound transducer on the maternal abdominal wall or an electrode attached to the fetal scalp has become the standard technique for collecting fetal heart rate data. With the scalp electrode, the cardiotachometer determines the time between each R wave (the R-R interval), and a rate in beats per minute is generated.

By convention, instantaneously calculated fetal heart rate and uterine activity are recorded on graph paper driven at a uniform speed. The paper speed is usually 3 cm/min. The vertical scaling is 30 to 240 bpm over 7 cm and 0 to 100 mm Hg (torr) over 4 cm. Thick vertical lines are placed at 1-minute intervals (Fig. 7-1). The heart rate tracing should be clearly labeled with the date, the patient's name, her identification number, and important clinical information. The tracing should be kept as a permanent part of the patient's medical record.

To evaluate uterine contractions or uterine activity, two methods have been developed. A tocodynamometer may be placed on the maternal abdomen overlying the gravid uterus and secured with a belt encircling the midsection of the body. The tocodynamometer detects alterations in the curvature of the abdomen resulting from changes in the configuration of the contracting uterus. Because no direct measurements are obtained, this system will not provide quantitative data on the strength or amplitude of contractions. However, the tocodynamometer will accurately record the frequency of contractions and show with reasonable accuracy the duration of the contractions. The second system for collecting information about uterine contractility requires the insertion of a small catheter filled with sterile water into the chorioamniotic sac after rupture of the membranes. The fluid-filled catheter is attached to a strain gauge and placed at a level that corresponds to the midpoint of the vertical axis of the uterus. Accurate pressure readings can then be obtained that indicate the onset, strength or amplitude, and duration of uterine contractions.

External Monitoring

In some cases, it may be clinically undesirable or impossible to rupture the membranes. Similarly, the obstetrician may not wish to use a fetal electrode or intrauterine pressure catheter. In these situations, the external form of fetal monitoring utilizing a tocodynamometer and ultrasound transducer can be applied (Fig. 7-2). An ultrasound transducer is affixed to the maternal abdomen at a position overlying the fetal heart so that sound waves can be transmitted toward the fetal heart valves. As the valves move, the reflected sound waves return to the transducer, permitting an accurate assessment of fetal heart rate activity. However, this process introduces a certain amount of "false" heart rate variability.

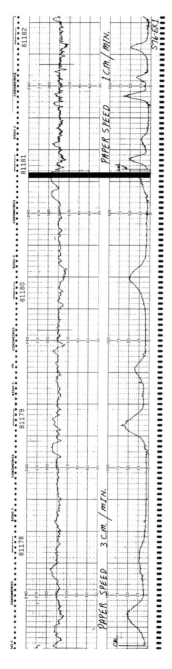

Fig. 7-1 Internal fetal heart rate data gathered at the standard recording speed of 3 cm/minute for the first portion. The same data are being recorded at a speed of 1 cm/minute in the last segment. Normal long-term and short-term variabilities are present. Note that the uterine activity channel has been calibrated so that the intrauterine pressure readings can be measured correctly.

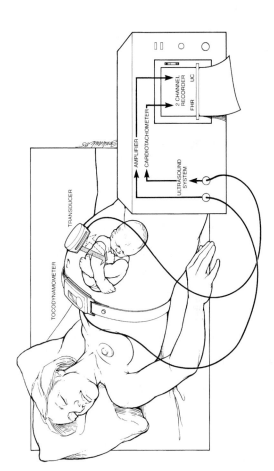

Fig. 7-2 Instrumentation for external monitoring. Contractions are detected by the pressure-sensitive tocodynamometer, amplified, and then recorded. Fetal heart rate is monitored using the Doppler ultrasound transducer, which both emits and receives the reflected ultrasound signal that is then counted and recorded.

There are few complications or side effects of external monitoring, although difficulty may be encountered in interpreting heart rate and uterine activity data if the recording is of poor quality.

Internal Monitoring

Internal monitoring requires the spontaneous or artificial rupture of the chorioamnion (Fig. 7-3). Usually, the cervix needs to be dilated 1 to 2 cm before the uterine pressure catheter can be inserted and the fetal electrode attached. The electrode is placed during a vaginal examination. With the examiner's finger inserted through the cervical os against the fetal scalp, a cartilaginous plate is first identified. The obstetrician must be certain the electrode will not be placed over the fetal face or fontanelle. An electrode introducer is next inserted along the finger to come to rest against the fetal vertex. Rotating the introducer 90 to 360 degrees will attach the spiral electrode to the fetal scalp. The introducer is removed, and the ends of the wires from the electrode are connected to a maternal leg plate that contains a ground lead and is attached to the fetal monitor. It is possible for the maternal electrocardiographic signal to be conducted through a dead fetus to the fetal electrode and be amplified and counted by the fetal monitor's cardiotachometer. The use of real-time ultrasonography to evaluate fetal cardiac valvular action can resolve this question quickly. The scalp electrode allows the patient more freedom of movement than does the ultrasound transducer, because maternal or fetal movement will not alter the quality of the signal.

Internal fetal heart rate monitoring involves breaking the skin or scalp to attach the electrode and may increase the risk of fetal infection with herpes and human immunodeficiency viruses.

After the electrode has been attached, a catheter for the determination of uterine activity can be inserted. The soft plastic intrauterine catheter is filled with sterile water to avoid corrosion of the pressure strain gauge, which may occur with dextrose and water or saline. The catheter should be filled with fluid before it is introduced to avoid the possibility of an air embolus.

An internal pressure catheter will not increase the risk of chorioamnionitis and postpartum endomyometritis. However, the longer an intrauterine catheter and electrode are in situ before a cesarean delivery is performed, the greater the likelihood of postpartum febrile morbidity.[27,28]

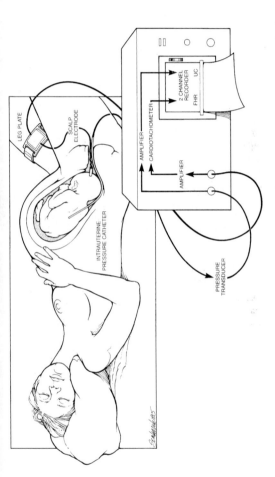

Fig. 7-3 Techniques used for direct monitoring of fetal heart rate and uterine contractions. Uterine contractions are assessed with an intrauterine pressure catheter connected to a pressure transducer. This signal is then amplified and recorded. The fetal electrocardiogram is obtained by direct application of the scalp electrode, which is then attached to a leg plate on the mother's thigh. The signal is transmitted to the monitor, where it is amplified, counted by the cardiotachometer, and recorded.

Physiologic Control of Fetal Heart Rate

Baseline Heart Rate

The human mean fetal heart rate varies between 110 and 160 bpm; however, rates as low as 90 or as high as 180 are not necessarily abnormal, especially if they are transient. Persistent periods (10 minutes or longer) of heart rate above 160 bpm are classified as baseline tachycardia. Persistent fetal heart rate below 110 bpm is known as fetal bradycardia. Persistent intervals of tachycardia or bradycardia are more likely to be associated with hypoxia than is a normal heart rate. Fetal tachycardia has also been identified in cases complicated by maternal fever, fetal infection, maternal thyrotoxicosis, fetal anemia, and fetal tachyarrhythmias. If the patient has received β-sympathomimetic drugs or parasympatholytic agents such as atropine, fetal tachycardia may also be observed.[29] Fetal bradycardia can be seen in patients treated with β-blockers such as propranolol. Damage to the conduction system of the fetal heart causing congenital heart block and a rate of 50 to 70 bpm can result from congenital heart malformation or maternal autoimmune disease.

Heart Rate Variability

Perhaps the most reliable indicator of fetal well-being is normal heart rate variability. Heart rate variability represents the interplay between the cardioinhibitory and cardioaccelerator centers in the fetal brain stem. It is unusual for a heart rate under normal central nervous system (CNS) control to be constant. Rather, there is considerable variation or variability, usually ranging from 6 to 25 bpm around an imaginary average heart rate. An expert panel convened recently by the National Institute of Child Health and Human Development recommended that a distinction no longer be made between "short-term" and "long-term" variability. The presence of normal fetal heart rate variability is one of the best indicators of intact integration between the CNS and heart of the fetus. By the time a fetus reaches 28 weeks' gestation or more, the CNS should be sufficiently mature to produce normal variability. The loss of heart rate variability often suggests fetal hypoxia, but other factors may be responsible, including a fetal sleep state, drugs that depress the CNS, a fetal tachycardia of more than 180 bpm, and anomalies of the heart and CNS.[31]

Although it occurs infrequently, a sinusoidal heart

rate (Fig. 7-4) may have great clinical importance. This baseline heart rate is usually within a normal range. However, it has a somewhat smooth, undulating pattern of uniform variability with an amplitude of 5 to 20 bpm that resembles a sine wave. The sinusoidal heart rate has often been associated with fetal anemia, as in Rh isoimmunization. Sinusoidal-like heart rate patterns can be seen following the administration of some narcotic analgesics and related agents. Whenever a persistent sinusoidal baseline heart rate pattern is noted intrapartum, it is advisable to collect fetal scalp capillary blood for an acid–base determination and hematocrit. The possibility of fetal anemia due to fetomaternal hemorrhage or hemolysis should also be considered.

Fetal Arrhythmias

While many fetal cardiac arrhythmias are transient and of little clinical significance, some have been associated with fetal compromise. Sustained fetal tachycardia at a rate above 200 bpm warrants investigation, and may lead to heart failure and hydrops. Atrial supraventricular tachycardia (rate 220 to 240) is most common. The fetus with complete heart block will usually demonstrate a rate of 50 to 70 bpm. Approximately 40 percent of these infants will have congenital heart disease, particularly a ventricular septal defect. Maternal autoantibodies associated with systemic lupus erythematosus are found in most of the others. Fetal heart failure and hydrops have also been associated with congenital heart block, albeit rarely.

Periodic Changes

Transient slowing of the fetal heart rate is known as a *deceleration*, while a transient increase is an *acceleration*. The four patterns of clinical significance are accelerations and early, variable, and late decelerations. Only two mechanisms alter fetal heart rate: (1) a reflex response secondary to the nervous control of the heart by direct nervous innervation or by humoral control of the autonomic nervous system and (2) transient slowing of the heart when fetal myocardial hypoxia is present.

Early Deceleration

With an early deceleration, the fetal heart rate demonstrates a gradual slowing or deceleration as a contraction begins, reaching its lowest point just as the acme of the contraction is reached and returning to baseline levels just as the contraction is finished. The heart rate

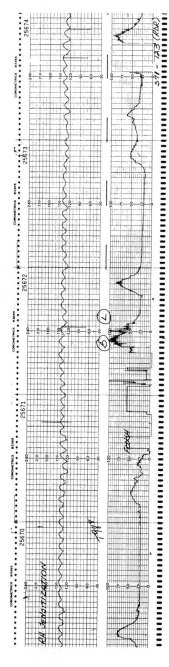

Fig. 7-4 The sinusoidal heart rate pattern with its even undulations is demonstrated. Internal monitoring shows the absence of beat-to-beat variability characteristic of true sinusoidal patterns.

never falls below 100 bpm (Fig. 7-5). This deceleration is known as an *early deceleration* because it starts early in the contraction. The early deceleration is thought to be due to pressure on the fetal head as it moves down the birth canal, and the mechanism is one of reflex slowing mediated by the vagus nerve. These early decelerative changes are innocuous and can be observed throughout labor without alteration in fetal condition.

Variable Deceleration

The variable deceleration is a reflex-mediated change in fetal heart rate, again mediated by the vagus nerve[2] but generally caused by umbilical cord compression (Fig. 7-6). This pattern is often seen in association with oligohydramnios. As the umbilical cord is compressed, fetal peripheral resistance increases. Fetal Po_2 falls and Pco_2 rises. Baroreceptors and chemoreceptors fire, causing an abrupt drop in heart rate, usually to a range below 100 bpm. The variable deceleration may begin before the onset of a contraction, with the onset of a contraction, or following the onset of a contraction. The variable deceleration is the most common periodic pattern noted during labor and generally can be corrected by changing maternal position to alleviate cord compression.

If the fetal heart rate does not fall below 80 bpm and the deceleration is brief, cord compression is usually of minimal clinical significance. However, with prolonged or deep variable decelerations (Table 7-1), a significant reduction in respiratory gas exchange may occur. Carbon dioxide accumulates in the fetal compartment, causing a transient respiratory acidosis. If the decelerations are severe and repetitive, hypoxia and metabolic acidosis may result. Fetal myocardial hypoxemia may then produce a delayed recovery to baseline. If this occurs, great care must be taken to eliminate this stress. If severe variables cannot be alleviated, the fetus may require early delivery.

Late Deceleration

A repetitive deceleration of the fetal heart rate noted to begin well after the contraction is under way is known as a *late deceleration* (Fig. 7-7). It reaches its lowest point after the acme of the contraction has been achieved and does not return to the baseline rate until after the contraction is over. Late decelerations indicate uteroplacental insufficiency and decreased intervillous exchange between mother and fetus with intermittent fetal hypoxia. As the uterine contraction peaks, limiting

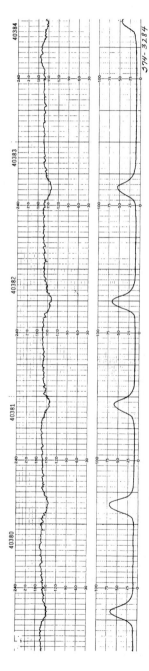

Fig. 7-5 Internal monitoring demonstrates a baseline heart rate of approximately 160 bpm, minimal to moderate short-term variability, and persistent early decelerations with each contraction.

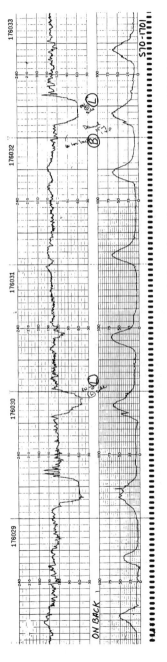

Fig. 7-6 Internal monitoring reveals uterine contractions every 2 to 3 minutes of 50- to 60-mm Hg intensity and a baseline of 5 to 10 mm Hg. Variable decelerations occur intermittently, providing adequate intervals between contractions for CO_2 and O_2 exchange and fetal recovery.

Table 7-1   Grading of Variable Decelerations

Grade	Nadir (bpm)	Duration (sec)
Mild	Any	<30
Moderate	70–80 bpm	>60
	<70 bpm	>30–<60
Severe	<70 bpm	>60

Modified from Kubli FW, Hon EM, Khazin EF et al: Observations on heart rate and pH in the human fetus during labor. Am J Obstet Gynecol 104:1190, 1969, with permission.

intervillous blood flow, fetal oxygenation is impaired, hence the late timing of the deceleration. In a setting of mild transient hypoxia, late decelerations represent a reflex vagally mediated response and are associated with normal heart rate variability. However, when hypoxia is prolonged and severe enough to produce acidemia, direct myocardial depression results in late decelerations with reduced or absent heart rate variability.

Late decelerations may occur with placental abruption, excessive uterine activity of either a spontaneous or pharmacologically induced nature, and maternal hypotension, anemia, or ketoacidosis. Shallow, repetitive late decelerations of only 5 to 10 bpm below baseline, especially in a setting of reduced beat-to-beat variability, are at least as ominous as deep ones. In the dying fetus, late decelerations give way to a marked bradycardia.

Mixed Patterns

Occasionally, two decelerative fetal heart rate patterns may be seen together. This combination has been called a *mixed pattern*. In managing such cases, clinical decisions should be based on the worst component of the mixed pattern.

Accelerations

Transient increases in fetal heart rate associated with uterine contractions or fetal movement are known as *accelerations* and are usually indicators of a fetus that is adequately oxygenated (Fig. 7-8).

Summary

A healthy fetus is characterized by a normal heart rate with normal heart rate variability and by the absence of significant repetitive late heart rate decelerations.

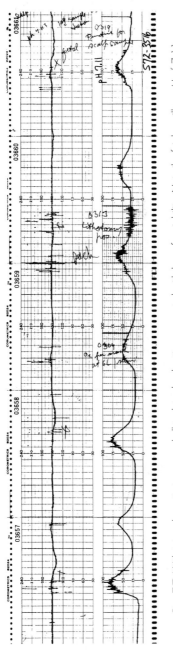

Fig. 7-7 With internal monitoring, very shallow late decelerations are noted with loss of variability. Note the fetal capillary pH of 7.11, indicative of a rather marked acidosis. Not surprisingly, scalp puncture did not produce a fetal heart rate acceleration.

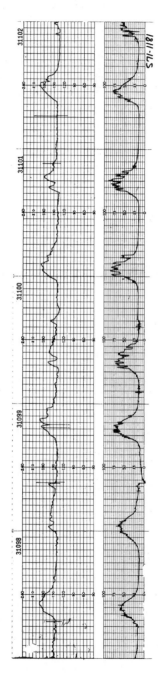

Fig. 7-8 Internal monitoring is used, and accelerations are noted with each contraction.

The presence of fetal heart rate accelerations strengthens the diagnosis of fetal well-being. In a potentially compromised fetus, the heart rate pattern is characterized by significant repetitive decelerations or by an abnormal baseline. Nonreassuring characteristics include the absence of fetal heart rate accelerations and the loss of fetal heart rate variability. The presence of repetitive late decelerations, repetitive moderate to severe variable decelerations, a sinusoidal pattern, or a baseline tachycardia, particularly when associated with diminished fetal heart rate variability, all indicate the need to evaluate fetal status further.

Fetal Acid–Base Evaluation

Blood Collection for Respiratory Gases

During labor, fetal acidosis may result from impaired fetomaternal exchange. A transient fall in fetal pH may be due to acute umbilical cord compression that leads to the rapid accumulation of carbon dioxide and a respiratory acidosis. Of greater concern is inadequate fetal oxygenation because of impaired respiratory gas exchange in the intervillous space. Lactic acidosis may result, with a fall in fetal pH. If sufficient hypoxia and acidosis develop, brain damage or death from asphyxia may occur. The collection of fetal blood for pH and respiratory gas evaluation, when performed at the appropriate time, may alert the obstetrician to impending fetal jeopardy and permit correction of the underlying problem or delivery by whatever route is safest for mother and fetus.

There is a linear correlation between the severity of heart rate patterns and the degree of acidosis present (Table 7-2).[39–43] Normal fetal capillary and umbilical blood pH and respiratory gas values are given in Tables 7-3 and 7-4. The fetal capillary scalp pH value will normally decline in early labor from approximately 7.30 to 7.25 at delivery. Traditionally a pH value of 7.25 or greater has been considered normal for the fetus during labor.[8,31] The pH range of 7.20 to 7.24 has been referred to as a preacidotic range. Many believe a fetal capillary pH value of 7.19 or less indicates potential fetal acidosis and, if substantiated on two collections 5 to 10 minutes apart, represents sufficient acidosis to warrant termination of labor. However, it is uncommon to find significant neonatal sequelae until a pH range of less than 7.10 is noted.

The base excess or deficit is an indication of fetal buffer reserves available to neutralize H^+ ions or fixed acids (see Table 7-5). With recurrent stress and a grow-

Table 7-2   Relationship of Fetal Heart Rate Pattern, Fetal Acid–Base Level, and 5-Minute Apgar Score

Cord pH Pattern	Fetal Scalp pH		5-Minute Apgar Score ≥7 (%)	
	Kubli[40]	Tejani[42]	pH ≥7[a]	pH ≥7.25[a]
Normal tracing	7.30 ± .04	7.33 ± .01	92	91
Accelerations		7.34 ± .01	91	97
Early decelerations	7.30 ± .04	7.33 ± .01	92	93
Variable decelerations (all)		7.30 ± .01	78	77
Moderate	7.26 ± .04			
Severe	7.15 ± .07			
Late decelerations (all)		7.29 ± .01	63	66
Moderate	7.21 ± .05			
Severe	7.12 ± .07			

[a] Data from Tejani N, Mann L, Bhakthavathsalan A: Correlation of fetal heart rate patterns and fetal pH with neonatal outcome. Obstet Gynecol 48:460, 1976, with permission.

Table 7-3   Normal Umbilical Cord Blood Gas Values

	Vein	Artery
pH	7.34 ± 0.15	7.28 ± 0.15
P_{O_2}	30 ± 15	15 ± 10
P_{CO_2}	35 ± 8	45 ± 15
Base deficit	5 ± 4	7 ± 4

ing base deficit, the interval before deterioration of fetal condition becomes progressively shorter despite apparently stable pH values.

In clinical practice, a trend of serial pH determinations correlated with the clinical setting is of greater importance than the absolute value of a single pH determination. The evaluation of base deficit as well as pH helps to distinguish between respiratory and metabolic acidosis and gives an indication of the duration of hypoxemia. Heart rate variability provides an important commentary on the severity of ominous periodic patterns. The fetus with normal heart rate variability and late decelerations will have a significantly higher scalp pH than will the fetus with decreased variability and late decelerations.

Maternal acidosis may occasionally cause fetal acidosis secondary to equilibration of H^+ ions across the placenta. Maternal respiratory alkalosis associated with hyperventilation has been reported to elevate fetal pH falsely.

To collect fetal blood, the chorioamnion must be ruptured and the cervix must be sufficiently dilated, approximately 2 to 3 cm, to provide exposure to the fetal scalp. The presenting part must be sufficiently low in the pelvis to remain reasonably immobile. A conical vaginal endoscope is passed through the vagina and cervix so that the small end of the endoscope comes to

Table 7-4   Fetal Capillary Blood Respiratory Gas Values

Normal	Respiratory Acidosis	Metabolic Acidosis
pH 7.25–7.40	Decreased	Decreased
P_{O_2} 18–22	Usually stable	Decreased
P_{CO_2} 40–50	Increased	Usually stable
Base deficit 0–11	Usually stable	Increased

Table 7-5   Base Deficit (Excess)[a] in Fetal Capillary Blood

Base (mEq/L)	Indication
0–9	Normal
9–11	Borderline
>11	Potential metabolic acidosis

[a] Base deficit and base excess have the same numerical value; however, a positive value is used for base deficit and a negative value for base excess (i.e., a base deficit of 6 is the same as a base excess of −6).

rest against the fetal scalp at a site not overlying a suture line or fontanelle. Once the scalp is cleaned, a small amount of silicone is spread over the exposed area. Using a microscalpel set in a plastic guard, the fetal scalp is punctured. To aid in the collection of blood, this puncture should be performed just at the beginning of a contraction so that scalp blood flow is facilitated. A long glass heparinized capillary tube is then introduced into the endoscope and, using gravity and capillary action, the fetal blood is collected into the capillary tube. Newer instruments require only 25 to 40 µl of fetal blood for determination of pH and respiratory gases. After the fetal blood sample has been collected, pressure should be applied to the puncture site through the completion of two contractions and the puncture site then observed through a third contraction to be certain there is no bleeding.

With the introduction of continuous fetal heart rate monitoring, fetal acid–base surveillance in labor is used mainly when the heart rate patterns are unclear or confusing or to gauge whether it is safe to continue to observe a fetus with a nonreassuring tracing whose delivery is expected to occur within a relatively short time.

Correlation of Stimulated Fetal Accelerations and Fetal pH

When the scalp is stimulated and an acceleration of 15 bpm lasting 15 seconds occurs, the fetal pH value is almost always 7.22 or greater. Unfortunately, the reverse does not hold true, and normal fetuses may not accelerate with scalp stimulation. Firm pressure on the fetal scalp during digital examination may be used in place of scalp blood sampling to evoke accelerations in normal fetuses.

Vibroacoustic stimulation is often used to evoke a fetal heart rate acceleration and clarify fetal status. An artificial larynx is placed on the maternal abdomen approximately one-third the distance from the symphysis pubis to the xiphoid process or over the fetal head. A stimulation interval of 2 to 5 seconds is used. Fetal heart rate accelerations in response to such stimulation have been associated with a fetus that is in good condition physiologically. However, about 50 percent of healthy fetuses will not respond with an acceleration.

Thus the use of scalp or acoustic stimulation can reduce the need for scalp pH testing. These techniques can be used earlier in labor than scalp sampling, since they do not require rupture of the membranes. In the presence of an ambiguous fetal heart rate tracing a scalp pH is usually unnecessary if the fetus responds to scalp or acoustic stimulation with accelerations. Scalp stimulation is especially useful to differentiate fetal sleep from acidosis when a fetal tracing shows reduced variability but no decelerations.

Umbilical Cord Acid–Base Analysis

Umbilical blood gas values are often used to relate intrapartum fetal heart rate data to acid–base status and neonatal condition at birth.[39] These data help to establish the state of fetal oxygenation at birth.[62,63] A doubly clamped, 10- to 30-cm segment of umbilical cord is obtained and, using preheparinized 1- to 2-ml syringes, samples of blood are collected from the umbilical artery or vein. When obtainable, the umbilical artery blood gas is preferable since it more closely reflects fetal status. Samples are then analyzed for respiratory gases (see Table 8-3). Cord blood gas studies are most helpful when a delivery is performed for fetal distress, when the newborn is depressed, and when one delivers an infant at greater risk for subsequent neurologic handicap, for example, a premature or growth-restricted infant.

Fetal Therapy

Amnioinfusion

Amnioinfusion, the transcervical instillation of fluid into the amnionic sac, is now widely used intrapartum to improve the intrauterine environment in settings of oligohydramnios. Amniotic fluid plays an important role in cushioning the umbilical cord from compression by contractions and fetal parts. Intrauterine infusion of saline can eliminate repetitive variable decelerations, reduce the incidence of cesarean delivery for fetal distress, and dilute meconium, decreasing the risk of meconium aspiration syndromes.

Normal saline is the fluid most commonly used for amnioinfusion. Initially 250 to 1,000 ml of fluid is infused at a rate of 10 to 15 ml/min via an intrauterine pressure catheter. Though some assess the amniotic fluid index by ultrasound to judge the adequacy of volume replacement, in clinical practice a predetermined volume or the resolution of variable decelerations is usually used as the endpoint. The initial fluid volume is followed by a continuous infusion of 100 to 200 ml/hr by pump or by gravity drainage to replace fluid leaking out during contractions. If fluid is administered more rapidly than 15 ml/min, it should be warmed to body temperature. Intrauterine pressure can be monitored via the same intrauterine pressure catheter,[66] a second one, or a double-lumen catheter.

Complications of amnioinfusion appear to be rare. Uterine tone may increase with amnioinfusion, and prolonged fetal bradycardia has been reported following rapid infusion (50 ml/min) of unwarmed fluid. Maternal respiratory failure and amniotic fluid embolism have been described in patients receiving amnioinfusion, via an infusion pump, but it is not clear whether these were the result of the infusion per se or other risk factors. A reduced risk for endometritis has been observed.

Tocolysis

The primary stress that the fetus must tolerate during labor is the contraction itself. When possible, resuscitation of the fetus in utero by reducing uterine activity to a level that the fetus is able to tolerate is preferable to operative delivery at a time when the pH may be low and the P_{CO_2} elevated. One or two parenteral injections of tocolytic agents such as 0.25 mg of subcutaneous terbutaline or 4 to 6 g of intravenous magnesium sulfate[78] can be used for this purpose. Using tocolysis in this manner, cesarean delivery may be avoided in some cases.

Management of Nonreassuring Fetal Heart Rate Patterns

General Principles

1. Patients at high risk for uteroplacental insufficiency (e.g., in settings of prolonged pregnancy, intrauterine growth retardation, oligohydram-

nios, meconium-stained fluid) should be monitored continuously. After rupture of the membranes, a fetal scalp electrode should be placed to assess fetal heart rate variability more accurately.

2. If an external technique is in use and there is flattening of the baseline or decelerations, an internal electrode should be placed to assess heart rate variability and to better correlate the timing of decelerations with uterine contractions.

3. For a mixed fetal heart rate pattern, the patient should be managed according to the most ominous pattern.

4. If there is an abnormal fetal heart rate pattern, such as a confusing pattern, late or severe variable decelerations, a baseline tachycardia, or loss of variability, a fetal stimulation test should be done. If the fetus does not respond with an acceleration or the abnormal pattern persists, a fetal scalp capillary blood sample should be obtained for acid–base determination.

Management of Specific Patterns

Late Deceleration

With repetitive late decelerations, the following steps to improve delivery of oxygen to the intervillous space should be initiated:

1. If oxytocin is in use, discontinue it. After appropriate reevaluation, if the pattern has corrected, oxytocin may be restarted.

2. Start oxygen at 6 to 8 L/min with a tight-fitting face mask.

3. Change the maternal position (e.g., supine to left or right lateral, elevate legs, knee–chest).

4. Check maternal blood pressure; if the mother is hypotensive, correct the hypotension as follows:
   a. Increase the rate of administration of electrolyte-containing intravenous fluids.
   b. If the hypotension is thought to be secondary to regional anesthesia, consult with an obstetric anesthesiologist regarding the possible use of a vasopressive agent (e.g., ephedrine 15 mg IV).

5. If the late decelerations are attributable to other maternal problems that adversely affect the fetus, such as maternal hypoxia, ketoacidosis, or sickle cell crisis, measures to correct the underlying condition should also be taken. If these are not promptly remediable, delivery may be indicated

(when safe for the mother) even if fetal pH proves normal.

The heart rate tracing should be assessed for variability during and between late decelerations. If variability is normal and accelerations are present or can be stimulated, the fetus is unlikely to be acidotic and time may be allowed for recovery of the tracing following the conservative maneuvers described above. If the fetal heart rate pattern does not normalize, or if there is poor variability, fetal capillary blood should be collected to assess fetal acid–base status:

1. If the fetal pH is in the pathologic range (less than 7.20), prompt delivery should be undertaken by the method that is quickest and safest for both mother and fetus.
2. If the fetal pH is in the prepathologic range (7.20 to 7.24) but the late deceleration pattern persists, another pH should be obtained in 15 to 20 minutes. If the pH is falling or the base deficit is large, the patient should be delivered promptly.
3. If the late deceleration pattern persists, but fetal acid–base status is satisfactory and it is decided to allow labor to continue, confirmation of satisfactory fetal acid–base status must be determined at 20-minute intervals as long as late decelerations are observed and scalp or acoustic stimulation does not produce accelerations. If repetitive scalp sampling cannot be done, delivery of the fetus is in order. The use of a tocolytic agent such as intravenous ritodrine or subcutaneous terbutaline to arrest labor and allow recovery of the fetus before delivery is often useful.

Variable Deceleration

When variable decelerations are mild and not repetitive, the pattern is usually associated with good fetal outcome. However, variable decelerations may worsen as labor progresses. Amnioinfusion should be initiated if variables are recurrent. It is preferable to begin an amnioinfusion before variables are severe because 20 to 30 minutes are needed to instill adequate fluid. If decelerations become repetitive, fall below 90 bpm at their nadir, and last longer than 60 seconds, fetal condition can deteriorate. This type of pattern most often occurs during the late first and the second stages of labor. When an ominous variable deceleration pattern is present, the following steps should be initiated:

1. If oxytocin is in use, discontinue it. When the pattern has been corrected and after appropriate re-evaluation, oxytocin may be restarted.
2. Unless clinically contraindicated (e.g., suspected placenta previa), a vaginal examination should be performed immediately to check for a prolapsed cord and to determine the progress of labor.
3. Maternal hypotension should be identified and corrected.
4. Maternal position should be changed (consider left lateral, right lateral, Trendelenburg, reverse Trendelenburg, or knee–chest).
5. Oxygen is started at 6 to 8 L/min with a tight-fitting face mask.
6. If uterine activity is excessive, the use of intravenous tocolysis with terbutaline or magnesium sulfate may be considered.
7. If the patient is in the second stage, postponing pushing for a few contractions may give the fetus a chance to recover.

If these management measures do not correct the pattern and if the variable decelerations worsen, the obstetrician should:

1. Prepare for delivery by the method that is quickest and safest for both mother and fetus (i.e., alert the operating room, shave the abdomen, and so forth).
2. Assess fetal acid–base status by a stimulation test or by analysis of fetal capillary blood. Care should be exercised to obtain the fetal capillary blood sample *after* the deceleration has returned to the baseline and just before the next contraction.
3. If the fetus does not have a metabolic acidemia, immediate delivery can be delayed if a safe vaginal delivery is expected within 20 to 30 minutes, unless the fetal heart rate pattern worsens acutely.

Prolonged Sudden Deceleration

Occasionally, an unexpected and often unexplained prolonged deceleration may occur. The fetal heart rate will drop below 80 bpm, and the deceleration can last several minutes. Though occasionally triggered by a vagal discharge in response to fetal manipulation, such sudden prolonged decelerations usually result from a mechanism that can cause fetal hypoxia, notably:

1. Uterine hyperactivity, usually oxytocin related
2. Conduction anesthesia with hypotension
3. Supine hypotension
4. Unrelieved cord compression
5. Uterine rupture
6. Maternal respiratory arrest (convulsions, high spinal anesthesia, intravenous narcotics)

Should a prolonged sudden deceleration occur, the following steps should be instituted:

1. Consider the causes of prolonged decelerations and attempt to correct them, including using tocolytic therapy for excessive uterine activity.
2. Change maternal position until an effective position is found.
3. Perform a vaginal examination, unless contraindicated, to check for cord prolapse and the progress of labor.
4. Institute oxygen at 6 to 8 L/min with a tight-fitting face mask.
5. Increase the infusion of intravenous fluids.

If these measures do not resolve the problem and vaginal delivery is not imminent after 5 minutes of a fetal heart rate at 60 bpm, cesarean delivery is indicated. If these steps do alleviate the deceleration, assessment of fetal acid–base status by a fetal stimulation test or by acid–base determinations should be obtained 10 to 15 minutes after the fetal heart rate has recovered. If the fetal pH is below 7.25, a second sample should be obtained within 15 minutes or until the pH is above 7.25.

After recovery, careful observation of the fetal heart rate should be maintained. If the deceleration should occur a second or third time, corrective measures need to be instituted and preparation for immediate delivery undertaken. If at all possible, delivery should be accomplished 10 to 15 minutes into the recovery period to allow the fetus to benefit from intrauterine resuscitation.

Risk Versus Benefit of Continuous Electronic Fetal Monitoring

While there are ample scientific data indicating that cord compression, fetal hypoxia, and acidosis can produce characteristic fetal heart rate patterns, and that these patterns can be more readily appreciated using continuous electronic monitoring rather than intermittent auscultation, it remains hotly debated whether the clinical application of continuous electronic fetal monitoring improves neonatal outcome. Transient episodes of fetal hypoxia, often associated with nonreassuring fetal heart rate tracing patterns, occur commonly during labor and are usually well tolerated by the fetus. Despite the enormous expectations for improvement in perinatal outcomes following the introduction of electronic fetal heart rate monitoring, and the observed decline of intrapartum stillbirths since that time, only 1 trial[25] of 12 randomized controlled trials[22-25,79-86] published over the past 20 years has shown a statistically significant reduction in perinatal mortality, and only a few have shown a reduction in neonatal morbidity in patients monitored continuously.

An increase in the frequency of cesarean delivery due to the introduction of fetal monitoring has been frequently cited in the lay as well as the scientific press. This has been attributed to the immobilization of the parturient imposed by the monitor, as well as to overzealous interventions in response to abnormal heart rate tracings. Although cesarean delivery rates have been higher in the monitored arm of several randomized controlled trials,[22,25,80,82,83] more detailed scrutiny suggests this is not an inevitable result of electronic monitoring.

The inability of randomized controlled trials to show statistically significant reduction in perinatal mortality does not adequately tell the story of electronic fetal monitoring's impact. Over the two decades since electronic monitoring became widely applied, perinatal mortality has fallen due to many changes in intrapartum and neonatal care.[92-95] Therefore, further reduction in the already low rates of death due to asphyxia will be difficult to achieve. It is interesting that perinatal outcomes were improved with electronic fetal monitoring in recent randomized controlled trials in less-developed nations.

Electronic fetal monitoring has altered our training of physicians and nurses and the staffing patterns of our labor floors. Though frequent intermittent auscultation performed well in many randomized controlled trials, nursing and midwifery support was also optimized in these studies. Thus, the studies document the potential efficacy of intermittent auscultation but may overestimate its effectiveness in clinical practice.

We have learned an enormous amount about fetal pathophysiology by the introduction of electronic fetal monitoring. It appears that the prevention of intrapartum stillbirths and depressed neonates is a reasonable goal for intrapartum monitoring of whatever type, but that the eradication of cerebral palsy is not. If we apply what has been discovered carefully, we should be able to use electronic monitoring in a selective and intelligent manner, minimizing unnecessary interventions while identifying most fetuses in jeopardy.

Key Points

- Normal fetal heart rate is between 110 and 160 bpm. The fetal heart rate is under CNS control through sympathetic and parasympathetic reflexes mediated through the vagus.
- Normal fetal heart rate variability consists of a variation in rate of 6 to 25 bpm.
- Labor presents a challenge to fetoplacental oxygen and carbon dioxide exchange because contractions reduce intervillous flow and may compress the umbilical cord.
- Normal fetal capillary pH is 7.25 to 7.40. During the course of normal labor there is a gradual decline in fetal pH.
- Loss of fetal heart rate variability can indicate hypoxia but may also be produced by fetal sleep, drugs that depress the CNS, fetal arrhythmias, and cardiac or CNS anomalies.
- In the presence of normal heart rate variability with spontaneous or induced accelerations of more than 15 bpm lasting at least 15 seconds, fetal acidemia is extremely unlikely regardless of the presence of decelerations.
- External fetal monitors use ultrasound detection of valve movement to assess fetal heart rate and may give a false impression of variability when little is present. The absence of variability in a tracing from an external monitor is reliable.
- In the presence of oligohydramnios or meconium, intrapartum amnioinfusion (instillation of fluid into the amniotic sac via an intrauterine pressure catheter) has been shown to reduce the rates of cesarean delivery for fetal distress and of meconium aspiration syndrome.
- Late decelerations are indicative of hypoxia produced by decreased intervillous exchange of respiratory gases during contractions. Variable decelerations

are drops in fetal heart rate caused by umbilical cord compression that increases vagal discharge. They are characterized by abrupt onset and resolution. If they are prolonged, a mixed pattern combining features of late deceleration with those of variables may be produced.
- Though there is correlation between abnormal fetal heart rate patterns and neurologic depression at birth, fetal heart rate patterns are poor predictors of long-term neurologic sequelae.

Obstetric Anesthesia

Joy L. Hawkins,
David H. Chestnut, and
Charles P. Gibbs

The word *anesthesia* encompasses all techniques used by anesthesiologists: general anesthesia, regional anesthesia, local anesthesia, and analgesia. In obstetrics, regional techniques include spinal and lumbar or caudal epidural and are usually administered by anesthesia personnel (see main text). In some cases, the anesthesiologist may combine a local anesthetic and opioid for epidural or spinal administration.

Psychoprophylaxis

Psychoprophylaxis is a nonpharmacologic method of minimizing the perception of painful uterine contractions. Relaxation, concentration on breathing, gentle massage (effleurage), and partner participation contribute to its effectiveness. In prepared childbirth classes patients learn about the physiology of pregnancy and the normal processes of labor and delivery. The couple visit the labor and delivery suites before labor, so that the fear of the unknown is largely mitigated.

Although psychoprophylactic techniques may discourage the use of drugs, not all patients are alike and not all will be satisfied with psychoprophylaxis.[32] The greatest disadvantage is the potential for believing the use of drug-induced pain relief is a sign of failure or will harm the child.

Systemic Opioid Analgesia

All opioids provide pain relief, but can also produce respiratory depression in the mother and newborn. Small doses of opioids (e.g., meperidine, fentanyl, butorphanol, and nalbuphine) are used and are administered via the more predictable intravenous route. Therefore, recent reports detail little neonatal depression.[43–46]

The immediate treatment for respiratory depression caused by opioids is ventilation. Infants depressed by opioids may be sleepy and may not breathe adequately. Initially they typically are not hypoxic, hypercarbic, or acidotic; however, if they are not ventilated, then these will result. If properly cared for, infants with opioid-induced depression will suffer no ill effects. Proper care includes ventilation, oxygenation, gentle stimulation, and the judicious use of the opioid antagonist naloxone. Positive-pressure ventilation is the single most effective measure and can be provided via face mask or intubation. Without ventilation, other measures are fruitless.

Naloxone, 0.1 mg/kg, should be given intravenously if possible, but it can be given intramuscularly or subcutaneously. This neonatal dose is higher than that previously recommended and should ensure an increased likelihood of effectiveness.[47] It may be repeated in 3 to 5 minutes if there is no immediate response. If there is no response after two or three doses, the depression is most likely not due to opioid effect.[48] Nursery personnel should be advised when naloxone has been given because it has a short duration of action, and therefore repeat administration may be necessary in the nursery.

An important and significant disadvantage of opioid analgesia is the prolonged effect of these agents on gastric emptying. If general anesthesia becomes necessary, the risk of aspiration is increased.[53–55]

Patient-Controlled Opioid Analgesia

In some centers opioids are administered by patient-controlled intravenous infusion. The infusion pump is programmed to give a predetermined dose of drug upon patient demand. The physician may program the pump to include a lock-out interval (that is, there is a minimum interval between doses of drug). Thus the physician may limit the total dose administered per hour.

Sedatives

Sedatives do not possess analgesic qualities and are most often used early in labor to relieve anxiety and reduce the nausea associated with opioids. All sedatives and hypnotics cross the placenta freely. Except for the benzodiazepines, they have no known antagonists. Because barbiturates and other sedatives are not analgesic, patients may be less able to cope with pain than if they had received no pharmacologic assistance at all; that is, normal coping mechanisms may be blunted.[71,72] The combination of barbiturate (100 mg secobarbital) with opioid (50 to 100 mg meperidine) increases the degree of newborn depression,[38] which may persist for a prolonged time. Thus these drugs should not be used during active labor.

Phenothiazines

Promethazine, promazine, and hydroxyzine are also commonly administered. When given in small doses in combination with an opioid, these drugs do not seem to produce additional neonatal depression.[74-76] However, these agents rapidly cross the placenta and, in large doses, can depress the fetus, and have no known antagonist.

Benzodiazepines

A major disadvantage of diazepam is that it renders newborns less able to maintain body temperature.[77] The drug may persist in the fetal circulation for as long as 1 week.[78] Sodium benzoate, a buffer in the injectable form of diazepam, competes with bilirubin binding to albumin and could be a threat to infants susceptible to kernicterus.[81] Midazolam is water soluble, and is shorter acting than diazepam.[82]

A disadvantage of all the benzodiazepines is their tendency to cause maternal amnesia. This can be a significant disadvantage if the drug is given near the time of delivery.[85] Flumazenil, a specific benzodiazepine antagonist, can reliably reverse benzodiazepine-induced sedation and ventilatory depression.[86]

Paracervical Block

Paracervical block analgesia is a simple, effective procedure. Usually, 5 to 6 ml of a dilute solution of local anesthetic without epinephrine is injected into the mucosa of the cervix at either 4 and 8 or 3 and 9 o'clock; an Iowa trumpet prevents deep penetration of the needle (Fig. 8-1). The block can only be applied during the first stage of labor and it must be reapplied frequently during the course of a long labor. Furthermore, it has the major disadvantage of fetal bradycardia, which occurs in 2 to 70 percent of applications. It occurs within 2 to 10 minutes and lasts from 3 to 30 minutes. Although

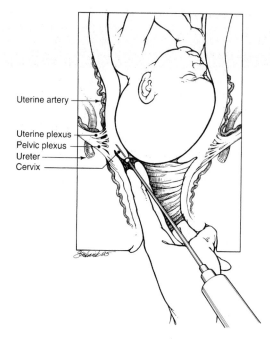

Fig. 8-1 Technique of paracervical block. Schematic coronal section (enlarged) of lower portion of cervix and upper portion of vagina shows relation of needle to paracervical region. (Modified from Banica JJ: Principles and Practice of Obstetric Analgesia and Anesthesia. Philadelphia, FA Davis, 1967, p 234, with permission.)

usually benign, it can be associated with fetal acidosis and occasionally with fetal death.[196–198]

There is no consensus regarding the mechanism of postparacervical block bradycardia. The theories include (1) high blood concentrations of local anesthetic in the fetus because the local anesthetic is injected close to the uterine artery, and could traverse its wall and pass directly to the fetus, (2) uterine artery vasoconstriction, secondary to a direct effect of the local anesthetic on the uterine artery,[199,200] and (3) postparacervical block increase in uterine activity.

Regardless of etiology, the severity and duration of the bradycardia correlate with the incidence of fetal acidosis. Freeman and colleagues[201] reported a significant fall in pH and a rise in base deficit only in those fetuses with bradycardia persisting more than 10 minutes. Paracervical block should not be used in mothers with fetuses in either acute or chronic distress.

Local Anesthesia

Spontaneous vaginal deliveries, episiotomies, and sometimes outlet forceps deliveries can be accomplished with perineal infiltration alone. Usually, 5 to 15 ml of 1 percent lidocaine suffices. Lidocaine passes to the fetus after perineal infiltration.

Pudendal Block

Pudendal block is a minor regional block that also is effective and safe. The obstetrician, using an Iowa trumpet and a 20-gauge needle, injects 5 to 10 ml of local anesthetic just below the ischial spine. Because the hemorrhoidal nerve may be aberrant in 50 percent of patients,[204] some physicians prefer to inject a portion of the local anesthetic somewhat posterior to the spine.

The technique is satisfactory for spontaneous vaginal deliveries and episiotomies and for some outlet forceps deliveries, but may not be sufficient for deliveries requiring additional manipulation.

More than with perineal infiltration, the potential for local anesthetic toxicity exists with pudendal block because of the proximity of large vessels close to the site of injection. Therefore, aspiration before injection is particularly important. Furthermore, the potential for large amounts of local anesthetic to be used increases when perineal infiltration is required in addition to the pudendal block. In these instances, it is important to monitor closely the amount of local anesthetic given.

Allergy to Local Anesthetics

There are two classes of local anesthetics: amides and esters. A true allergic reaction to an amide-type local anesthetic (e.g., lidocaine, bupivacaine, mepivacaine, etidocaine) is extremely rare. Allergic reactions to the esters (2-chloroprocaine, procaine, tetracaine) are also rare but occur more often. Generally, when a patient says she is "allergic" to local anesthetics, she is referring to what may have been a reaction to the epinephrine that is occasionally added to local anesthetics, particularly by dentists. Epinephrine can cause increased heart rate, pounding in the ears, and nausea, symptoms that may be interpreted as an allergy. Was there a rash? Hives? Difficulty breathing? If so, which local anesthetic was used? If a specific local anesthetic can be identified, choosing one from the other class should be safe.

Lumbar Epidural Analgesia/Anesthesia

Epidural blockade is a major regional anesthetic technique in which local anesthetic is injected into the epidural space. Epidural blockade may be used to provide *analgesia* during labor or surgical *anesthesia* for vaginal or cesarean delivery. A large-bore needle is used to locate the epidural space. Next, a catheter is inserted through the needle, and the needle is removed over the catheter. Local anesthetic is injected through the catheter, which remains taped in place to the mother's back to enable subsequent injections throughout labor. Thus it is often called *continuous epidural analgesia*. A test dose of local anesthetic is given first to check for the possibility that the catheter was unintentionally placed in the subarachnoid (spinal) space or in a blood vessel.

Two forms of epidural analgesia are used for labor: lumbar and caudal. The catheter is placed via a lumbar interspace in the former and via the sacral hiatus in the latter. More local anesthetic is necessary for the caudal technique, because the local anesthetic must fill the entire sacral canal before filling the epidural space up to T10.

Most anesthesiologists now prefer the lumbar approach and use a technique described as *segmental epidural analgesia*. Only the smallest amount and the weakest effective concentration of local anesthetic is injected via the L2–L3, L3–L4, or L4–L5 interspace. Thus both sensation and motor function of the perineum and lower extremities remain mostly intact. The patient can move about and perceive the impact of the presenting part on the perineum. If perineal anesthesia is needed for delivery, a larger concentration and dose of local anesthetic can be administered at that time through the catheter.

Disadvantages of epidural anesthesia include hypotension, local anesthetic toxicity, allergic reaction, high or total spinal anesthesia, neurologic injury, spinal headache, and, in some cases, adverse effects on progress of labor.

Key Points

- Use of parenteral opioids for labor analgesia can produce respiratory depression in the mother and newborn and delayed gastric emptying in the mother. However, when used appropriately, opioids are safe and effective.
- The pain of labor can be managed by obstetric personnel by systemic opioid analgesia, paracervical and pudendal blocks, although these are not as effective as lumbar epidural blocks.

Chapter 9

Malpresentations

John W. Seeds and
Margaret Walsh

Near term or during labor, the fetus normally assumes a vertical orientation or lie and a cephalic presentation with the fetal vertex flexed on the neck (Fig. 9-1). In about 5 percent of cases, however, deviation occurs from this normal lie, presentation, and flexion attitude, and such deviation constitutes a fetal malpresentation. *Malpresentations* are associated with increased risk to both the mother and the fetus.

This chapter examines malpresentations, possible etiologies, and the mechanics of labor and vaginal delivery unique to each situation.

Clinical Circumstances Associated With Malpresentation

Factors associated with malpresentation include (1) diminished vertical polarity of the uterine cavity, (2) increased or decreased fetal mobility, or (3) obstructed pelvic inlet. The association of great parity with malpresentation is presumably related to laxity of maternal abdominal muscular support and therefore loss of the normal vertical orientation of the uterine cavity. Placentation either high in the fundus or low in the pelvis is another factor that diminishes the likelihood of a fetus comfortably assuming a longitudinal axis. Uterine myomata, intrauterine synechiae, and müllerian duct abnormalities such as septate uterus or uterus didelphys are also associated with a higher than expected rate of malpresentation. Both prematurity and hydramnios permit increased fetal mobility; thus, there is an increased probability of a noncephalic presentation if labor or rupture of membranes occurs. In contrast, such conditions as autosomal trisomies, myotonic dystrophy, and fetal neurologic dysfunction that result in decreased fetal muscle tone, strength, or activity are

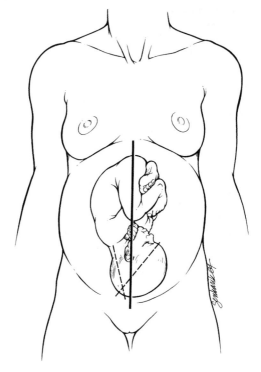

Fig. 9-1 Frontal view of a fetus in a longitudinal lie with fetal vertex flexed on the neck.

also associated with an increased incidence of malpresentation. Furthermore, preterm birth involves a fetus that is small relative to the maternal pelvis and results in increased fetal mobility. In these cases, pelvic engagement and descent with labor or rupture of membranes can occur despite malpresentation. Finally, the cephalopelvic disproportion associated with severe fetal hydrocephalus or with a frankly contracted pelvis is frequently implicated as an etiology of malpresentation because normal engagement of the fetal head is prevented.

Abnormal Axial Lie

The fetal "lie" indicates the orientation of the fetal spine relative to that of the mother. The normal fetal lie is longitudinal and by itself does not indicate whether the presentation is cephalic or breech. If the fetal spine or long axis crosses that of the mother, the fetus may be said to occupy a transverse or oblique lie (Fig. 9-2) resulting in a shoulder or arm presentation. The presentation is termed *unstable* if the fetal membranes are intact and there is great fetal mobility.[1]

Abnormal fetal lie is diagnosed on average in approximately 1/300 cases.[2–8] Prematurity is often a factor, with abnormal lie reported to occur in about 2 percent of pregnancies at 32 weeks, or six times the rate found at term.[9] Persistence of a transverse, oblique, or unstable lie beyond 37 weeks requires a systematic clinical assessment and plan for management, since rupture of membranes without a fetal part filling the inlet of the pelvis imposes a high risk of cord prolapse, fetal compromise, and maternal morbidity if neglected.

Great parity, prematurity, pelvic contracture, and abnormal placentation are the most commonly reported clinical factors associated with abnormal lie,[2,5–9] although many cases show none of these.

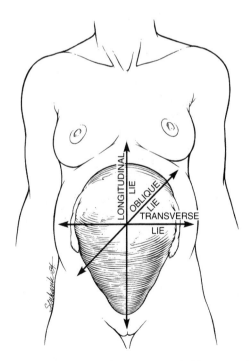

Fig. 9-2 A fetus may occupy a longitudinal, oblique, or transverse axis, as illustrated by these vectors. The lie does not indicate whether the vertex or the breech is closest to the cervix.

Management

The normally grown infant at term cannot undergo a safe vaginal delivery from an axial malpresentation.[4,7] Furthermore, a careful search for a potentially dangerous or compromising etiology is indicated. A transverse/oblique or unstable lie late in the third trimester necessitates ultrasound examination to exclude major fetal malformation and abnormal placentation. Elective hospitalization facilitates observation and early recognition of cord prolapse.[6,11] Active intervention at or beyond 37 weeks or after confirmation of fetal lung maturity may be of benefit.

External cephalic version followed by induction of labor after 37 weeks in the case of abnormal lie is a reasonable alternative to both expectant management and elective cesarean delivery.

If external version is unsuccessful or unavailable, if spontaneous rupture of membranes occurs, or if active labor has begun with an abnormal lie, cesarean delivery is the treatment of choice for the potentially viable infant.[1,3,14] There is no place for internal podalic version and breech extraction in the management of transverse or oblique lie or unstable presentation in singleton pregnancies because of the unacceptably high rate of fetal and maternal complications.[2]

A persistent abnormal axial lie, particularly if accompanied by ruptured membranes, also alters the choice of uterine incision at cesarean delivery. Although a low transverse cervical incision has many surgical advantages, up to 25 percent of transverse incisions require vertical extension for delivery of an infant from an abnormal lie to allow access to and atraumatic delivery of the vertex entrapped in the muscular fundus.[3,14] Furthermore, the lower uterine segment is often poorly developed. Therefore, in cases of transverse or oblique lie with ruptured membranes or a poorly developed lower segment, a vertical incision is more prudent. Intraoperative cephalic version may allow the use of a low transverse incision, as reported by Pelosi et al.,[14] but ruptured membranes with oligohydramnios makes this unlikely.

Deflection Attitudes

The normal "attitude" of the fetal vertex during labor is one of full flexion on the neck, the fetal chin against the upper chest. Deflection attitudes include various degrees of deflection or even extension of the fetal head on the neck (Fig. 9-3). Spontaneous conversion to a more normal flexed attitude or further extension of an

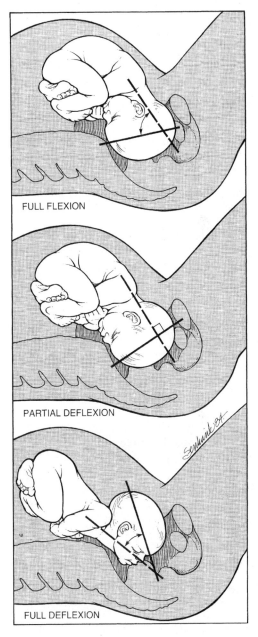

FULL FLEXION

PARTIAL DEFLEXION

FULL DEFLEXION

Fig. 9-3 The normal "attitude" (top view) shows the fetal vertex flexed on the neck. Partial deflexion (middle view) shows the fetal vertex intermediate between flexion and extension. Full deflexion (lower view) shows the fetal vertex completely extended, with the face presenting.

intermediate deflection to a fully extended position will commonly occur as labor progresses. Although safe vaginal delivery is possible in most cases, experience indicates that cesarean delivery is the only appropriate alternative when arrest of progress is observed.

Face Presentation

A face presentation is characterized by a longitudinal lie and full extension of the fetal head on the neck, with the occiput against the upper back. The fetal chin is chosen as the point of designation at vaginal examination. For example, a fetus presenting by the face whose chin is in the right posterior quadrant of the maternal pelvis would be called a *right mentum posterior* (Fig. 9-4). The reported incidence of face presentation is 1/500 live births overall. Reported perinatal mortality, corrected for nonviable malformations and extreme prematurity, is 2 to 3 percent.

All clinical factors known to increase the general rate of malpresentation (see box) have been implicated in face presentation, but as many as 60 percent of infants with a face presentation are malformed. Anencephaly, for instance, is found in about one-third of cases of face presentation.[5,25,26] Frequently observed maternal factors include a contracted pelvis or cephalopelvic disproportion.[17,20,23]

Etiologic Factors in Malpresentation

Maternal
 Great parity
 Pelvic tumors
 Pelvic contracture
 Uterine malformation
Fetal
 Prematurity
 Multiple gestation
 Hydramnios
 Macrosomia
 Hydrocephaly
 Trisomies
 Anencephaly
 Myotonic dystrophy
 Placenta previa

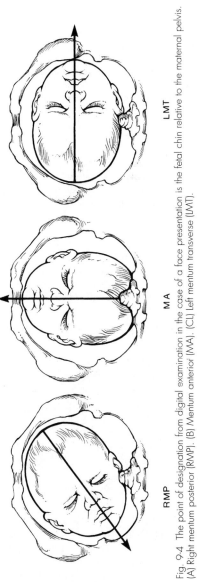

RMP

MA

LMT

Fig. 9.4 The point of designation from digital examination in the case of a face presentation is the fetal chin relative to the maternal pelvis. (A) Right mentum posterior (RMP). (B) Mentum anterior (MA). (C) Left mentum transverse (LMT).

Mechanism of Labor

Knowledge of the early mechanism of labor for the face presentation is incomplete. Many infants with a face presentation probably begin labor in the less extended brow position. With descent into the pelvis, the forces of labor press the fetus against maternal tissues, and either flexion or full extension of the head on the spine occurs. The labor of a face presentation must involve engagement, descent, internal rotation generally to a mentum anterior position, and delivery by flexion under the symphysis (Fig. 9-5). However, flexion of the

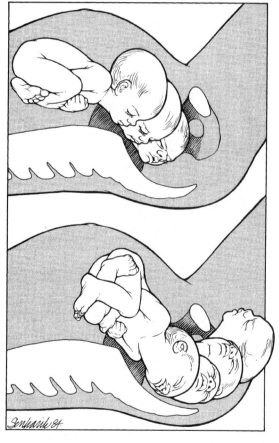

Fig. 9-5 Engagement, descent, and internal rotation remain cardinal elements of vaginal delivery in the case of a face presentation, but successful vaginal delivery of a term-size fetus presenting a face generally requires delivery by flexion under the symphysis from a mentum anterior position as illustrated here.

occiput may not always occur. Delivery in the full extended attitude may be common.

The prognosis for labor with a face presentation depends on the orientation of the fetal chin. At diagnosis, 60 to 80 percent of infants with a face presentation are mentum anterior,[5,20,22,29] 10 percent are mentum transverse,[5,22,29] and 20 to 25 percent are mentum posterior.[5,20,22,29] Almost all average-sized infants presenting mentum anterior with adequate pelvic dimensions will achieve spontaneous or easily assisted vaginal delivery.[5,22,30,31] Furthermore, most mentum transverse infants will rotate to the mentum anterior position and deliver vaginally, and even 25 to 33 percent of mentum posterior infants will rotate and deliver vaginally in the mentum anterior position.[5,16,20] Schwartz et al.[29] found that the mean birth weight of those infants in mentum posterior who did rotate and deliver vaginally was 3,425 g, compared with 3,792 g for those infants who did not rotate and deliver vaginally. Persistence of mentum posterior with an infant of normal size, however, makes safe vaginal delivery less likely. Overall, 70 to 80 percent[5,20,22,23] of infants with face presentation can be delivered vaginally, either spontaneously or by low forceps. Manual attempts to convert the face to a flexed attitude or to rotate a posterior position to a more favorable mentum anterior are rarely successful and increase both maternal and fetal risks.[16,22,26,32] Internal podalic version and breech extraction as a remedy for face presentation is contraindicated. Fetal losses are up to 60 percent with this maneuver. Maternal deaths from uterine rupture and trauma after version with extraction have also been documented. Spontaneous delivery or cesarean delivery are therefore the preferred routes for maternal safety as well.[16,22,26]

Prolonged labor is a common feature of face presentation[5,8] and has been associated with an increased number of intrapartum deaths.[17] Therefore, prompt attention to an arrested labor pattern is recommended. The choice between augmentation of a dysfunctional labor or primary cesarean delivery rests on an assessment of uterine activity, pelvic adequacy, and fetal condition. In the case of an average or small fetus, adequate pelvis, and hypotonic labor, oxytocin may be considered. Fetal compromise is common, with a 10-fold increase associated with face presentation. Abnormal fetal heart rate patterns occur more often with face presentation.[16,18] Continuous intrapartum electronic fetal heart rate monitoring of a fetus with face presentation is mandatory, but extreme care must be exercised in the placement of an electrode to avoid ocular and cosmetic damage. If external Doppler heart rate monitoring is inadequate and an internal electrode is considered necessary, placement of the electrode on the fetal chin is often recommended.

Laryngeal and tracheal edema resulting from pressures of the birth process might require immediate nasotracheal intubation.[33] Nuchal teratomas or simple goiter, fetal anomalies that might have caused the malpresentation, require expert neonatal management.

No absolute contraindication to oxytocin augmentation of hypotonic labor in the case of a face presentation exists, but an arrest of progress despite adequate labor or a nonreassuring fetal heart rate pattern should call for cesarean delivery.[8] Although cesarean delivery has been reported in up to 60 percent of cases of face presentation,[18,27] safe vaginal delivery may often be accomplished. A trial of labor with careful monitoring of fetal condition and progress is not contraindicated unless macrosomia or a small pelvis is identified.

Brow Presentation

An infant in a brow presentation occupies a longitudinal axis, with a partially deflexed cephalic attitude, midway between full flexion and full extension[24] (Fig. 9-6). The frontal bones are the point of designation. If the anterior fontanelle is on the mother's left side, with the sagittal suture in the transverse pelvic axis, the fetus

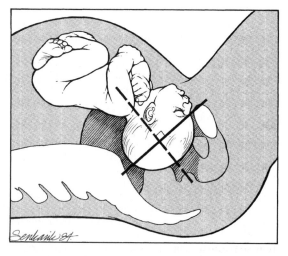

Fig. 9-6 This fetus is a brow presentation in a frontum anterior position. The head is in an intermediate deflexion attitude.

would be in a left frontum transverse position. The incidence of brow presentation is about 1/1,500 deliveries. Brow presentation will be detected more often in early labor before flexion occurs to a normal attitude. Less frequently, further extension results in a face presentation.

Corrected perinatal mortality rates for fetuses presenting by the brow depended on the mode of delivery. The highest rate, 16 percent, was associated with manipulative vaginal birth.[37]

Factors that delay engagement are associated with persistent brow presentation. Cephalopelvic disproportion, prematurity, and great parity are often found and have been implicated in more than 60 per cent of cases of persistent brow presentation.[5,35,38,39]

A persistent brow presentation requires engagement and descent of the largest (mento-occipital) diameter or profile of the fetal head.[40] This maneuver is possible only with a large pelvis or a small infant. However, brow presentations convert spontaneously by flexion or further extension to either a vertex or a face presentation and are then managed accordingly.[34,35] The earlier the diagnosis, the more likely conversion is to occur spontaneously. Fewer than half of infants with persistent brow presentations undergo spontaneous vaginal delivery, but in most cases a trial of labor is not contraindicated.[5,36]

Prolonged labors have been observed in half of brow presentations,[5,20,35,38,39] and secondary arrest is not uncommon.[34] Forced conversion of the brow to a more favorable position with forceps is contraindicated,[34,35,38] as are attempts at manual conversion. One unexpected cause of persistent brow presentation may be an open fetal mouth pressed against the vaginal wall, splinting the head and preventing either flexion or extension.[28,35]

In most cases of brow presentation, minimal manipulation yields the best results[35,41] if the fetal heart rate pattern remains reassuring. However, expectancy is justified only with a large pelvis, a small infant, and adequate progress. If a brow presentation persists with a large baby, successful vaginal delivery is unlikely, and cesarean delivery may be most prudent.[20] Regardless of pelvic dimensions, consideration of a trial of labor with careful monitoring of maternal and fetal condition may be appropriate. As in the case of a face presentation, oxytocin may be used cautiously to correct hypotonia, but prompt resumption of progress toward delivery should follow.

Compound Presentation

Whenever an extremity is found prolapsed beside a major presenting fetal pole, the situation is referred to as a compound presentation.[42] The combination of an upper extremity and the vertex is the most common compound presentation.

This diagnosis should be suspected with any arrest of labor in the active phase or failure to engage during active labor.[44] The diagnosis is made by vaginal examination that discovers an irregular mobile tissue mass adjacent to the larger presenting part. Diagnosis late in labor is common, and as many as 50 percent of persisting compound presentations are not diagnosed until the second stage.[42] Delay in diagnosis may not be detrimental because it is likely that only the persistent cases require significant intervention.

Although maternal age, race, parity, and pelvic size have all been associated with compound presentation,[43,44] prematurity is the most consistent clinical finding.[5,42] It is primarily the very small fetus that is at great risk of persistent compound presentation. In late pregnancy, external cephalic version of a fetus in breech position may increase the risk of a compound presentation.[46]

Fetal risk in the case of compound presentation is specifically associated with birth trauma and cord prolapse. Cord prolapse occurs in 10 to 20 percent of cases[5,43,44] and is the most frequent single complication of this malpresentation. Cord prolapse probably occurs because the prolapsed extremity splints the presenting part and results in an irregular fetal aggregate that incompletely fills the pelvic inlet. In addition to the hypoxic risk of cord prolapse, common fetal morbidity includes neurologic and musculoskeletal damage to the involved extremity.

Labor is not necessarily contraindicated with a compound presentation, but the prolapsed extremity should not be manipulated.[42–44,47] As the major presenting part descends, the accompanying extremity usually retracts; 75 percent of vertex/upper extremity combinations deliver spontaneously. Occult or undetected cord prolapse is possible, and therefore continuous electronic fetal heart rate monitoring is recommended.

The primary indications for surgical intervention are cord prolapse, nonreassuring fetal heart rate patterns, and failure to progress.[5] Cesarean delivery is the only appropriate clinical intervention,[42] since both version extraction and attempts to reposition the prolapsed extremity are associated with high fetal and maternal morbidity and mortality and are to be avoided.[43,44] Protraction of the second stage of labor occurs more frequently with persistent compound presentation, and dysfunctional labor patterns are common.[42] Again, as in other malpresentations, spontaneous resolution occurs more often and surgical intervention is less frequently necessary in those cases diagnosed early in labor. Persistent compound presentation is more likely with a small infant, as is the prognosis for successful vaginal delivery. Persistent compound presentation with a term-sized infant has a poor prognosis for safe vaginal delivery, and cesarean delivery is usually necessary.

Breech Presentation

The infant presenting as a breech occupies a longitudinal axis with the cephalic pole in the uterine fundus. Breech presentation occurs in 3 to 4 percent of labors overall, although it is found in 7 percent of pregnancies at 32 weeks and in 25 percent of pregnancies of less than 28 weeks' duration.[48] There are three types of breech (Table 9-1). The infant in the frank breech position is flexed at the hips with extended knees. The complete breech is flexed at both joints, and the footling breech has one or both hips extended (Fig. 9-7).

The diagnosis of breech presentation may be made by abdominal palpation or vaginal examination with confirmation by ultrasound. Prematurity, fetal malformation, and polar placentation are commonly observed causative factors. High rates of breech presentation are noted in certain genetic disorders, including trisomies 13, 18, and 21, Potter syndrome, and myotonic dystrophy.[49] Thus conditions that alter fetal muscular tone and mobility also increase the frequency of breech presentation.

Table 9-1   Breech Categories

	Risk (%)	
Type	Cord Prolapse	Premature
Frank Breech	0.5[64]	40[48]
Complete	5[64]	10[48]
Footling	15[64]	50[48]

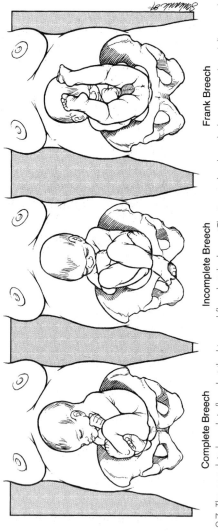

Complete Breech   Incomplete Breech   Frank Breech

Fig. 9-7 The complete breech is flexed at the hips and flexed at the knees. The incomplete breech shows incomplete deflexion of one or both knees or hips. The frank breech is flexed at the hips and extended at the knees.

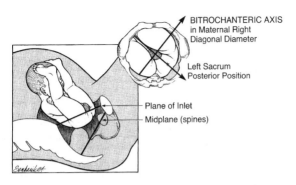

Fig. 9-8 The breech typically enters the inlet with the bitrochanteric diameter aligned with one of the diagonal diameters, with the sacrum as the point of designation in the other diagonal diameter. This is a case of left sacrum posterior (LSP).

Mechanism and Conduct of Labor and Vaginal Delivery

The two most important elements for the safe conduct of vaginal breech delivery are continuous electronic fetal heart rate monitoring and noninterference until spontaneous delivery of the breech to the umbilicus has occurred. Early in labor, the capability for immediate cesarean delivery should be established. Anesthesia should be available, the operating room readied, and appropriate informed consent obtained. Two obstetricians should be in attendance as well as a pediatric team. Appropriate training and experience with vaginal breech delivery are fundamental to success. The instrument table should be prepared in the customary manner, with the addition of Piper forceps and extra towels. There is no contraindication to epidural analgesia once labor is well established, and many view epidural anesthesia as an asset in the control of the second stage.

The infant presenting in the frank breech position usually enters the pelvic inlet in one of the diagonal pelvic diameters (Fig. 9-8). Engagement has occurred when the bitrochanteric diameter of the fetus has passed the plane of the inlet, although by vaginal examination the presenting part may only be palpated at −2 to −4 station (out of 5) relative to the ischial spines. As the breech descends and encounters the levator ani muscle sling, internal rotation usually occurs to bring the bitrochanteric diameter into the anteroposterior (AP) axis of the pelvis. The point of designation in a breech labor is the fetal sacrum, and, therefore, when the bitrochanteric diameter is in the AP axis of the pelvis, the fetal sacrum will lie in the transverse pelvic diameter.

If normal descent occurs, the breech will present at the outlet and begin to emerge first as a sacrum transverse, then rotate to a sacrum anterior. Crowning occurs when the bitrochanteric diameter passes under the pubic symphysis. An episiotomy in the midline to but not through the anal sphincter will facilitate delivery but should be delayed until crowning begins. Some argue that a mediolateral episiotomy offers more room and less risk of extension through the anal sphincter, but considerable skill and experience are required to repair a mediolateral episiotomy properly, and this incision is associated with greater blood loss and pain. Premature episiotomy will contribute to unnecessary blood loss and to the level of anxiety and perhaps a tendency to rush the delivery. As the infant emerges, rotation begins, usually toward a sacrum anterior position. This direction of rotation may reflect the greater capacity of the hollow of the posterior pelvis to accept the fetal chest and small parts. It is important to emphasize that operator intervention is not yet needed or helpful other than to cut the episiotomy and encourage maternal expulsive efforts.

Premature or aggressive assistance may adversely affect the breech birth in at least two ways. First, cervical dilatation must be maximized and complete dilatation sustained for sufficient duration to retard retraction of the cervix and entrapment of the aftercoming fetal head. Rushing the delivery of the trunk may significantly diminish the effectiveness of this process. Second, the safe descent and delivery of the breech infant must be the result of expulsive forces from above to maintain flexion of the fetal vertex. Any traction from below in an effort to speed delivery would encourage deflexion of the vertex and result in the presentation of the larger occipitofrontal fetal cranial profile to the pelvic inlet. Such an event could be catastrophic. Rushed delivery also increases the risk of a nuchal arm, with one or both arms trapped behind the head above the pelvic inlet. Entrapment of a nuchal arm makes safe vaginal delivery much more difficult as it dramatically increases the size of the aggregate object that must pass through the birth canal. The safe breech delivery of an average-size infant, therefore, depends predominantly on maternal expulsive forces, not on traction from below.

As the frank breech emerges further, the fetal thighs are typically pressed firmly against the fetal abdomen, often splinting and protecting the umbilicus and cord. As the umbilicus appears over the maternal perineum, the operator may align his or her fingers medial to one thigh, then the other, pressing

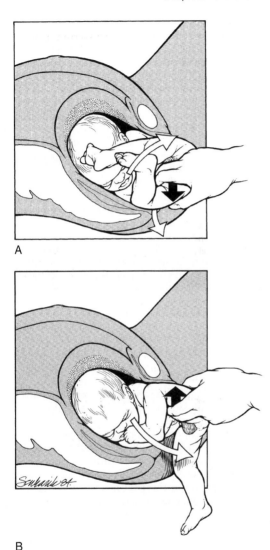

A

B

Fig. 9-9 After spontaneous expulsion to the umbilicus, external rotation of each thigh (A) combined with opposite rotation of the fetal pelvis results in flexion of the knee and delivery of each leg (B).

laterally as the fetal pelvis is rotated away from that side (Fig. 9-9). This results in external rotation of the thigh at the hip, flexion of the knee, and delivery of one and then the other leg. The dual movement of counterclockwise rotation of the fetal pelvis as the operator externally rotates the right thigh and clock-wise rotation of the fetal pelvis as the operator externally rotates the fetal left thigh is most effective in facilitating delivery. The fetal trunk is then wrapped with a towel to provide secure support of the body while further descent results from expulsive forces from the mother. The operator primarily facilitates the delivery of the fetus. The operator is not applying outward traction on the fetus that might result in deflexion of the fetal head or nuchal arm.

When the scapulae appear at the outlet, the operator may slip a hand over the fetal shoulder from the back (Fig. 9-10), follow the humerus, and, with a lateral movement, sweep first one and then the other arm across the chest and out over the perineum. Gentle rotation of the fetal trunk counterclockwise to assist de-livery of the right arm, and clockwise to assist delivery of the left arm, may be applied in a manner similar to that used for delivery of the legs (Fig. 9-11). If the ver-tex has remained flexed on the neck, the chin and face will appear at the outlet; the airway may be cleared and suctioned (Fig. 9-12).

With further maternal expulsive forces alone, sponta-neous controlled delivery of the fetal head will often occur. If not, delivery may be accomplished with a sim-ple manual effort to maximize flexion of the vertex using pressure on the fetal maxilla (not mandible) along with suprapubic pressure and gentle downward traction (Fig. 9-13). Although maxillary pressure will maximize cephalic flexion, the main force effecting de-livery remains the mother.

Alternatively, the operator may apply Piper forceps to the aftercoming head to facilitate delivery. The ap-plication requires slight elevation of the fetal trunk by the assistant, while the operator kneels and applies the Piper forceps directly to the fetal head in the pelvis. Hyperextension of the fetal neck from excessive eleva-tion of the fetal trunk should be avoided. In Piper for-ceps the pelvic curvature characteristic of most forceps has been eliminated. This modification allows direct application to the fetal head and avoids conflict with the fetal body that would occur with the application of standard instruments from below. The forceps are inserted into the vagina from beneath the fetus. The right blade is inserted with the operator's right hand along the right maternal sidewall and placed against the left fetal parietal bone. The left blade is then in-serted by the left hand along the left maternal sidewall and placed against the right fetal parietal bone. Forceps application controls the fetal head and prevents exten-sion of the head on the neck. Gentle downward traction

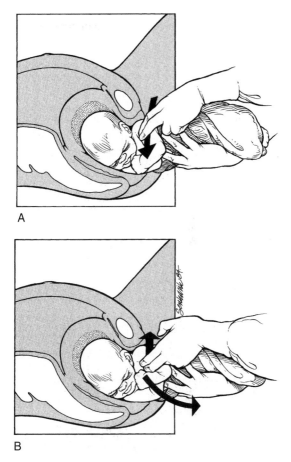

Fig. 9-10 When the scapulae appear under the symphysis, the operator reaches over the left shoulder, sweeps the arm across the chest (A), and delivers the arm (B).

on the forceps with the fetal trunk supported on or near the forceps shanks results in controlled delivery of the vertex. Routine use of Piper forceps to the aftercoming head may be advisable both to ensure control of the delivery and to maintain optimal operator proficiency in anticipation of deliveries that require their use.

Any arrest of spontaneous progress in labor necessitates consideration of cesarean delivery. Any evidence of fetal compromise or sustained cord compression based on continuous electronic fetal monitoring also

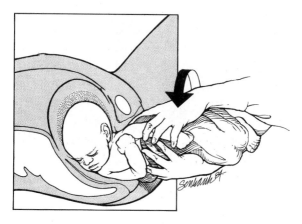

Fig. 9-11 Gentle rotation of the shoulder girdle facilitates delivery of the right arm.

requires consideration of cesarean delivery. Vaginal interventions directed at facilitating delivery of the breech complicated by an arrest of spontaneous progress are discouraged, because fetal and maternal morbidity and mortality are both greatly increased.

The mechanisms of descent and delivery of the footling and the complete breech are not unlike those of the frank breech described above, except one or both

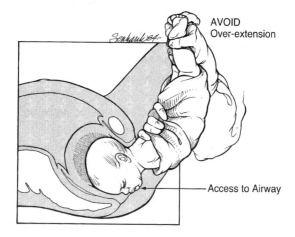

Fig. 9-12 Following delivery of the arms, the fetus is wrapped in a towel for control and slightly elevated. The fetal face and airway may be visible over the perineum. Excessive elevation of the trunk is avoided.

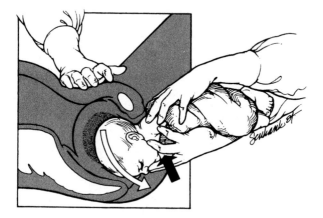

Fig. 9-13 Cephalic flexion is maintained by pressure (heavy arrow) on the fetal maxilla (not mandible!). Often delivery of the head is easily accomplished with continued expulsive forces from above and gentle downward traction.

legs might already be extended and thus not require attention. The risk of cord prolapse or entanglement is greater, hence the increased possibility of emergency cesarean delivery. Furthermore, the footling and complete breech are not as effective a dilator of the cervix as either the vertex or the larger aggregate profile of the thighs and buttocks of the frank breech, which might increase the risk of entrapment of the aftercoming head, and, as a result, primary cesarean delivery is often advocated for nonfrank breech presentations.

Management of the Term Breech

The reported perinatal mortality associated with breech presentation is three to five times that of the nonbreech infant at term.[52-54] The excess deaths are largely due to lethal anomalies and complications of prematurity, both of which are found more frequently among breech infants. Excluding anomalies and extreme prematurity, the corrected perinatal mortality reported by some investigators approaches zero regardless of the method of delivery, while others find that, even with exclusion of these factors, the term breech infant is at higher risk for birth trauma and asphyxia.[55-57] The major dangers facing the breech infant are summarized in Table 9-2.

At least a portion of the striking increase in the rate of cesarean deliveries over the past two decades is a

Table 9-2   Complications Seen with Breech
             Presentation

Intrapartum fetal death
Intrapartum asphyxia
Cord prolapse
Birth trauma
Arrest of aftercoming head
Spinal cord injuries with extended head
Major anomalies
Prematurity
Hyperextension of head

---

response to the risk of morbidity and mortality associated with the breech presentation.[58–61]

In some series, improved perinatal survival has been reported for breeches born by cesarean delivery,[51,54,63,68,69] and there is evidence, though inconsistent, that the method of delivery may also impact on the quality of survival. Some authors conclude that breech outcome relates to degree of prematurity, impact of pregnancy complications, and presence of malformations as well as birth trauma or asphyxia. The benefit of arbitrary cesarean delivery in the case of breech presentation therefore remains uncertain.

Associated Risks

The various categories of breech presentation clearly demonstrate dissimilar risks, and management plans might vary among these situations.[72,73]

Low birth weight (less than 2,500 g) is a confounding factor in about one-third of all breech presentations.[50,56,59,65,74,75] While the benefit of cesarean delivery to the perinatal mortality rate of the 1,500- to 2,500-g breech infant remains controversial,[11,35,51,74,76–81] improved survival with abdominal delivery has often been found in the 1,000- to 1,500-g weight group.[56,78]

Hyperextension of the fetal head has been consistently associated with a high (21 percent) risk of spinal cord injury if the breech is delivered vaginally.[30,88,89] In such cases, it is important to differentiate simple deflexion of the head from clear hyperextension, since simple deflexion carries no excess risk.

Finally, the footling breech carries a prohibitively high (16 to 19 percent) risk of cord prolapse during labor. In many cases, cord prolapse is manifest only late in labor, after commitment to vaginal delivery has been made.[56,77] Cord prolapse necessitates prompt cesarean delivery. Furthermore, the footling breech is a

Management of the Breech

Trial of labor may be considered if
  Estimated fetal weight (EFW) = 2,000 to 3,800 g
  Frank breech
  Adequate pelvis
  Flexed fetal head
  Fetal monitoring
  Zatuchni-Andros score ≥4
  Rapid cesarean possible
  Good progress maintained in labor
  Experience and training available
  Informed consent possible
Cesarean delivery may be prudent if
  EFW less than 1,500 or over 4,000 g
  Footling presentation
  Small pelvis
  Hyperextended fetal head
  Zatuchni-Andros score under 4
  Absence of expertise
  Nonreassuring fetal heart rate pattern
  Arrest of progress

poor cervical dilator, and cephalic entrapment becomes more likely.

Breech Second Twin (See Chapter 16, Multiple Gestations)

External Cephalic Version

External cephalic version is a third alternative to vaginal delivery or cesarean delivery for the breech infant.[15,50,52,108-111] External cephalic version significantly reduces the incidence of breech presentation in labor and is associated with few complications such as cord compression or placental abruption.[15,111] Reported success with external version varies from 60 to 75 percent, with a similar percentage of these remaining vertex to labor.[15,112-115]

Gentle constant pressure applied in a relaxed patient with frequent fetal heart rate assessments are elements of the method stressed by all investigators.[50,52,108] Methodology varies, although the "forward roll" is more widely supported than the "back flip" (Fig.

9-14).[108] The mechanical goal is to squeeze the fetal vertex gently out of the fundal area to the transverse and finally into the lower segment of the uterus.

Tocolysis and ultrasound during the procedure may also be helpful, but benefit from tocolysis remains unproven. Factors associated with failure of version included obesity, deep pelvic engagement of the breech, oligohydramnios, and posterior positioning of the fetal back.[114] Fetal–maternal transfusion has been reported to occur in up to 6 percent of patients undergoing external version[119]; thus Rh-negative

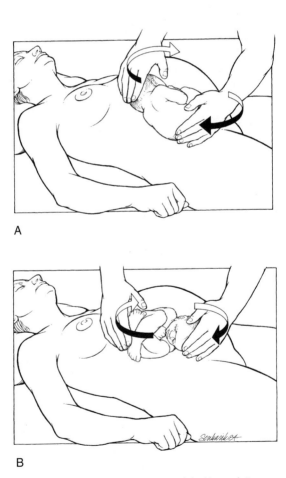

A

B

Fig. 9-14 External cephalic version is accomplished by gently "squeezing" the fetus out of one area of the uterus and into another. Here, the "forward roll," often the most popular, is illustrated.

unsensitized women should receive Rh immune globulin.

Shoulder Dystocia

Shoulder dystocia is diagnosed when, after delivery of the fetal head, further expulsion of the infant is prevented by impaction of the fetal shoulders within the maternal pelvis. Specific efforts are necessary to facilitate delivery.

Although a difficult shoulder dystocia occurs infrequently, the clinician does not soon forget the experience. Often, but not always, at the end of a difficult labor, the fetal head may be delivered spontaneously or by forceps, but the neck then retracts. Often, the fetal head appears to be drawn back with the chin against the maternal thigh. It may be difficult to suction the infant's mouth because of its close approximation to the perineum. As maternal expulsive efforts are encouraged, the fetal head becomes plethoric, and the danger to the infant is apparent if delivery cannot be promptly accomplished.

Shoulder dystocia is associated with increased perinatal morbidity and mortality.[120,121] Severe asphyxia was observed in 143/1,000 births with shoulder dystocia compared with 14/1,000 overall.[122] About 30 percent of infants born with shoulder dystocia demonstrate some neuropsychiatric dysfunction at 5- to 10-year follow up. Fewer than one-half of these children had immediate morbidity.

The relative probability of shoulder dystocia in the 7 percent of infants over 4,000 g was 11 times greater than the average; in the 2 percent of infants over 4,500 g the risk was 22 times greater. With macrosomia or continued fetal growth beyond term, the trunk and particularly the chest grow larger relative to the head. The chest circumference exceeds the head circumference in 80 percent of cases.[124] The arms also contribute to the greater dimensions of the upper body. Within a barely adequate pelvis, such bulk might easily block fetal rotation from a disadvantageous AP to the more desirable oblique outlet diameter. Macrosomia shows the strongest correlation with shoulder dystocia of any clinical factor and occurs more often with gestational diabetes and twice as often in postdate pregnancies. Postdate pregnancy also correlates with decreased amniotic fluid volume and perhaps decreased lubricating properties. Other clinical factors associated with shoulder dystocia appear to be related to macrosomia as well and include maternal obesity,[122,126] previous birth of an infant weighing over 4,000 g,[122,124,126] diabetes mellitus,[126,127] prolonged second stage of labor,[126] prolonged deceleration phase (8 to 10 cm),[118] and instrumental midpelvic delivery.[127] Increased maternal age and excess maternal weight gain have been found by some but not all investigators[122,126,127] to increase the risk of macrosomia and shoulder dystocia.

Clinical efforts to detect macrosomia prenatally could be helpful in anticipating problems with delivery of the shoulders. Such efforts, however, have had imperfect results. There is a growing trend to consider cesarean delivery of any infant with an estimated weight over 4,500 g or of any infant of a diabetic mother with an estimated weight over 4,000 g.[125,127] Any consideration of elective abdominal delivery based on estimated fetal weight alone, however, must consider the technical error of estimating fetal weight.

Successful treatment follows anticipation and preparation. Deliveries are best managed in a delivery room. Deliveries in bed increase the difficulty of reducing a shoulder dystocia because the bedding precludes fullest use of the posterior pelvis and outlet. Strong consideration for cesarean delivery is recommended when a prolonged second stage occurs in association with macrosomia.

Once a vaginal delivery has begun, the obstetrician must resist the temptation to rotate the head forcibly to a transverse axis. Maternal expulsive efforts should be used rather than traction. Gentle manual pressure on the fetal head inferiorly and posteriorly will push the posterior shoulder into the hollow of the sacrum, increasing the room for the anterior shoulder to pass under the pubis (Fig. 9-15). This pressure is not outward traction and must be symmetric. If the head is pressed asymmetrically, as if to "pry" the anterior shoulder out, brachial injury is more likely.

If delivery is not accomplished, a deliberate, planned sequence of efforts should then be initiated. One must not pull desperately on the fetal head. Fundal expulsive efforts, including maternal pushing and any fundal pressure, should be temporarily stopped. Aggressive fundal pressure prior to disimpaction or rotation of the shoulders will not facilitate delivery and may work against rotation and disimpaction. The McRoberts maneuver,[132] a simple, logical, and usually successful measure to promote delivery of the shoulders, involves hyperflexion of maternal legs on the maternal abdomen that results in flattening of the lumbar spine and ventral rotation of the maternal pelvis and symphysis (Fig. 9-16). This maneuver may increase the useful size of the posterior outlet, resulting in easier disimpaction of the anterior shoulder. The McRoberts maneuver significantly

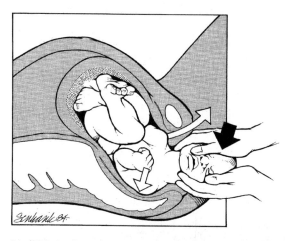

Fig. 9-15 Gentle, symmetric pressure on the head will move the posterior shoulder into the hollow of the sacrum and encourage delivery of the anterior shoulder. Care should be taken not to "pry" the anterior shoulder out asymmetrically, as this might lead to trauma to the anterior brachial plexus.

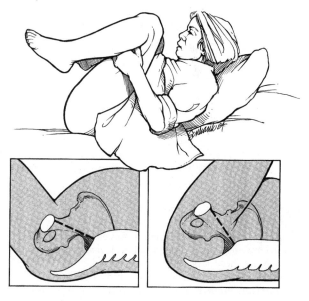

Fig. 9-16 The least invasive maneuver to disimpact the shoulders is the McRoberts maneuver. Sharp ventral flexion of the maternal hips results in ventral rotation of the maternal pelvis and an increase in the useful size of the outlet.

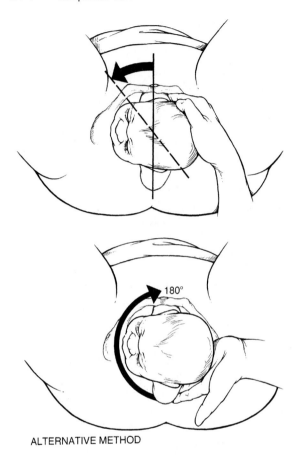

ALTERNATIVE METHOD

Fig. 9-17 Rotation of the anterior shoulder forward through a small arc or the posterior shoulder forward through a larger one will often lead to descent and delivery of the shoulders. Forward rotation is preferred as it tends to compress and diminish the size of the shoulder girdle, while backward rotation would open the shoulder girdle and increase the size.

reduces shoulder extraction forces, brachial plexus stretching, and the likelihood of clavicular fracture.

If the shoulders remain undelivered, often only moderate suprapubic pressure is required to disimpact the anterior shoulder and allow delivery. If this is not effective, the operator's hand may be passed behind the occiput into the vagina, and the anterior shoulder may be pushed forward to the oblique, after which, with maternal efforts and gentle posterior pressure, delivery should occur (Fig. 9-17).[119] Alternatively, the posterior shoulder may be rotated forward, through a 180 degree arc, and passed under the pubic ramus as in turning a screw (Wood screw maneuver). As the posterior shoulder rotates anteriorly, delivery will often occur.[134]

Many advocate delivery of the posterior arm and shoulder should the above methods fail. The operator's hand is passed into the vagina, following the posterior

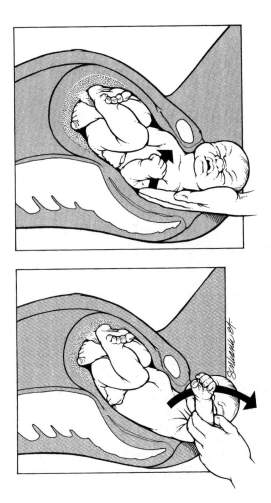

Fig. 9-18 The operator here inserts a hand and sweeps the posterior arm across the chest and over the perineum. Care should be taken to distribute the pressure evenly across the humerus to avoid unnecessary fracture.

arm of the fetus to the elbow. The arm is flexed and swept out over the chest and the perineum (Fig. 9-18). In some cases, delivery will now occur without further manipulation. In others, rotation of the trunk, bringing the freed posterior arm anteriorly, is required.[119,124]

Deliberate fracture of the clavicle is possible and will facilitate delivery by diminishing the rigidity and size of the shoulder girdle. It is best if the pressure is exerted in a direction away from the lung to avoid puncture. Sharp instrumental transsection of the clavicle is not recommended, since lung puncture is common with such a method, and infection of the bone through the open wound is a serious possible complication.

Two techniques rarely used in the United States include vaginal replacement of the fetal head with cesarean delivery (Zavanelli maneuver) and subcutaneous symphysiotomy.

Key Points

- The "fetal lie" indicates the orientation of the fetal spine relative to that of the mother. Normal fetal lie is longitudinal and by itself does not indicate whether the presentation is cephalic or breech.
- Cord prolapse occurs 20 times as often with an abnormal axial lie as it does with a cephalic presentation.
- Fetal malformations are observed in more than half of infants with a face presentation.
- Fetal malpresentation requires timely diagnostic exclusion of major fetal malformation and/or abnormal placentation.
- With few exceptions, a closely monitored labor and vaginal delivery is a safe possibility with most malpresentations.
- With few exceptions, cesarean delivery is the only acceptable alternative if normal progress toward spontaneous vaginal delivery is not observed.
- External cephalic version of the infant in breech presentation near term is a safe and often successful management option.
- Appropriate training and experience is a prerequisite to the safe vaginal delivery of selected infants in breech presentation.
- Shoulder dystocia cannot be precisely predicted or prevented but is often associated with macrosomia, maternal obesity, gestational diabetes, and postdates.
- The clinician must be prepared to deal with shoulder dystocia at every vaginal delivery with a deliberate, controlled sequence of interventions.

Chapter 10

Obstetric Hemorrhage

Thomas J. Benedetti

The normal pregnant patient frequently loses 500 ml of blood at the time of vaginal delivery and 1,000 ml at the time of cesarean delivery. Appreciably more blood can be lost without clinical evidence of a volume deficit as a result of the 40-percent expansion in blood volume that occurs by the 30th week of pregnancy.

The pregnant patient does not exhibit early signs of volume loss. When 1,000 ml is rapidly removed from the circulatory blood volume, however, vasoconstriction occurs in both the arterial and venous compartments in order to preserve essential body organ flow (Fig. 10-1). Blood pressure is initially maintained by increases in systemic vascular resistance. As volume loss exceeds 20 percent, the fall in cardiac output accelerates and blood pressure can no longer be maintained by increases in resistance. Blood pressure and cardiac output then fall in parallel. In addition, if the volume loss has occurred more than 4 hours earlier, significant fluid shifts from the interstitial space into the intravascular space will partially correct the volume deficit. This movement of fluid, termed *transcapillary refill,* can replace as much as 30 percent of lost volume. In more chronic bleeding states, the final blood volume deficit may amount to as little as 70 percent of the actual blood lost.

Classification of Hemorrhage

A standard classification for volume loss secondary to hemorrhage is illustrated in Table 10-1. Hemorrhage can be classified into one of four groups, depending on the volume lost. The determination of the class of hemorrhage reflects the volume deficit, which may not be the same as the volume loss. The average 60-kg pregnant woman has a blood volume of 6,000 ml at 30

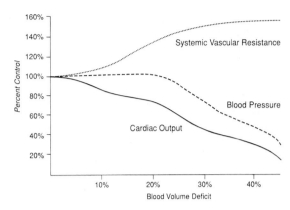

Fig. 10-1 Relationships among systemic vascular pressure, cardiac output, and blood pressure in the face of progressive blood volume deficit.

weeks, and an unreplaced volume loss of less than 900 ml falls into class 1. Such patients rarely exhibit signs or symptoms of volume deficit.

A blood loss of 1,200 to 1,500 ml is characterized as a class 2 hemorrhage. These individuals will begin to show expected physical signs, the first being a rise in pulse rate and/or a rise in respiratory rate. Tachypnea is a nonspecific response to volume loss and, although a relatively early sign of mild volume deficit, is frequently overlooked. A doubling of the respiratory rate may be observed in this circumstance. If the patient appears to

Table 10-1   Classification of Hemorrhage in the Pregnant Patient[a]

Hemorrhage Class	Acute Blood Loss[b]	Percentage Lost
1	900	15
2	1,200–1,500	20–25
3	1,800–2,100	30–35
4	2,400	40

[a] Total blood volume = 6,000 ml.

[b] In the usual clinical setting, very few episodes of volume loss occur without some infusion of intravenous fluids, usually crystalloid-containing solutions such as Ringer's lactated solution, or normal saline. Therefore, the amount of blood loss preceding physical signs and symptoms will usually exceed the values listed.

Adapted from Baker R: Hemorrhage in obstetrics. Obstet Gynecol Annu 6:295, 1977, with permission.

be breathing rapidly, the minute ventilation is usually twice its normal value. This finding should not be interpreted as an encouraging sign, but rather one of impending problems.

Patients with class 2 hemorrhage will frequently have orthostatic blood pressure changes and may have decreased perfusion of the extremities. However, this amount of blood loss will not usually result in the classic cold, clammy extremities. Rather, a more subtle test is needed to document this phenomenon. One can simply squeeze the hypothenar area of the hand for 1 to 2 seconds and then release the pressure. A patient with normal volume status will have an initial blanching of the skin, followed within 1 to 2 seconds by a return to the normal pink coloration. A patient who has a volume deficit of 15 to 25 percent will have delayed refilling of the blanched area of the hand.

Narrowing of the pulse pressure is another sign of class 2 hemorrhage. Blood loss results in sympathoadrenal stimulation, which causes a rise in diastolic pressure. Since the systolic pressure is usually maintained with small volume deficits (15 to 25 percent), the first blood pressure response seen with volume loss is narrowing of the pulse pressure (120/70 to 120/90 mm Hg). That is, pulse pressure changes from 50 to 30 mm Hg. When pulse pressure drops to 30 mm Hg or less, the patient should be carefully evaluated for other signs of volume loss.

Class 3 hemorrhage is defined as blood loss sufficient to cause overt hypotension. In the pregnant patient, this usually requires a blood loss of 1,800 to 2,100 ml. These patients exhibit marked tachycardia (120 to 60 bpm) and may have cold, clammy skin and tachypnea (respiratory rate of 30 to 50 per minute).

In class 4 patients, the volume deficit exceeds 40 percent. These patients are in profound shock and frequently have no discernible blood pressure. They may have absent pulses in their extremities and are oliguric or anuric. If volume therapy is not quickly begun, circulatory collapse and cardiac arrest will soon result.

After acute blood loss, the hematocrit will not change significantly for at least 4 hours, and complete compensation requires 48 hours. Infusion of intravenous fluids can alter this relationship, resulting in earlier lowering of measured hematocrit. When significant hemorrhage is thought to have occurred, a hematocrit should always be obtained. If this result shows a significant fall from a previous baseline value, a large amount of blood has been lost. Measures should immediately be taken to evaluate the source of the loss and whether the hemorrhage is ongoing but unrecognized.

Cesarean delivery is a frequent cause of excessive blood loss. It must be remembered that narcotics, which are frequently used for pain relief in the immediate postoperative period, can significantly reduce the ability of the sympathetic nervous system to effect vasoconstriction of the arterial and venous compartments. If these medications are given to a hypovolemic patient, serious hypotension can result. Signs and symptoms of hypovolemia should always be sought before the postoperative patient is given narcotic analgesics on the first postpartum day.

Urine Output—"The Window of Body Perfusion"

In hypovolemic patients, urine output must be carefully monitored. In many cases, the urine output will fall before other signs of impaired perfusion are manifest. In contrast, adequate urine volume in patients who have not received diuretics strongly suggests perfusion to vital body organs is adequate.

There is reasonable correlation between renal blood flow and urine output. If the urine output is low, renal blood flow is often low as well. When there is a rapid decrease in renal blood flow, there is usually a reduction in urine output. Urine will become more concentrated and will have a lower concentration of sodium and a higher osmolarity. With a gradual fall in renal blood flow, the urine sodium and osmolarity will often be affected before any significant fall in urine output. A urine sodium concentration of less than 10 to 20 mEq/L or a urine/serum osmolar ratio of greater than 2 usually indicates reduced renal perfusion.

Treatment

Patients showing signs of class 2 or greater volume loss should receive crystalloid intravenous fluids pending the arrival of blood and blood products. The infusion rate should be rapid, between 1,000 and 2,000 ml in 30 to 45 minutes, or faster if the patient is obviously hypotensive. This infusion may serve as a therapeutic trial to help determine the amount of blood loss. If the physical signs and symptoms return to normal and remain stable after this challenge, no further therapy may be needed. If blood loss has been severe and the patient continues to bleed, however, this favorable response may be only transient. In this situation, typed and cross-matched blood should be given. The initial administration of a balanced salt solution will reduce the amount of whole blood needed to restore an adequate blood volume.[2]

Blood and Blood Products

The use of whole blood has been discouraged by blood banking centers around the United States. In obstetrics, the main indication for whole blood rather than component therapy is massive blood loss requiring more than a 4,000-ml replacement (see Table 10-2).

The storage of whole blood has significant effects on its cellular elements as well as coagulation factors. After 24 hours, white blood cells (WBCs) and platelets are either absent or nonfunctional. After 7 days, levels of factors V and VIII have fallen 50 percent or more. There remains a large amount of plasma protein in stored blood, however, for which reason it remains the agent of choice for transfusion in the face of major hemorrhage.

Massive Blood Transfusion

The essentials of management of the patient requiring massive transfusion (10 units) are maintenance of circulation, blood volume, oxygen-carrying capacity, hemostasis, colloid osmotic pressure, and biochemical balance. As soon as it is apparent that more than two units of blood will be required, preparations should be made to have a significant quantity of blood products available. After four units of packed red cells are given, whole blood will provide both the coagulation factors and proteins needed to maintain hemostasis and colloid osmotic pressure. If whole blood is not available, earlier laboratory testing for coagulation deficiencies should be performed because more component therapy will probably be required. As soon as it becomes apparent that massive transfusion therapy is required, baseline coagulation tests should be ordered and the laboratory notified that more tests will be coming on a periodic basis. These tests should include complete blood count, platelet count, fibrinogen, prothrombin time (PT), and partial thromboplastin time (PTT). The laboratory must be alerted regarding the life-threatening nature of the problem and top priority. A turnaround time of 15 minutes should be the goal.

In general, microvascular oozing will be apparent at platelet counts below 50,000. This drop usually requires the replacement of one and a half blood volumes. However, counts may drop to this level or below in the face of the consumptive process of disseminated intravascular coagulation (DIC) prior to the loss of 15

Table 10-2 Blood Replacement

Product	Contents	Volume (cc)	Effect
Whole blood (WB)	Red blood cells (2,3-DPG) White blood cells (not functional after 24 hours) Coagulation factors (50%—V, VIII after 7 days) Plasma proteins	500	Increase volume (ml/ml) Increase hematocrit 3%/unit
Packed red cells	Red blood cells—same as whole blood White blood cells—less than whole blood Plasma proteins—few	240	Same red blood cells as whole blood Less risk of febrile or WBC transfusion reaction Increase hematocrit 3%/unit
Platelets	55×10^6 platelets/unit, few white blood cells	50	Increase platelet count 5,000–10,000 µl/unit Give 6 packs minimum
Fresh frozen plasma	Clotting factors V and VIII, fibrinogen	250	Only source of factors V, XI, XII Increase fibrinogen 10 mg/dl/unit
Cryoprecipitate	Factor VIII 25% Fibrinogen von Willebrand's factor	40	Increase fibrinogen 10 mg/dl/unit
Albumin 5%	Albumin	500	
Albumin 25%	Albumin	50	

units of blood. In addition, platelet function itself may be impaired in patients undergoing massive transfusion. If there is continued surgical evidence of microvascular bleeding in the face of laboratory tests near the critical levels, more replacement should be given.

If whole blood is available, there will often be no need for the transfusion of fresh frozen plasma because many of the coagulation factors are present in stored blood. However, if packed cells are used, frequent monitoring of the PT should be performed. When the PT is prolonged by greater than 5 seconds, fresh frozen plasma should be used. In the face of DIC there will also be prolongation of the PTT and fall in fibrinogen. In this case, cryoprecipitate should also be used as a source of factor VIII and fibrinogen.

Metabolic derangements are frequently mentioned when massive transfusion is discussed. However, traditional formulas for using alkylating agents or calcium supplements are probably unnecessary. Hypocalcemia is a theoretic problem, but clinical symptoms from this problem are infrequently described and the possible complications of prophylactic calcium infusion may be more harmful than hypocalcemia. The one time hypocalcemia can be clinically important is when it is combined with hyperkalemia and hypothermia, a triad that can lead to cardiac arrhythmias. Hypothermia can be a problem if recently refrigerated blood is administered at a rate of one unit every 5 to 10 minutes. If this rate of administration is required, attempts should be made to warm the blood above 4°C before transfusion. Close attention should be paid to the electrocardiogram. If arrhythmias are noted, supplemental calcium should be considered.

Acid–base problems may arise in the event of massive transfusion due to citrate toxicity. However, this is rarely a problem because the healthy liver can metabolize the citrate in a unit of blood in 5 minutes. Unless transfusion rates exceed one unit per 5 minutes or the liver is diseased, citrate toxicity should not be a problem. Although stored blood has an acid pH, acidosis is uncommon because the metabolism of citrate produces alkalosis. Prolonged acidosis is more often the result of hypoperfusion and shock rather than blood replacement. Blood gas measurement should guide the therapy with bicarbonate in this instance.

Packed Red Blood Cells

Packed red blood cells (PRBCs) are the most effective and efficient way to provide increased oxygen-carrying capacity to the anemic patient. Unless a patient has suffered massive blood loss, PRBCs and crystalloid will satisfy most clinical needs. Oxygen-carrying capacity may become impaired in the euvolemic patient when the hemoglobin level drops below 7 g/dl. If adequate volume replacement has not been accomplished, patients may exhibit orthostatic blood pressure changes or other signs of impaired oxygen-carrying capacity at hemoglobin levels above 7 g/dl. Because PRBCs have only small amounts of WBCs and isohemagglutinins (anti-A and anti-B), its use reduces the incidence of non-hemolytic transfusion reactions compared with that of one unit of whole blood. However, care should be taken to administer PRBCs with normal saline rather than Ringer's lactated or dextrose solutions. These solutions can cause the blood to clot or the red cells to lyse.

Platelets

A unit of platelets is derived from a single unit of whole blood and has a shelf life of 72 hours. Transfusion of a single unit of platelets can be expected to raise the platelet count between 5,000 and 10,000/μl. Platelets should be administered rapidly, over 10 minutes, with repeat laboratory evaluation performed 2 hours after infusion. For the obstetric patient, it is important that the platelets be ABO and Rh specific, since the platelet concentrate usually contains some RBCs that can potentially sensitize an Rh-negative woman. Sensitization can be prevented by concomitant administration of Rh immune globulin. One 300-μg dose will prevent sensitization for 30 platelet packs. It must also be remembered that six packs of platelets have a volume effect if multiple doses are used. Each unit of platelets carries the transfusion risk of a single unit of blood.

Platelet administration is frequently considered for patients with DIC, massive hemorrhage, severe preeclampsia, and idiopathic thrombocytopenia (ITP). In each of these conditions, the absolute levels at which a platelet transfusion is indicated may vary depending on the time course of the thrombocytopenia (more chronic forms will result in less hemostatic defects than acute loss), the need to perform a surgical procedure, the etiology of the inciting event producing thrombocytopenia, and the level of blood pressure elevation and the bleeding time. In general, platelet counts below 50,000/μl will require transfusion prior to or during surgery. However, when the need for a cesarean delivery arises in patients with platelet counts ranging from 20,000 to 50,000 platelets, transfusion may be avoided or the amount reduced if the transfusion is delayed until the need becomes apparent. This is usually evident from bleeding from skin edges, as hemostasis in the uterus is primarily a function of uterine muscle contraction, not platelet function.

Cryoprecipitate

Prepared by warming fresh frozen plasma and collecting the precipitate, cryoprecipitate contains significant amounts of factor VIII fibrinogen and von Willebrand factor. Cryoprecipitate is used primarily in patients with von Willebrand disease and in patients with a normal blood volume who require factor replacement. Except for factor VIII, the same coagulation factors are available in this product as in fresh frozen plasma but in only 15 percent of the volume. As with platelets, cryoprecipitate should be ABO and Rh specific. One unit of cryoprecipitate will raise the serum fibrinogen level 10 mg/dl. This preparation should be used when significant hypofibrinogenemia must be treated.

Fresh Frozen Plasma

Fresh frozen plasma contains all the coagulation factors present in cryoprecipitate, including appreciably higher levels of factor VIII. Fresh frozen plasma should be administered when both volume replacement and coagulation factors are needed. The main clinical indication for this therapy is the massively hemorrhaging patient. If bleeding continues after the transfusion of four to five units of blood, a coagulation screen should be checked to see whether the replacement of clotting factors and platelets is indicated. If the coagulation parameters and PTT are abnormal, two units of fresh frozen plasma should be administered. Subsequent therapy should be determined by clinical response and follow-up laboratory testing.

Transfusion Risks

PRBCs, fresh frozen plasma, cryoprecipitate, and platelets have the same risk of transmitting infectious diseases as a unit of whole blood. Table 10-3 lists the common risks of blood transfusion when blood is procured from volunteer donors. Significant progress has been made in historical and laboratory screening for common infectious diseases. The risks of serious complications from blood transfusion have fallen to very low rates. Blood obtained from paid sources can be expected to have higher rates of many of the complications listed in the table.

Table 10-3   Risks of Blood Transfusion

Complication	Incidence of Complication	Incidence of Death
Human immunodeficiency virus	1/270,000	1/270,000
Hepatitis B	1/100,000	1/2,000,000
Hepatitis C	1/5,000	Less than 1/500,000
Hemolytic transfusion reaction	1/6,000	1/100,000
Nonhemolytic transfusion reaction	1/100	1/10,000,000

Autologous Transfusion

Primarily as the result of fear of acquiring the acquired immunodeficiency syndrome virus from blood transfusion, interest in autologous blood transfusion for pregnant patients has been heightened in recent years. Autologous transfusion can be accomplished in two ways. In the most common approach, blood is collected and stored during the weeks before delivery. This presents some logistic problems for the pregnant patient since 3 weeks is the longest time that the blood can be stored. Most patients are unable to maintain a hematocrit above 33 percent with a donation frequency of less than 2 to 3 weeks. Although predelivery autologous blood donation is generally safe for both mother and fetus, the low incidence of blood transfusion in patients at the time of childbirth and the safety of allogeneic transfusion has limited enthusiasm on the part of health care professionals.

A second type of autologous donation, intraoperative blood salvage, can occur at the time of excessive blood loss. Intraoperative autotransfusion has been reported in obstetric patients at the time of ruptured ectopic pregnancy and recently after delayed cesarean hysterectomy. This technique has some limitations in the obstetric setting. Heavy bacterial contamination is a contraindication, and use during cesarean delivery should also be avoided because of the possibility of amniotic fluid, fetal debris, and bacterial contamination. However, in the case of cesarean hysterectomy with massive bleeding or delayed re-operation because of continued bleeding this technique can be considered.[5]

Antepartum Hemorrhage

Abruptio Placenta

The premature separation of the normally implanted placenta from its attachment to the uterus is called *abruptio placenta* or *placental abruption*. This event occurs with a frequency of approximately 1/120 births but accounts for nearly 15 percent of perinatal mortality. Diagnosis of placental abruption is certain when inspection of the placenta shows an adherent retroplacental clot with depression or disruption of the underlying placental tissue; however, this frequently is not found if the abruption is of recent onset. Clinical findings indicating placental abruption include the triad of external or occult uterine bleeding, uterine hypertonus and/or hyperactivity, and fetal distress and/or fetal death. Placental abruption can be broadly classified into three grades that correlate with clinical and laboratory findings.

Grade 1: Slight vaginal bleeding and some uterine irritability are usually present. Maternal blood pressure is unaffected, and the maternal fibrinogen level is normal. The fetal heart rate pattern is normal.

Grade 2: External uterine bleeding is mild to moderate. The uterus is irritable, and tetanic contractions may be present. Maternal blood pressure is maintained, but the pulse rate may be elevated and postural blood volume deficits may be present. The fibrinogen level is usually reduced to 150 to 250 mg/dl. The fetal heart rate often shows signs of fetal distress.

Grade 3: Bleeding is moderate to severe but may be concealed. The uterus is tetanic and painful. Maternal hypotension is frequently present and fetal death has occurred. Fibrinogen levels are often reduced to less than 150 mg/dl; other coagulation abnormalities (thrombocytopenia, factor depletion) are present.

Etiology

Maternal hypertension (>140/90 mm Hg) seems to be the most consistently identified factor predisposing to placental abruption.[17] This relationship is true for all grades of placental abruption but is most strongly associated with grade 3 abruption, in which 40 to 50 percent of cases are found to have hypertensive disease of pregnancy.[16,17] Intrapartum hypertension significantly increases the risk of abruption, but one study failed to show a relationship between the antenatal detection of hypertension and placental abruption.

Blunt external maternal trauma is an increasingly important cause of placental abruption. Two conditions account for the majority of blunt abdominal trauma leading to placental abruption: motor vehicle collision and maternal battering. Historically 1 to 2 percent of grade 3 abruptions have been attributed to maternal trauma.[17,18] However, recent epidemiologic studies show an alarmingly high incidence of maternal battering in some populations.[19] The physical evidence of trauma may be minimal and still be associated with placental abruption that can progress from grade 1 to 3 within 24 hours.

Rapid decompression of the overdistended uterus is an uncommon cause of placental abruption. The two clinical situations in which this may occur are patients with multiple gestations and those with polyhydramnios. There is a significant recurrence rate for placental abruption. This figure has been reported to vary from 5 to 17 percent.[9,13,17] If a patient has suffered an abruption in two pregnancies, the chance for recurrence is 25 percent.

Diagnosis and Management

Vaginal bleeding in the third trimester of pregnancy is the hallmark of placental abruption and should always prompt an investigation to determine its etiology. The other common and potentially life-threatening cause of third-trimester bleeding, placenta previa, should be recognized in nearly all cases in which it is present. If ultrasound examination fails to show a placenta previa and if other local causes of vaginal bleeding (including cervical or vaginal trauma, labor, or malignancy) have been ruled out, placental abruption becomes a more likely diagnosis.

Ultrasound can identify three predominant locations for placental abruption. These are subchorionic (between the placenta and the membranes), retroplacental (between the placenta and the myometrium), and preplacental (between the placenta and the amniotic fluid). Hematomas identified by ultrasound during the early phases of vaginal bleeding and pain are most likely to be hyperechoic or isoechoic compared with the placenta. As the hematoma resolves, it will become hypoechoic within a week and sonolucent within 2 weeks.[22] Retroplacental hematomas carry a worse prognosis for fetal survival than subchorionic hemorrhages. The size of the hemorrhage is also predictive of fetal survival. Large retroplacental hemorrhages (>60 ml/>50 percent) are associated with a 50 percent or greater fetal mortality, whereas similar-sized subchorionic hemorrhages are associated with a 10 percent mortality.[23]

Gestational age at the time of presentation is an important prognostic factor. Among patients who present at less than 20 weeks, 82 percent can be expected to have a term delivery despite evidence of placental separation. If the presentation occurs after 20 weeks' gestation, only 27 percent will deliver at term.

Nearly 80 percent of patients who eventually prove to have a placental abruption will present with vaginal bleeding. The remaining 20 percent of patients fail to exhibit external signs of bleeding. These patients have a concealed abruption and are commonly given the diagnosis of premature labor. Such cases must be watched very carefully. On some occasions, the abruption may progress despite successful tocolysis, and fetal death may result. Other classic signs of placental abruption include increased uterine tenderness and tone. These findings are uncommon (17 percent) unless the abruption is grade 2 or 3.[9]

Once the diagnosis of placental abruption has been entertained, precautions should be taken to deal with the possible life-threatening consequences for both mother and fetus. At least 4 units of blood should be available for maternal transfusions. A large-bore (16-gauge) intravenous line must be secured and the infusion of a crystalloid solution begun. Blood should be drawn for hemoglobin and hematocrit determinations and coagulation studies (fibrinogen, platelet count, fibrin degradation products, PT, PTT). A red-topped tube should also be obtained and used to perform a clot test. If a clot does not form within 6 minutes or forms and lyses within 30 minutes, a coagulation defect is probably present and the fibrinogen level is less than 150 mg/dl. Because fetal distress will develop in as many as 60 percent of patients who present with a live fetus, continuous fetal monitoring should be used to record fetal heart rate and document uterine activity.

In the patient with a term fetus in whom the diagnosis of grade 1 abruption is made, close observation for signs of fetal or maternal compromise is essential. If the fetus is known to be mature, controlled delivery should be accomplished by induction of labor while the mother and fetus are in stable condition.

The occurrence of a grade 1 placental abruption with a preterm fetus presents greater challenge. A small placental abruption may stimulate uterine irritability, further separating the placenta until fetal compromise becomes evident. In carefully selected cases, it may be possible to inhibit uterine contractions as long as there are no signs of acute fetal distress and no ultrasonographic evidence of intrauterine growth retardation. Magnesium sulfate has fewer adverse cardiovascular side effects than β-sympathomimetic agents and has been used in this circumstance.

In many cases of placental abruption, delivery will be the treatment of choice. During labor, careful attention must be paid to several maternal and fetal parameters. Because 60 percent of fetuses may exhibit signs of intrapartum fetal distress, continuous fetal heart rate monitoring is essential. In a similar manner, continuous monitoring of maternal volume status is important. An indwelling Foley catheter will permit accurate assessment of maternal urine output. Serial maternal hematocrit determinations should be made regularly at intervals of 2 to 3 hours. The goal of therapy should be to maintain a maternal urine output of 1 ml/min and a hematocrit of at least 30 percent. An updated flow sheet at the bedside permits the clinician to follow maternal vital signs, urine output, laboratory values, and critical clotting parameters.

Placental abruption frequently stimulates the clotting cascade, resulting in DIC. Intravascular fibrinogen is converted to fibrin by activation of the extrinsic clotting cascade. In the usual clinical setting, platelets and clotting factors V and VIII are also depleted. Serial measurements of plasma fibrinogen provide valuable information regarding the coagulation status of the patient and will help estimate the volume of blood loss that has occurred.

The normal maternal fibrinogen concentration in the third trimester is 450 mg/dl. In grade 1 abruptions, there is often no alteration in this value and no evidence of DIC. However, when the fibrinogen value drops below 300 mg/dl, significant coagulation abnormalities are usually present. Most women with significant falls in fibrinogen will require blood transfusion to maintain a normal circulating volume. If the presenting fibrinogen level is less than 150 mg/dl, most patients will have already lost 2,000 ml of blood. The signs and symptoms of such blood loss may not be obvious because, as noted earlier, the normal hypervolemia of pregnancy protects the mother from a volume loss that a nonpregnant individual could not tolerate. In the case of grade 3 placental abruption, the mean blood loss is 2,500 ml or more.[27] In patients with grade 2 and grade 3 abruption, rapid crystalloid infusion of at least 1,000 ml pending the availability of whole blood should be done. Two to 3 ml of crystalloid should be given for each 1 ml of blood lost to maintain euvolemia.

If urine output fails to reach 30 ml/hr despite adequate volume replacement, then consideration should be given to inserting a central venous pressure (CVP) catheter to determine the adequacy of intravascular volume. This catheter is best inserted through a site in the arm rather than the neck or subclavian area because of the severe coagulopathy that is often present. The absolute level of CVP is less important than the response of the CVP to volume infusion, as long as the CVP is less than 7 cm H_2O in response to the preceding 250-ml aliquot. If this response has been achieved but the urine output is still inadequate, consideration should be given to replacing the CVP catheter with a pulmonary artery catheter. This circumstance is uncommon unless there is intrinsic heart disease or severe preeclampsia or the patient has already suffered critical renal ischemia and is in acute renal failure.

Extravasation of blood into the uterine muscle to produce red to purple discoloration of the serosal surface will be found in 8 percent of patients. This finding, known as a Couvelaire uterus, has been feared to result in a high incidence of uterine hemorrhage secondary to atony. However, atony is the exception rather than the rule, and most patients with a Couvelaire uterus demonstrate an appropriate response to the infusion of oxytocin. Hysterectomy should be reserved for cases of atony and hemorrhage unresponsive to conventional uterotonics.

Placenta Previa

Placenta previa is defined as the implantation of the placenta over the cervical os. There are three recognized variations of placenta previa: total, partial, and marginal. In total placenta previa, the cervical os is completely covered by the placenta. This type presents the most serious maternal risk, as it is associated with greater blood loss than either marginal or partial placenta previa. Partial placenta previa is defined as the partial occlusion of the cervical os by the placenta and occurs in 31 percent of diagnosed cases. A marginal placenta previa is characterized by the encroachment of the placenta to the margin of the cervical os. It does not cover the os. The differentiation of the latter two degrees of placenta previa is dependent on the dilatation of the cervix and the method of diagnosis (ultrasound or direct examination).

A leading cause of third trimester hemorrhage, placenta previa presents classically as painless bleeding. Bleeding is thought to occur in association with the development of the lower uterine segment in the third trimester. Placental attachment is disrupted as this area gradually thins in preparation for the onset of labor.

When this occurs, bleeding occurs at the implantation site, as the uterus is unable to contract adequately and stop the flow of blood from the open vessels.

Significant risk factors are maternal age above 35 years (risk ratio 4.7) and black or other minority races (risk ratio 1.3). Whether the increased risk for older mothers is related to parity or to an independent risk factor is still uncertain. The most important obstetric risk factor in the development of placenta previa is previous cesarean delivery. The risk for placenta previa occurring in the pregnancy following a cesarean delivery has been reported to be between 1 and 4 percent.[33,36–39] There is a linear increase in placenta previa risk with the number of prior cesarean deliveries. In patients with four or more cesarean deliveries, the risk of placenta previa approaches 10 percent.[36]

Once the diagnosis of placenta previa is made, management decisions depend on the gestational age, amount of bleeding, fetal condition, and presentation. In the patient who is unequivocally at 37 weeks' gestation with evidence of uterine activity or with persistent bleeding, delivery is the treatment of choice. In previous years a double setup examination was the initial step in this process. With the advent of rapid and reliable ultrasound availability and interpretation, including transvaginal sonography, this technique is necessary much less often. In the patient in whom there is unequivocal evidence of placenta previa, cesarean delivery is the method of choice.

In some patients vaginal delivery may still be considered. Patients with marginal or partial placenta previa who present in labor with minimal bleeding are ideal candidates. It can also be considered for patients with pre-viable gestations or intrauterine fetal demise. Appropriately conducted labor in these selected instances can be safe for both mother and fetus.[42]

For the patient who is remote from term (24 to 36 weeks' gestation), expectant management is the treatment of choice. The essence of this approach is maintenance of the fetus in a healthy intrauterine environment without jeopardizing maternal condition. Maternal blood loss should be replaced in order to maintain the maternal hematocrit between 30 and 35 percent. This RBC volume will provide a margin of safety in the event of a large hemorrhage. Even an initial blood loss in excess of 500 ml can be expectantly managed with adequate volume replacement.

Although obstetricians are most concerned about maternal hemorrhage, they must remember that fetal blood can also be lost during the process of placental separation. Rh immune globulin should be given to all at-risk patients with third-trimester bleeding who are Rh negative and unsensitized. A Kleihauer-Betke preparation of maternal blood should also be performed in all Rh-negative women. This test will detect the occasional patient with a fetomaternal hemorrhage of greater than 30 ml. Thirty-five percent of infants whose mothers require antepartum transfusion will themselves be anemic and require transfusion when delivered.[34]

Because of the reduced risk of cardiovascular complications, magnesium sulfate has become the agent of choice for the treatment of patients in preterm labor with placenta previa at many institutions. Infusion of a 6-g loading dose followed by 3 g/hr or more are often necessary to control uterine irritability because of the increased maternal glomerular filtration rate. Once the patient has been stabilized on magnesium sulfate, the use of oral β-mimetics therapy is an appropriate choice provided that euvolemia has been achieved.

If the mother responds to conservative management, she should be treated with bedrest, preferably in the hospital setting. Blood should always be available for maternal transfusion in the event of sudden hemorrhage.

Approximately 25 to 30 percent of patients can be expected to complete 36 weeks' gestation without labor or repetitive bleeding forcing earlier delivery. In these patients, amniocentesis should be performed and, if the analysis of amniotic fluid documents pulmonary maturity, cesarean delivery planned.

When encountering a patient with placenta previa, the possibility of a placenta accreta or one of its variations, placenta percreta or placenta increta, should be considered (Fig. 10-2).[53] In this condition, the placenta forms an abnormally firm attachment to the uterine wall. There is absence of the decidua basalis and incomplete development of the fibrinoid layer. The placenta can be attached directly to the myometrium (accreta), invade the myometrium (increta), or penetrate the myometrium (percreta).

Prior cesarean delivery and other uterine surgery are the factors most often associated with placenta accreta. In patients with multiple cesarean deliveries and placenta previa, the risk of accreta is 60 to 65 percent. At least two-thirds of the patients with placenta previa/ placenta accreta will require cesarean hysterectomy.[34,56,57] However, in cases where uterine preservation is highly desired and no bladder invasion has occurred, bleeding after placental removal has been successfully controlled with a variety of surgical techniques. Packing of the lower uterine segment with sub-

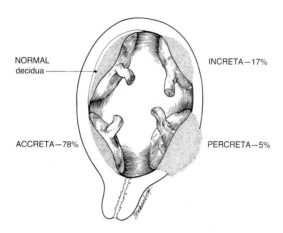

NORMAL decidua

INCRETA—17%

ACCRETA—78%

PERCRETA—5%

Fig. 10-2 Uteroplacental relationships found in abnormal placentation.

sequent removal of the pack through the vagina within 24 hours[57] has been successful. Interrupted circular suture of the lower uterine segment on the serosal surface of the uterus has also been reported to be successful.[58] Predelivery placement of catheters for angiographic embolization of pelvic vessels is another technique recently described.[59,60]

Suspicion or confirmation of complete placenta accreta before attempted placental removal may permit other treatment options. Bleeding may be minimal unless the placenta has partially separated. If no cleavage plane is identified and a placenta accreta is suspected, one should first make preparations for the possibility of major postpartum blood loss. At least 4 units of blood should be on hand and an anesthesiologist present in the delivery room. If vaginal delivery has occurred, the patient should be in a suite in which a laparotomy can be performed, and surgical instruments for hysterectomy should be sterilized and ready. Whenever possible, the obstetrician should discuss the likely diagnosis with the patient and review possible treatment options.

Five therapeutic plans may be considered. If uterine preservation is not important, or if maternal blood loss is excessive, hysterectomy offers the best chance for survival and will minimize morbidity.[61] If uterine preservation is important, four treatment options are available: (1) placental removal and oversewing the uterine defects—after removing as much of the placenta as possible, the bleeding defects are oversewed and the patient treated with oxytocics and antibiotics (this option is probably most useful when there is significant bleeding from a partially separated placenta with only a focal accreta); (2) localized resection and uterine repair; (3) curettage of the uterine cavity; and (4) leaving the placenta in situ. For the patient who wishes to maximize her chances for uterine preservation and who is not actively bleeding, the placenta may be left in situ. The umbilical cord should be ligated and cut as close to its base as possible. The patient should then be treated with antibiotics. This approach has been successful when bleeding has not necessitated more aggressive surgical procedures.[62] Some authors have advocated treatment with methotrexate in this instance, but there is presently no consensus on whether this therapy is any more effective than observation.

In rare cases placenta accreta invades the maternal bladder. In this instance, it is probably best to treat in a manner similar to abdominal pregnancy and avoid placental removal. However, this may not obviate the need for eventual hysterectomy and cystectomy.[63,64]

Postpartum Hemorrhage

Acute blood loss is the most common cause of hypotension in obstetrics. Hemorrhage usually occurs immediately preceding or after delivery of the placenta. Excessive blood loss most commonly results when the uterus fails to contract after the delivery of its contents. Effective hemostasis after separation of the placenta is dependent on contraction of the myometrium to compress severed vessels. Failure of the uterus to contract can usually be attributed to myometrial dysfunction and retained placental fragments. Factors predisposing to myometrial dysfunction include overdistention of the uterus as in multiple pregnancy, fetal macrosomia, hydramnios, oxytocin-stimulated labor, uterine relaxants (magnesium, β-mimetics), and amnionitis.

Prevention

The need to deal with excessive blood loss after vaginal birth or cesarean delivery can be limited by recognizing high-risk factors for postpartum hemorrhage (Table 10-4) and by applying proven methods to limit blood loss after delivery. Dilute solutions of oxytocin in addition to gentle cord traction reduce cesarean delivery associated blood loss by 31 percent compared with manual removal of the placenta.[67] Similarly, umbilical cord clamping within 30 seconds of delivery and gentle cord traction followed by administration of intramuscular or dilute solutions of intravenous oxytocin before delivery of the placenta reduce postpartum blood loss and postpartum transfusion requirements.[68] Adminis-

Table 10-4   Risk Factors for Obstetric Hemorrhage of Greater Than 1,000 ml

Factor	Risk Increase
Placental abruption	12.6
Placenta previa	13.1
Multiple pregnancy	4.5
Obesity	1.6
Retained placenta	5.2
Induced labor	2.2
Episiotomy	2.1
Birth weight >4 kg	1.9

From Stones RW, Paterson CM, Saunders NJ: Risk factors for major obstetric hemorrhage. Eur J Obstet Gynecol Reprod Biol 48:15, 1993, with permission.

tration of oxytocin before delivery of the placenta is associated with a reduction in the length of the third stage of labor (mean 5 minutes) and a low incidence of manual removal of the placenta (2 percent) compared with physiologic management of the third stage of labor (15 minutes and 2.5 percent, respectively).[68] When the placenta is retained for 30 minutes or longer, randomized studies have shown that injection of the umbilical cord with either saline or oxytocin has no significant benefit in effecting spontaneous delivery of the placenta. In the absence of significant maternal hemorrhage, an additional 30 minutes of expectant management can be allowed because half of the retained placentas will deliver spontaneously during this time, avoiding the need for manual removal, anesthesia, and excessive blood loss.

Upon encountering postpartum hemorrhage, manual digital exploration of the uterus should be quickly accomplished to rule out the possibility of retained placental fragments. If retained tissue is not detected, manual massage of the uterus should be started (Fig. 10-3). Simultaneously, pharmacologic methods should be employed to control uterine bleeding. Initial therapy includes the administration of a dilute solution of oxytocin, usually 10 to 20 units of oxytocin in 1,000 ml of physiologic saline solution. The solution can be administered in rates as high as 500 ml in 10 minutes without cardiovascular complications. However, an intravenous bolus injection of as little as 5 units of oxytocin may be associated with maternal hypotension, further stressing an already compromised maternal cardiovascular system.

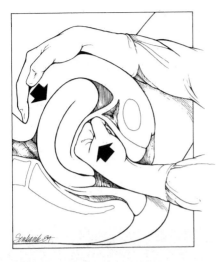

Fig. 10-3 Manual compression and massage of the uterus to control bleeding from uterine atony.

When oxytocin fails to produce adequate uterine contraction, most clinicians now administer synthetic 15-methyl-$F_{2\alpha}$-prostaglandin (Prostin). Although ergonovine (0.2 mg IM) has been a standard second-line drug for many years, the efficacy and safety of prostaglandin medications in this instance have obviated the need to use ergonovine in most instances. Initial studies with prostaglandin medications for postpartum hemorrhage were performed with the naturally occurring $F_{20\alpha}$ prostaglandin compound, which required direct intrauterine injection. The total dose used was 1 to 2 mg diluted in 10 to 20 ml of saline.[69] Subsequently, clinical trials of the synthetic 15-methyl-$F_{2\alpha}$-prostaglandin produced promising results.[70] This compound should be given in 0.25-mg doses in the deltoid muscle every 1 to 2 hours. As many as five doses may be administered without adverse effect.

When pharmacologic methods fail to control hemorrhage from atony, surgical measures should be undertaken to arrest the bleeding before it becomes life threatening. However, before laparotomy, a careful inspection of the vagina and cervix should be made to confirm that the uterus is the source of the bleeding.

If the uterus is found to be contracted appropriately and no placental fragments are retained within the uterus, a laceration of maternal soft tissues is the likely cause of continued vaginal bleeding. Careful inspection of the cervix and vagina will often indicate the source of the bleeding. Figures 10-4 through 10-6 illustrate

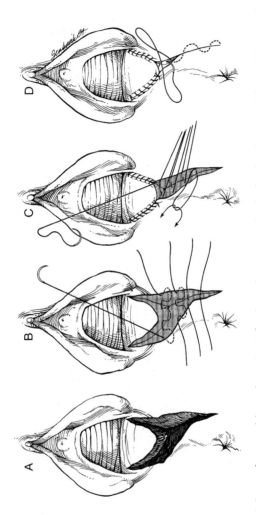

Fig. 10-4 Repair of a second-degree laceration. A first-degree laceration involves the fourchet, the perineal skin, and the vaginal mucous membrane. A second-degree laceration also includes the muscles of the perineal body. The rectal sphincter remains intact.

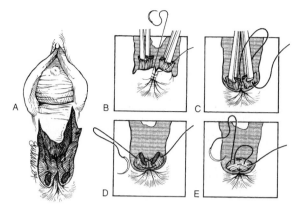

Fig. 10-5 Repair of the sphincter after a third-degree laceration. A third-degree laceration extends not only through the skin, mucous membrane, and perineal body, but includes the anal sphincter. Interrupted figure-of-eight sutures should be placed in the capsule of the sphincter muscle.

second-, third-, and fourth-degree lacerations of the perineum and techniques for their repair. Adequate exposure for the repair of such lacerations is critical and, if needed, assistance should be summoned to aid in retraction.

In cervical laceration, it is important to secure the base of the laceration, which is often a major source of bleeding. However, this area is frequently the most difficult to suture. Valuable time can be lost trying to expose the angle of such a laceration. A helpful technique to use in these cases, especially when help is limited or slow in responding, is to start to suture the laceration at its proximal end, using the suture for traction to expose the more distal portion of the cervix until the apex is in view (Fig. 10-7). This technique has the added advantage of arresting significant bleeding from the edges of the laceration.

When uterine bleeding is not responsive to pharmacologic methods and no vaginal or cervical lacerations are present, surgical exploration may be necessary. Laceration of uterine vessels during the birth process will occasionally be found, most commonly after forceps delivery. Substantial episodic hemorrhage followed by periods of relatively little blood flow is often a sign of uterine vessel laceration. In this case, unilateral ligation and repair will stop the blood loss.

If hemorrhage is secondary to atony, vascular ligation will often be necessary to control bleeding. Hypogastric artery ligation, a technique recommended for

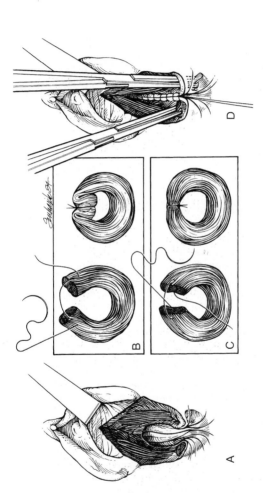

Fig. 10-6 Repair of a fourth-degree laceration. This laceration extends through the rectal mucosa. (A) The extent of this laceration is shown, with a segment of the rectum exposed. (B) Approximation of the rectal submucosa. This is the most commonly recommended method for repair. (C) Alternative method of approximating the rectal mucosa in which the knots are actually buried inside the rectal lumen. (D) After closure of the rectal submucosa, an additional layer of running sutures may be placed. The rectal sphincter is then repaired.

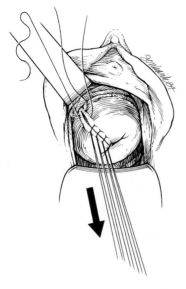

Fig. 10-7 Repair of a cervical laceration, which begins at the proximal part of the laceration, using traction on the previous sutures to aid in exposing the distal portion of the defect.

many decades to control postpartum hemorrhage, has fallen out of favor because of the prolonged operating time, technical difficulties associated with its performance, and an inconsistent clinical response. Instead, a stepwise progression of uterine vessel ligation should be rapidly accomplished. Ligation of the ascending branch of the uterine arteries should be attempted as a first step if hemorrhage is unresponsive to oxytocin or prostaglandin.[71,72] The uterine artery should be located at the border between the upper and lower uterine segment and suture ligated with No. 0 or 1 chromic suture. The suture should be placed 2 cm medial to the uterine artery and the needle driven from the anterior surface of the uterus posteriorly and tied. Because the suture is placed high in the lower uterine segment, the ureter is not in jeopardy and the bladder usually does not need to be mobilized. In approximately 10 to 15 percent of cases of atony, unilateral ligation of the uterine artery is sufficient to control hemorrhage. Bilateral ligation will control an additional 75 percent.[72]

If bleeding continues, attention should next be paid to interrupting the blood flow to the uterus from the infundibulopelvic ligament (Fig. 10-8). There are a number of techniques to accomplish this. The easiest

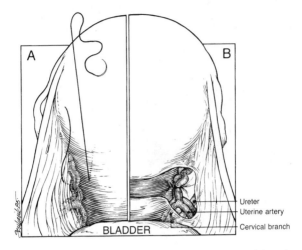

Fig. 10-8 View of sutured uterus: ligated uterine artery, and ligated utero-ovarian artery.

involves ligation of the anastomosis of the ovarian and uterine artery, high on the fundus, just below the utero-ovarian ligament. A large suture on an atraumatic needle can be passed from the uterus, around the vessel, and tied. If bilateral utero-ovarian vessel ligation does not stop the bleeding, temporary occlusion of the infundibulopelvic ligament vessels may be attempted. This can be accomplished with digital pressure or with rubber-sleeved clamps. It may be an especially useful technique if the patient is of low parity and future child-bearing is of great importance. If this appears to control hemorrhage, ligation of the infundibulopelvic ligament can be performed by passing an absorbable suture from anterior to posterior through the avascular area inferior to and including the ovarian vessels. Although the ovarian blood supply may be decreased, successful pregnancy has been reported after all major pelvic vessels were ligated to arrest postpartum hemorrhage.[72,73]

Pelvic Hematomas

Vulvar Hematoma

This type of hematoma results from laceration of vessels in the superficial fascia of either the anterior or posterior pelvic triangle. The usual physical signs are subacute volume loss and vulvar pain. The blood loss in this case is limited by Colle's fascia and the urogenital diaphragm. In the posterior area, the limitations are the anal fascia. Because of these fascial boundaries, the mass will extend to the skin and a visible hematoma will result.

Treatment in these cases requires the volume support outlined previously. Surgical management calls for wide linear incision of the mass through the skin and evacuation of blood and clots. As this condition is often the result of bleeding from small vessels, the lacerated vessel will not usually be identified. Once the clot has been evacuated, the dead space can be closed with sutures. The area should then be compressed by a large sterile dressing and pressure applied. Efforts to pack the cavity are usually futile and only serve to create further bleeding. An indwelling catheter should be placed in the bladder at the start of the surgical evacuation and left in place for 24 to 36 hours. Compression can be removed after 12 hours.

Vaginal Hematoma

Vaginal hematomas may result from trauma to maternal soft tissues during delivery. These hematomas are frequently associated with a forceps delivery but may occur spontaneously. They are less common than vulvar hematomas. In this instance, blood accumulates in the plane above the level of the pelvic diaphragm. It is unusual for large amounts of blood to collect in this space. The most frequent complaint in such cases is severe rectal pressure. Examination will reveal a large mass protruding into the vagina.

Vaginal hematomas should be treated by incision of the vagina and evacuation. As with vulvar hematomas, it is uncommon to find a single bleeding vessel as the source of bleeding. The incision need not be closed, as the edges of the vagina will fall back together after the clot has been removed. A vaginal pack should be inserted to tamponade the raw edges. The pack is then removed in 12 to 18 hours.

Inversion of the Uterus

Occasionally the third stage of labor is complicated by partial delivery of the placenta followed by rapid onset of shock in the mother. These events characterize uterine inversion. Hypotension usually results before significant blood loss has occurred. The inexperienced obstetrician may mistake an inversion of the uterus for a partially separated placenta or aborted myoma. Uterine inversion usually occurs in association with a fundally inserted placenta.

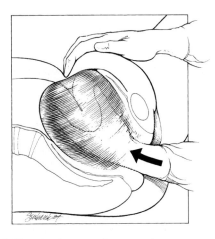

Fig. 10-9 Manual replacement of an inverted uterus.

Treatment of uterine inversion should include fluid therapy for the mother and restoration of the uterus to its normal position. This latter is best accomplished using the technique illustrated in Figure 10-9 and should be attempted immediately upon recognition of the inversion. Separation of the placenta before replacement of the uterus will only increase maternal blood loss.[77] If possible, the uterus should be replaced without removing the placenta. Initial efforts to replace the uterus should be made without the use of uterine relaxing agents. If initial efforts fail, the use of either β-mimetic agents or magnesium sulfate should be tried. In the case of severe maternal hypotension, magnesium sulfate is probably the best choice.

Occasionally, it is impossible to reposition the subacutely inverted uterus vaginally and laparotomy is necessary.

Once the uterine inversion has been corrected, the anesthetic agents used for uterine relaxation should be discontinued and oxytocic agents given to produce uterine contraction. If oxytocin fails to contract the uterus, prostaglandin $F_{2\alpha}$ should be used. The same dosage and intervals used to arrest postpartum hemorrhage with uterine atony are appropriate in this circumstance.

Coagulation Disorders

Continued bleeding in the third stage of labor that is unresponsive to usual treatment should cause the clinician to consider uncommon but serious maternal coagulation disorders. The most frequent is von Willebrand's disease (VWD), a hemorrhagic disorder that affects both men and women. This coagulopathy is inherited in an autosomal dominant pattern and is characterized by the following laboratory abnormalities: prolonged bleeding time, decreased factor VIII activity, decreased factor VIII–related antigen, and decreased von Willebrand factor. The latter is a plasma factor that is essential for proper platelet function and aggregation.

VWD is quite variable in its clinical course, severity, and laboratory abnormalities, even in the same patient. It is therefore possible for a patient with this disorder to go undetected throughout pregnancy until bleeding problems develop postpartum. The usual increase in factor VIII coagulant activity associated with pregnancy may also mask VWD. Only those patients with very low levels (<5 percent) before gestation fail to exhibit this rise.

When VWD is diagnosed before parturition, factor VIII activity should be monitored serially and transfusion with cryoprecipitate given to keep the factor VIII activity near term at 40 percent. If factor VIII levels are inadequate, the patient should be given one bag of cryoprecipitate per 10 kg body weight 24 hours before the planned induction of labor or cesarean delivery. This infusion will immediately restore the factor VIII activity level, but it will take 24 hours for the associated platelet defect to be corrected. If one suspects this disorder in a patient with unexplained postpartum hemorrhage, coagulation studies should be ordered and a hematologist consulted. However, since time is often limited, it would be prudent to notify the blood bank that cryoprecipitate may be needed emergently. In this situation, at least 6 units of cryoprecipitate are required, to be given every 12 hours for the next 3 to 5 days.[79]

Amniotic Fluid Embolism/Anaphylactoid Syndrome of Pregnancy

Amniotic fluid embolism (AFE) is a rare but frequently fatal obstetric emergency. The classic clinical presentation of the syndrome has been described by five signs that often occur in the following sequence: (1) respiratory distress, (2) cyanosis, (3) cardiovascular collapse, (4) hemorrhage, and (5) coma. Important new findings are the certainty of fetal distress accompanying this syndrome and the high incidence of maternal coagulopathy. In many cases, fetal distress is the initial presenting symptom, rapidly followed by maternal distress.

Only scanty information is available on which to base the treatment. Early airway control usually necessitating endotracheal intubation has been stressed in the few patients surviving the full-blown syndrome.[85,86] Once maximal ventilation and oxygenation have been achieved, attention should be paid to restoration of cardiovascular equilibrium. Recent data suggest that the hypotension results from myocardial failure and that efforts should be used to provide myocardial support.[83] These would include inotropic agents such as dopamine, as well as volume therapy.[87] If the patient survives the initial cardiorespiratory collapse, there is a high likelihood that coagulopathy will develop if it has not been previously clinically apparent. DIC results in the depletion of fibrinogen, platelets, and coagulation factors, especially factors V, VIII, and XIII. The fibrinolytic system is activated as well.[88] Supportive coagulation and volume therapy (blood, fresh frozen plasma, or cryoprecipitate) should be administered as soon as they are available.

The neonatal outcome in patients suffering this catastrophe is better than the maternal outcome. Among fetuses alive at the time of the event, nearly 80 percent will survive the delivery. Unfortunately, 50 percent of the survivors will incur neurologic damage.[82]

Disseminated Intravascular Coagulation

DIC results from the loss of local control of the body's clotting mechanisms. Normally, there are four essential elements in the maintenance of local control of the hemostatic system: vascular integrity, platelet function, the coagulation system, and clot lysis.[89] The body must maintain vascular integrity for the survival of the organism. To minimize blood loss, any break in this system initiates the entire hemostatic cascade.

During DIC, the body is forming and lysing fibrin clots throughout the circulation rather than in the ubiquitous localized physiologic process. Therefore, the loss of localization of the clotting process is the main defect in DIC. The lytic process may be activated as well but occurs only in response to the activation of the clotting system.

In obstetrics, DIC causing hemorrhage may involve any of the four mechanisms involved in the localization process. However, it is uncommon for DIC to be initiated by a failure of vascular integrity. Similarly, a platelet abnormality leading to diffuse platelet aggregation is an unlikely cause of hemorrhage in obstetrics.

Rather, activation of the coagulation cascade by the presence of large amounts of tissue phospholipid is a common stimulus for DIC in obstetrics. Such conditions include abruptio placenta, retained dead fetus, and AFE. These tissue phospholipids contribute to the utilization of large amounts of clotting factors and lead to a consumption coagulopathy. Once this widespread coagulation has taken place, the lytic process is called into action. The degradation of large amounts of fibrin produces fibrin split products, or fibrin degradation products. These factors have their own physiologic activity and, when present in large amounts, contribute to bleeding by inhibiting fibrin cross-linking and producing platelet dysfunction.

The platelet count and fibrinogen level are the most clinically useful tests in evaluating the patient with DIC. Because platelets and fibrinogen have a half-life of 4 to 5 days, they are not immediately replaced by the body's own mechanisms and will give an accurate reflection of ongoing consumption as well as the effectiveness of factor replacement.

The sine qua non of successful management of DIC is treatment of the initiating event. Once the cause has been located and treated, the process should resolve. However, depleted factors must be restored to permit orderly repair of injured tissues. Successful therapy involves the replacement of essential factors faster than the body is consuming them. These factors are platelets, coagulation factors derived from fresh frozen plasma or cryoprecipitate, and fibrinogen supplied by cryoprecipitate of fresh frozen plasma.

Key Points

- The rapid assessment of volume loss is dependent on basic vital signs and physical findings.
- Blood product use should be based on objectively determined needs rather than predetermined formulas.
- Platelet transfusions should be ABO and Rh specific.
- An action plan should be developed for situations in which massive blood transfusion is anticipated or arises unexpectedly.
- In patients with abruptio placenta, cesarean delivery usually should be performed for obstetric or fetal indications, not maternal coagulopathy.
- Expectant management of patients with abruptio placenta or placenta previa can be safely accomplished in many patients.
- In patients with postpartum hemorrhage secondary to uterine atony, dilute solutions of oxytocin (IV) and

15-methyl-$F_{2\alpha}$-prostaglandin (IM) should be the first two drugs administered.

- The maternal risks from heterologous blood transfusion have decreased significantly in the last 5 years.
- The clinical presentation of amniotic fluid embolism is more heterogeneous than previously described.
- When uterine inversion is encountered, the uterus should be replaced and reinverted before placental removal is attempted.
- Oxytocin should be given before placental expulsion and separation to minimize postpartum blood loss.

Cesarean Delivery

Richard Depp

Cesarean birth has become the most common hospital-based operative procedure in the United States, accounting for more than 23.5 percent of all live births in 1993.[1,2] The increase has been attributed to the liberalization of indications for "fetal distress," cephalopelvic disproportion/failure to progress, and breech presentations, as well as elective repeat cesarean delivery.[3] In many medical centers the present overall rate would be significantly higher were it not for a recent change in attitude facilitating acceptance of vaginal birth after cesarean birth.[4]

As the percentage of laboring patients presenting with a prior cesarean birth has increased, there has been an associated increase in more difficult repeat cesarean deliveries and complications, including a higher incidence of placenta previa, placenta accreta, symptomatic uterine rupture, hemorrhage, requirement for transfusion, and need for unplanned hysterectomy.

Cesarean Birth Rates

The reported rate of cesarean delivery in the United States increased in dramatic fashion from 4.5 percent in 1965 to 16.5 percent in 1980, finally peaking at 24.7 percent in 1988.[20] At least 90 percent of the increase between 1980 and 1985 was attributable to three factors: repeat cesarean deliveries (48 percent), dystocia (29 percent), and "fetal distress" (16 percent).

In 1979, the National Institutes of Health established a Task Force on Cesarean Childbirth.[24] The task force recommended that efforts be made to diminish the impact of elective repeat cesarean delivery and the diagnosis of "dystocia" because these indications were the two major causes of the increase in cesarean birth rates that were likely to be susceptible to reduction.

Benefits and Risks of Cesarean Birth

Maternal Mortality

Maternal mortality as a result of cesarean delivery fortunately is an infrequent occurrence, but the overall rate is estimated to be severalfold higher than that following vaginal delivery. Approximately 300 maternal deaths occur annually in the United States out of slightly more than 4 million deliveries of all types per year, an overall rate less than 10/100,000 live births. The cesarean delivery–associated maternal mortality can be estimated to range from 6.1[5] to 22/100,000 live births. Approximately one-third[42] to one-half[5] of maternal deaths of cesarean patients can be attributed directly to the cesarean procedure itself.[5,42]

Perinatal Morbidity and Mortality

The hypothesis that cesarean birth offers a major opportunity to improve perinatal outcome has, with few exceptions, not been proven.

Indications for Cesarean Delivery

Fetal Indications

Fetal indications for cesarean birth are in large part designed to minimize neonatal morbidity and possibly long-term consequences of profound intrapartum acidemia and/or delivery-related trauma or transmission of infection.[50,51] Accepted indications, often employed selectively, include the following: "significant" nonremediable and nonreassuring FHR patterns, especially when associated with progressive loss of variability; various categories of breech presentation at risk for head entrapment and/or cord prolapse; the VLBW fetus; and active genital herpes.

Maternal–Fetal Indications

Placental abnormalities such as placenta previa or placental abruption in which hemorrhage poses a significant risk to both mother and fetus, as well as labor "dystocia," are indications for which cesarean delivery offers a potential benefit to both mother and fetus.

Dystocia is a term used to describe indications for cesarean birth arising from one or more of the three "Ps": relatively large fetus (passenger), relatively small "passage" (pelvis), or relatively insufficient or inefficient uterine contractions (power). Included in "dystocia" are "failure to progress," relative "cephalopelvic disproportion" (CPD), and absolute CPD on the rare occasion when the latter can be diagnosed. Some include "failed inductions" under this designation. CPD is almost always a relative term; the CPD diagnosis is made only after application of a number of diagnostic and therapeutic measures, including oxytocin. In most instances it involves a normal-sized fetus.[55]

Maternal Indications

There are only a few indications for cesarean delivery that are solely maternal. They include mechanical obstructions of the vagina from large vulvovaginal condylomata, advanced lower genital tract malignancy, and placement of a permanent abdominal cerclage with a desire for future pregnancies.

Hospital Requirements for Cesarean Delivery

Any hospital that provides labor and delivery services should be equipped to perform an "emergency" cesarean delivery. A hospital offering obstetric services should provide the professional and institutional resources to respond to "acute obstetric emergencies" (i.e., a cesarean delivery) within 30 minutes, when indicated, from the time a decision is made until the procedure is begun.[58] The nursing, anesthesia, neonatal resuscitation, and obstetric personnel required must be either in the hospital or readily available. Should vaginal birth after cesarean–trial of labor (VBAC-TOL) be considered a physician who is capable of evaluating the labor and performing the cesarean should be "readily" available.[59]

Abdominal Incisions

Selection of Incision Type

The surgeon may choose either a vertical or a transverse skin incision (Fig. 11-1) when performing a cesarean delivery. The ultimate choice hinges on factors such as the urgency of the procedure, the presence of prior abdominal scars, and associated nonobstetric pathology, if any. The midline vertical, transverse Maylard, and transverse Pfannenstiel incisions are the three most commonly employed types.

In general, vertical incisions allow more rapid access to the lower uterine segment, have less blood loss, pro-

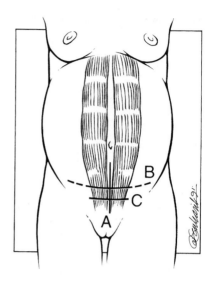

Fig. 11-1 The obstetrician most commonly uses one of three abdominal incisions: (A) midline, (B) Maylard, and (C) Pfannenstiel. Hatched lines indicate possible extension. (Modified from Baker C and Shingleton HM: Incisions. Clin Obstet Gynecol 31:701, 1988, with permission.)

vide greater feasibility for incisional extension around the umbilicus, and allow easier examination of the upper abdomen. In pregnancy, speed of entry through a midline vertical incision is facilitated by the common occurrence of diastasis of the rectus muscles.

Transverse incisions are somewhat more time consuming; the difference in time of entry between the two incision types is approximately 30 to 60 seconds in the hands of an experienced clinician. Transverse incisions are preferred cosmetically, are generally less painful, have been associated with a lower risk of subsequent herniation, and yet provide equal, if not better, visualization of the pelvis.

The Maylard incision (Fig. 11-1) differs from the Pfannenstiel incision in that it involves transverse incision of the anterior rectus sheath and the rectus muscles bilaterally.[82] The Pfannenstiel incision (Fig. 11-1) is a curvilinear incision that is best suited for the nonobese patient. The incision is generally made approximately 3 cm above the symphysis pubis within the pubic hairline at its midpoint. The determination of its lateral extension should, to some extent, be a function of the estimated fetal size.

Selection of Lower Uterine Incision

The most commonly employed uterine incisions (Fig. 11-2) are the low transverse incision and the low vertical incision. A low transverse (Kerr) incision is employed in more than 90 percent of all cesarean births. The low transverse incision has the following advantages over a vertical incision: less risk of entry into the upper uterine segment, greater ease of entry, less bladder dissection, less operative blood loss, less repair, easier reperitonealization, and less likelihood of adhesion formation to bowel or omentum should it not be possible to apply the bladder flap above the top of the incision line. Importantly, in subsequent pregnancies the obstetrician can feel more comfortable offering a VBAC trial because there is less likelihood of uterine rupture.[88]

In contrast, a vertical incision (classic or low vertical) may be advantageous if the patient has not been in labor and the lower uterus is narrow and poorly developed or if the fetus is other than in a cephalic presentation, particularly a back-down transverse lie or preterm breech. Should a transverse incision be performed under such circumstances, there is a greater likelihood of lateral extension of the incision into the vessels of the broad ligament. However, individualization is reasonable. Other possible indications for a vertical incision include leiomyomata obstructing exposure to the lower segment and structural uterine anomalies.

The classic uterine incision involves the upper active uterine segment. More commonly encountered complications associated with classic incisions include subsequent adhesion formation and greater risk of uterine rupture with later pregnancies.[90] Patients who have had a prior classic incision should consider an appropriately timed elective repeat cesarean birth because of the risk of uterine rupture even before labor has started.

Performing the Cesarean Delivery

Development of Bladder Flap

In most instances the uterus is dextrorotated such that the left round ligament may be visualized more anteriorly and closer to the midline than is the right. The uterovesical peritoneum (serosa) is grasped in the midline and undermined with Metzenbaum scissors inserted between the peritoneum and underlying myometrium to develop bluntly a retroperitoneal space bilaterally to the lateral margins of the lower uterine segment. The peritoneal reflection is then incised bilat-

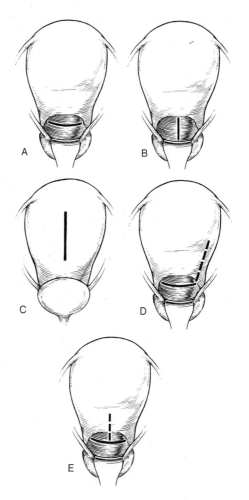

Fig. 11-2 Uterine incisions for cesarean delivery. (A) Low transverse incision. The bladder is retracted downward, and the incision is made in the lower uterine segment, curving gently upward. If the lower segment is poorly developed, the incision can also curve sharply upward at each end to avoid extending into the ascending branches of the uterine arteries. (B) Low vertical incision. The incision is made vertically in the lower uterine segment after reflecting the bladder, avoiding extension into the bladder below. If more room is needed, the incision can be extended upward into the upper uterine segment. (C) Classic incision. The incision is entirely within the upper uterine segment and can be at the level shown or in the fundus. (D) J incision. If more room is needed when an initial transverse incision has been made, either end of the incision can be extended upward into the upper uterine segment and parallel to the ascending branch of the uterine artery. (E) T incision. More room can be obtained in a transverse incision by an upward midline extension into the upper uterine segment.

erally in an upward direction and the vesicouterine fold is grasped with forceps and the bladder lifted anteriorly, allowing blunt separation of the bladder from the underlying lower uterine segment. Once the dissection is complete in the midline, the fingers may be carefully swept laterally in each direction to free the bladder more completely. After the bladder flap is adequately developed, a universal retractor or bladder blade is used to retract the bladder anteriorly and inferiorly to facilitate exposure of the intended incision site.

Low Transverse Cesarean Incision

The lower uterine segment incision (Fig. 11-2A) is begun 1 to 2 cm above the site of the original upper margin of the bladder. A small midline incision is first made with a scalpel through the lower uterine segment to the fetal membranes. Continuous suction should be available to facilitate visualization of the operative field. Care should be taken to avoid laceration of the fetus.

After suctioning, the incision may be extended laterally and slightly upward (cephalad) to the lateral margin of the lower uterine segment so as to maximize incisional length and avoid extension into the uterine vessels. Extension of the incision may be accomplished by either of two methods: (1) sharp dissection, taking care to avoid fetal fingers and toes; or (2) blunt dissection by spreading the incision with each index finger.

Low Vertical Incision

Should the fetus present as a breech or transverse lie, particularly back down, there is often advantage to a low vertical (Fig. 11-2B) uterine incision, particularly if the lower uterine segment is not well developed. The bladder is displaced downward to expose the lower uterine segment more inferiorly so that the low vertical incision will be less likely to extend into the upper segment. Once the anticipated site is exposed, an incision is made at the inferior margin of the lower segment and extended cephalad with either bandage scissors or a knife.

Although vertical cesarean incisions are traditionally categorized into low vertical and classic types, the performance of a true low vertical incision that does not enter the upper contractile portion of the uterus is actually uncommon. The clinical implication is that the low vertical incision poses considerably less risk in a subsequent VBAC trial than would be the case with a classic incision; the risk of rupture is nonetheless probably somewhat greater than that of a low transverse incision.

Classic Cesarean Incision

The initial incision (Fig. 11-2C) is made with a scalpel 1 to 2 cm above the bladder reflection. Once the fetus or membranes are visualized, the incision is extended cephalad with bandage scissors, the size of the incision varying with the estimated size of the fetus. The patient should also be advised of this occurrence and its importance to future pregnancies should a VBAC trial be considered.

Delivery of the Fetus

Upon completion of the incision, the retractors are removed and a hand is inserted into the uterine cavity to elevate and flex the fetal head through the uterine incision. Should the head be deeply wedged within the pelvis, it can be dislodged by an assistant applying upward pressure vaginally. Once the occiput presents into the incision, moderate fundal pressure may facilitate expulsion. On occasion the head may be delivered with shorthandled Simpson forceps or vacuum. Once delivery of the fetal head is completed, the nose and oropharynx are suctioned with a bulb syringe. If meconium is present, suction can be accomplished with continuous wall suction. When suctioning is complete, expulsion of the remainder of the newborn is facilitated by moderate uterine fundal pressure. The cord is then doubly clamped and cut, and the infant is transferred to the resuscitation team.

Operative Techniques for the Preterm Fetus

The uterine incision to be used for the delivery of the preterm fetus is best selected after entry into the maternal abdomen. At least 50 percent of cases will require a low vertical or classic incision for indications such as malpresentation or a poorly developed lower uterine segment.

Manual Versus "Spontaneous" Placental Expulsion

Following delivery of the fetus, 20 to 40 units of oxytocin can be administered in an isotonic crystalloid solution. Subsequent removal of the placenta is commonly done manually. Following its removal, the placenta should be inspected for missing cotyledons.

Repair of the Uterine Incision

Closure of the uterine incision may be aided by manual delivery of the uterine fundus through the abdominal incision.[97]

Delivery of the uterine fundus through the abdominal incision facilitates uterine massage and observation of uterine tone, as well as routine examination of the adnexa and tubal ligation. The fundus may be covered with a moistened laparotomy pad and the uterine incision inspected for obvious bleeding points, which are controlled with either Ring forceps or Allis clamps until suture closure can be accomplished. The uterine cavity may then be inspected and wiped clean with a dry laparotomy sponge to remove fetal membranes and placental fragments.

Midline placement of a ring forceps or Allis clamp may be used to elevate the lower portion of the low transverse uterine incision, facilitating visualization of the field and approximation of the incision. Allis clamps can be routinely placed at the angles of the incision to control bleeding and to identify the end of the incision.

Reapproximation of the lower uterine incision (Fig. 11-3) may be performed using zero or double-zero chromic suture or similar absorbable synthetic suture such as Vicryl, the second layer inverting the first. The initial suture should be placed lateral to the angle of a

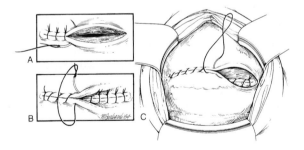

Fig. 11-3 Closure of low transverse incision. (A) The first layer can be either interrupted or continuous. A continuous locking suture is less desirable, despite its reputed hemostatic abilities, because it may interfere with incision vasculature and, hence, with healing and scar formation. (B) A second inverted layer created by using a continuous Lembert's or Cushing's stitch is customary but is really needed only when apposition is unsatisfactory after application of the first layer. Inclusion of too much tissue produces a bulky mass that may delay involution and interfere with healing. (C) The bladder peritoneum is reattached to the uterine peritoneum with fine suture.

transverse incision or inferior to the lower margin of a vertical incision. Subsequent stitches may be run in a continuous manner to the opposite end of the incision. The sutures may be placed through the entire myometrium. Reapproximation of the visceral (vesicouterine) and parietal peritoneum is not necessary.

Closure of a classic cesarean incision involving the more thickened upper segment most often will require a two-layer closure. Should the uterine wall be unusually thick, it may be necessary to use a third layer.

Abdominal Closure

Once the uterine incisional reapproximation is completed, the incision should once again be inspected for bleeding points, which can be individually ligated, coagulated, or controlled with figure-of-eight sutures. Before closing the abdomen, the uterus, fallopian tubes, and ovaries should be examined for unsuspected pathology. Some surgeons routinely examine the appendix. The pelvis and lower abdomen may be irrigated, especially if there is coexistent chorioamnionitis or if there has been heavy spillage of meconium outside the operative field. The operating team should confirm that the needle and sponge counts are correct.

There is no need to reapproximate the parietal peritoneum or rectus muscles. The rectus fascia may be closed with either interrupted or continuous (nonlocking) sutures. Suture choice is important in fascial healing. Chromic suture should be avoided when possible. Unlike their chromic counterparts, synthetic braided sutures maintain tensile strength throughout fascial healing. They are predictably broken down by hydrolysis. If the surgeon is dealing with a patient at risk for wound breakdown (from chronic corticosteroid therapy), delayed absorbable material such as PDS or polyglyconate (Maxon) or permanent material such as nylon or polypropylene (Prolene) may have merit.

Large bites using larger gauge suture material are less likely to transect tissue than are small bites with narrow-gauge suture material. Suture entry and exit sites should be well beyond the 1-cm inner zone of collagenolysis at the margin of the wound. Sutures should be placed at approximately 1-cm intervals approximately 1.5 cm from the incision line.

It is acceptable to use a running suture in closing the fascia in patients with a clean incision.[108] Should a patient be at high risk for wound dehiscence, it is preferable that the fascia not be closed with continuous suturing, particularly on a vertical incision. If the patient is at high risk for abdominal distention and wound

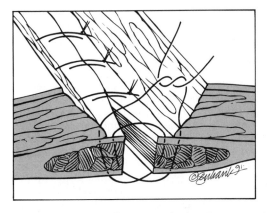

Fig. 11-4 Modification of far-near, near-far Smead-Jones suture. Suture passes deeply through lateral side of anterior rectus fascia and adjacent fat, crosses the midline of the incision to pick up the medial edge of the rectus fascia, then catches the near side of the opposite rectus sheath, and, finally, returns to the far margin of the opposite rectus sheath and subcutaneous fat. (Modified from American College of Obstetricians and Gynecologists: Prolog. *In* Gynecologic Oncology and Surgery. Washington, DC, American College of Obstetricians and Gynecologists, 1991, p 187, with permission.)

breakdown, a mass or Smead-Jones (Fig. 11-4) closure is preferable.

It is generally not necessary to reapproximate the subcutaneous tissue unless the patient is markedly obese, in which case subcutaneous closure may facilitate skin closure. Skin may be closed with staples or a subcuticular stitch. If staples are used, they may be replaced with Steristrips 3 or 4 days after surgery, depending on regional practice, to decrease scarring.

Intraoperative Complications

Uterine Lacerations

Lacerations of the lower uterine incision are more common when a low transverse incision is used in the presence of a macrosomic fetus or a noncephalic presentation. Fortunately, these lacerations are usually easily sutured as long as they only extend laterally to the margin of the myometrium or inferiorly into the vagina. Care must be taken to avoid ligation of the ureters.

Bladder Injuries

Should a bladder laceration be encountered, the bladder may be repaired with a two-layer closure with 2-0 or 3-0 chromic. After the bladder has been repaired, a catheter can be left in place for 7 to 10 days.[113,116]

Uterine Atony

Initial efforts to control uterine atony include uterine massage and medical therapy with (1) intravenous oxytocin, 20 to 40 units/L; (2) methergotamine, 0.2 mg, or ergonovine administered intramuscularly; or (3) 15-methylprostaglandin $F_{2\alpha}$ (Hemabate), which can be administered either intramuscularly or directly into the myometrium. Should the initial dose of prostaglandin be insufficient, successive dosages of 250 μg, up to a total dose of 1.0 to 1.5 mg, can be used. Should medical treatment fail, the surgeon must decide among ligation of the uterine arteries, hypogastric artery ligation, and hysterectomy. Uterine or hypogastric artery ligation may be the desirable approach should the patient be stable cardiovascularly and desirous of future pregnancy. Hypogastric artery ligation can be accomplished by ligation of the ascending branch, which can usually be found at the inferior and lateral extreme of the low transverse incision ascending retroperitoneally within the broad ligament (Fig. 11-5). Unfortunately, even hypogastric artery ligation is actually successful in less than one-half of the cases.[20] Should uterine or hypogastric artery ligation also fail to control the hemorrhage, it may be necessary to proceed to hysterectomy.

Placenta Accreta

Placenta accreta is now the most common indication for postcesarean hysterectomy. Approximately 25 percent of patients having a cesarean delivery for placenta previa in the presence of a prior uterine incision subsequently require cesarean hysterectomy for placenta accreta. The risk of placenta accreta appears to increase with the number of prior incisions. This obstetric complication may be increasing in frequency because of the increasing incidence of previous cesarean sections.[121,122]

If the accreta is focal and the patient desires future pregnancies, it may be possible to excise the site of trophoblastic invasion, oversewing bleeding areas with several figure-of-eight sutures. If that is not possible, hysterectomy should be initiated. A complete hysterectomy will usually be required because a placenta accreta commonly involves the lower uterine segment, and, in such cases, a supracervical hysterectomy will not be effective in controlling the bleeding.

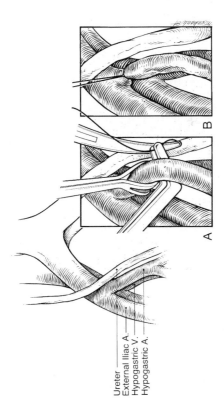

Ureter
External Iliac A.
Hypogastric V.
Hypogastric A.

Fig. 11-5 Hypogastric artery ligation. Approach to the hypogastric artery via the peritoneum, parallel and just lateral to the ovarian vessels, exposing the interior surface of the posterior layer of the broad ligament. The ureter will be found attached to the medial leaf of the broad ligament. The bifurcation of the common iliac artery into its external and internal (hypogastric) branches is exposed by blunt dissection of the loose overlying areolar tissues. Identification of these structures is essential. (A,B) To avoid traumatizing the underlying hypogastric vein, the hypogastric artery is elevated by means of a Babcock clamp before passing an angled clamp to catch a free tie. (Adapted from Breen J, Cregori CA, Kindzierski JA: Hemorrhage in Gynecologic Surgery. New York, Harper & Row, 1981, p 438, with permission.)

Preoperative and Intraoperative Fluid Guidelines

Extracellular (interstitial and intravascular) water constitutes approximately one-third of total body water and 20 percent of total body weight. Ordinary daily physiologic fluid needs approximate 2,000 to 2,500 ml. In the pregnant patient, daily physiologic fluid losses are estimated to be 1,000 ml in excess of urinary output and include urinary output (800 to 1,500 ml), insensible loss (800 ml) from both skin and lungs, and stool loss (200 ml). Insensible loss in the laboring patient can be considerably greater.

There will be little problem with dehydration if intravenous fluid intake has been maintained at 100 to 125 ml/hr. Should this not be the case, fluid losses can be estimated based on the average hourly need (100 to 125 ml) times the cumulative number of hours since the time of last fluid intake.

Fluid and Electrolyte Replacement

Should the patient be only mildly hypovolemic in the first 24 hours, normal isotonic saline or Ringer lactate solution in 5 percent dextrose is preferable to more hypotonic solutions because there is greater retention of fluids in the intravascular space providing volume expansion. In contrast, infusion of a 5 percent dextrose in water solution will result in distribution of fluid evenly throughout all water spaces, two-thirds being in the intracellular space.

Intraoperative Fluids

Intraoperative fluid requirements, apart from blood replacement, range from 500 to 1,000 ml/hr, up to a maximum of 3 L in a 4-hour interval under ordinary surgical conditions.

Postoperative Complications

Maternal Morbidity and Mortality

Even when morbidity and mortality arising from the indication leading to cesarean delivery have been excluded, maternal morbidity and mortality remain severalfold higher for cesarean delivery than for vaginal delivery.[5,42,132] In a review of approximately 400,000 cesarean births performed between 1965 and 1978, maternal death occurred in 1/1,635 (mortality rate was

6.1/100,000) procedures; approximately one-half of the deaths were attributable to the procedure.[5,42]

Major sources of morbidity and associated mortality relate to complications of maternal sepsis, anesthesia, and thromboembolic disease and its complications.

Endomyometritis and Wound Infection

For a discussion of endomyometritis and wound infection, see Chapter 22.

Fascial Dehiscence

Dehiscence of a wound through the fascia is infrequent, occurring in approximately 5 percent of wound infections.[145] Dehiscence is suggested by the presence of a large amount of discharge from the wound. If loops of small bowel protrude through the incision, the small bowel should be immediately covered with wet sterile dressings. The wound should be opened and inspected and emergency closure performed in the operating room under sterile conditions. If a dehiscence is confirmed, the wound should be cleansed, debrided, and closed with either Smead-Jones or retention sutures (Fig. 11-4).

Urinary Complications

Urinary tract infections are second to endomyometritis as a cause of postcesarean febrile morbidity. The reported incidence varies from as low as 2 percent to as high as 16 percent.[161] Attention to detail in terms of proper preparation and insertion of the catheter and the use of a closed drainage system have decreased this risk.

Gastrointestinal Complications

Most patients undergoing cesarean delivery have little if any gastrointestinal problems postoperatively. However, anesthesia and narcotics employed to treat postoperative pain may contribute to bowel dysfunction. As a result, an occasional patient may have postoperative nausea or mild transient abdominal distention in the first 24 hours.

Ileus should be suspected if prolonged nausea or vomiting together with signs such as abdominal distention, absence of bowel sounds, and failure to pass flatus are persistent. Distended loops of bowel with or without air–fluid levels on x-ray will provide confirmatory evidence. In most instances simply withholding oral intake, providing adequate fluid replacement, and being observant are sufficient. If the ileus is persistent, nasogastric suction may be required.

Thromboembolic Disorders

The risk of deep venous thrombophlebitis (DVT) after cesarean delivery is approximately three to five times greater than after vaginal delivery.[165] Compounding risk factors include obesity, inability to ambulate, advanced maternal age, and higher parity. Should the DVT go untreated, approximately 15 to 25 percent of patients will develop pulmonary emboli, and 15 percent will sustain a fatal pulmonary embolus (PE). However, if recognized early and treated appropriately, the risks of PE and death are reduced to 4.5 and 0.7 percent, respectively.[164,166]

Classic symptoms for DVT include unilateral leg pain, tenderness, and swelling. A 2-cm difference in leg circumference between the affected and normal limbs is generally required for diagnosis. Other clinical signs include edema, a palpable cord, and a change in limb color. A positive Homan sign (calf pain on passive dorsiflexion of the foot) suggests DVT.

Unfortunately, the first sign of DVT may be the occurrence of a PE, which can present with symptoms of tachypnea (90 percent), dyspnea (80 percent), pleuritic chest pain with or without splinting (more than 70 percent), apprehension (approximately 60 percent), tachycardia (40 percent), and cough (more than 50 percent).[167,168] Other findings include atelectatic rales, a friction rub, accentuated second heart sound, and a gallop. Patient evaluation is complicated in the postcesarean delivery patient, since splinting from incisional pain and tachypnea are not unusual findings. Doppler studies have a sensitivity of 90 percent for popliteal, femoral, or iliac thromboses but only 50 percent for calf involvement because of abundant collateral vessels. Impedance plethysmography (IPG) is sensitive in approximately 95 percent of proximal thromboses, but is not as effective as Doppler for pelvic vessel thrombosis and will generally identify most cases, especially above the calves. Should Doppler and IPG be inconclusive, ascending venography, the most accurate of the three tests, should be performed. IPG can be used as a first-line test postpartum in the nonlactating mother. Should PE be suspected, a baseline arterial blood gas, chest x-ray, and electrocardiogram, as well as prothrombin time and partial thromboplastin time, should be obtained. Oxygen therapy should also be administered. Once the diagnosis has been established, heparin therapy should be started (see Ch. 21).

Septic Pelvic Thrombophlebitis

For a discussion of septic pelvic thrombophlebitis, see Chapter 22.

Postoperative Management

Postoperative Analgesia

Analgesia should be provided in a dose and at a frequency that will neither obtund nor cause respiratory depression and yet allow the patient (1) to avoid the consequences of extremes in analgesic blood levels resulting in unnecessary pain and (2) to cooperate with normal postoperative management. The patient receiving inadequate analgesia may, in an effort to protect her wound, maintain a shallow breathing pattern without deep breaths and, hence, develop atelectasis.[170]

Commonly employed analgesics include meperidine (50 to 75 mg) and morphine (10 mg, depending on maternal size), administered intravenously or intramuscularly every 3 to 4 hours. Intrathecal or epidural narcotic administration employed with agents such as morphine can also be used for postoperative anesthesia, which may last as long as 30 hours following delivery, providing an advantage to a patient who has undergone a regional block.[171]

Ambulation

Early ambulation is important in reinstitution of inflation of the most dependent alveoli and the prevention of pulmonary complications, particularly in the patient who has had general anesthesia. Early ambulation also promotes the return of normal urinary and bowel activity. Under most circumstances, the uncomplicated patient can be allowed to sit up within 8 to 12 hours following the procedure, even after epidural anesthesia. The patient generally can ambulate within the first day after surgery and by the second day can shower without fear of injury to the incision.

Oral Intake

Active bowel sounds are commonly not observed until the second postoperative day. Nonetheless, in most instances the patient will easily tolerate oral fluids the day after surgery. Only rarely, when the patient has been septic or there has been extensive intra-abdominal manipulation, will there be a need to withhold oral fluids, even though the patient may have diminished bowel sounds and not pass gas. Most clinicians feel comfortable in providing clear liquids and ice chips with only a small amount of liquid as soon as nausea subsides to relieve complaints of a dry mouth. The progression of the diet also varies according to clinician. Some advance the patient rapidly to a regular diet, whereas others institute a progression to a full liquid diet by 48 hours, awaiting the return of normal bowel sounds and passage of flatus to indicate return of colonic function. Few wait beyond the third postoperative day to institute a regular diet.

Bladder Management

The urinary catheter is ordinarily removed within 12 to 24 hours following surgery unless there have been intraoperative complications.

Postoperative Wound Care

The incision is generally covered for the first day with a light dressing, until the wound is sealed. The dressing is removed after the first postoperative day.

Laboratory Studies

Blood loss arising from an uncomplicated cesarean delivery is approximately 1,000 ml.[172] As a consequence of blood loss as well as intra- and postoperative hydration, the postoperative hematocrit may be expected to drop by approximately 2 to 3 percentage points during the initial 2 days following surgery, independent of hydration status.

Postoperative Fluids

The normal postpartum period is generally characterized by mobilization of the physiologic accumulation of fluid during pregnancy. As a consequence, large volumes of intravenous fluids are seldom required after cesarean delivery. In the low-risk patient, fluid replacement needs during a 24-hour interval are generally only 1,000 ml above urinary output. Three liters of a salt-containing solution will thus generally suffice during the first 24 hours unless urinary output falls below 30 ml/hr. Under certain circumstances there may be increased requirements for fluids: following prolonged labor, febrile illness, vomiting and diarrhea, or even prior use of diuretics or salt restriction. More complex patients may have additional needs. Potassium is ordinarily not required during the first 24 hours by uncomplicated patients because of intracellular potassium release from cell destruction. After the first 24 hours, intravenous fluid replacement with 5 percent dextrose in 0.45 percent sodium chloride is commonly employed, unless volume expansion is an issue. If it is anticipated that the patient will require prolonged intravenous fluids, potassium may be administered as 60 to 80 mEq/day. Should the patient be oliguric, potassium is generally not given until the patient has normal urinary output.

Average Length of Stay

Depending on postoperative morbidity/complications and availability of care at home, hospital discharge may occur as early as the second to fifth postoperative day.

Discharge Management

The mother's activities at home for the first week should be limited to personal care and to care of the newborn. By the third to fourth week, the patient can generally resume most activities at home. The length of hospitalization associated with cesarean birth, like that associated with vaginal delivery, has declined dramatically.[1,23]

Reducing the Current Cesarean Birth Rate

Table 11-1 summarizes potential clinical strategies to reduce the current cesarean rate. The strategy most likely to have a significant impact is one that strongly encourages VBAC-TOL.

Table 11-1   Potential Approaches to Reduce Cesarean Births

Vaginal birth after cesarean trial of labor (VBAC-TOL)

Dystocia/CPD/FTP
  Disciplined approach to labor management
  Active management of labor

Breech presentation/transverse lie
  External version
  Selective vaginal delivery of breech

Fetal hypoxia/acidosis
  Develop more predictive markers for acidosis
  Fetal capillary blood gases for reassurance
  Fetal stimulation for reassurance

Data from Taffel SM, Placek PJ, Moien M, Kosary CL: 1989 US cesarean section rate steadies—VBAC rises to nearly one in five. Birth 18:73, 1991, with permission.

Vaginal Birth After Cesarean Birth

Benefits and Risks of VBAC-TOL

VBAC-TOL is successful in 60 to 80 percent of acceptable candidates.[194-197] If applied to all patients presenting with a prior cesarean procedure (8.2 to 8.5 percent), there is a potential to increase the rate of overall vaginal delivery by approximately 5 percent. Furthermore, there is evidence VBAC-TOL reduces the incidence of postpartum infection, the need for postpartum transfusion, and maternal length of stay; as a result, there is significant cost savings.

One of the first questions to be raised by a patient when considering a VBAC-TOL is, what is the likelihood for a successful vaginal birth according to the indication for the prior cesarean birth? Obstetric history regarding preexisting conditions is helpful in the prediction of VBAC success. Women who have previously given birth vaginally or women whose prior cesarean delivery was for nonrecurring conditions are more likely to succeed.[196,218,220]

The likely success of a VBAC trial will depend to some degree on whether the indication for the prior cesarean is a recurring or nonrecurring one. Patients with a nonrecurring indication (breech presentation, so-called fetal distress–nonreassuring FHR pattern, and conditions such as placenta previa, abruption, or maternal hemorrhage) are more likely (82 to 86 percent) to achieve success than is the patient who has undergone a prior cesarean for a potentially recurring condition (70 percent) such as dystocia (failure to progress and/or CPD), approximating the success rate for the so-called low-risk nulliparous patient.[208,218,225]

Recent American College of Obstetricians and Gynecologists (ACOG) guidelines do not specify a maximum number of prior cesarean births as a criterion for VBAC.[58,214] The safety of VBAC-TOL in women having had two or more cesareans is now well established; they can be managed in a manner similar to that for patients with only one prior incision, with few complications.[4,193,201,208-211,213,214,220,229] Women who have had more than one prior cesarean before a trial of labor are 30 percent less likely to be successful. Although uterine rupture is more likely in this group, there is no appreciable increase in perinatal mortality.

Considerations in Management of VBAC-TOL

Management of the patient undergoing a VBAC-TOL is similar to that of patients attempting to achieve a vaginal delivery.[234] As a consequence, it is appropriate to use oxytocin and epidural anesthesia as one would in other labors. Potential problems such as suspected fetal macrosomia will be encountered, and management will be no different from that in normal labor. The major difference will arise from some heightening of concern for uterine dehiscence and/or rupture. Uterine dehiscence is generally defined as asymptomatic separation of the uterine scar with an intact uterine serosa remaining, whereas in, uterine rapture, the peritoneal and uterine cavities are not separated. Patients with uterine rupture require acute intervention, while those with uterine dehiscence usually do not. Dehiscence is uncommon (2 percent or less) and rupture is relatively rare (less than 1 percent). Routine uterine exploration of the lower uterine segment following a successful VBAC is no longer considered necessary.

Prior Low Vertical Incision

A trial of labor in a patient with a prior low vertical scar is controversial.

Prior Classic Incision

It is likely that we will continue on occasion to be confronted with patients who have had a prior classic incision. A trial of labor should be strongly discouraged in such cases.[58] Patients with a prior classic incision have an associated 12 percent risk of symptomatic uterine rupture during labor.[212,236] Since approximately one-third of ruptures occur prior to labor, it is currently recommended that women who have a prior classic cesarean delivery be delivered by repeat cesarean procedure upon achieving fetal pulmonary maturity prior to the onset of labor. Such patients should be warned of the hazards of an unintended labor and the signs of possible uterine rupture.[237]

Known Versus Unknown Incision Type

In an era when prior medical records are not always readily available, it is reassuring that the overall risk of dehiscence or rupture is low even among women undergoing a trial of labor with an unknown prior cesarean incision type. Overall, 90 to 95 percent of women with unknown scars will have had a low transverse incision.[202]

Fetal Monitoring

In most cases a significant alteration in FHR pattern is the presenting sign of uterine rupture; on occasion, an alteration (increased frequency and/or intensity) in uterine contraction pattern (if monitored externally) or a loss of intrauterine pressure (if monitored with an internal pressure catheter) is the presenting sign.[199] Unfortunately, use of intrauterine pressure catheters does not reliably assist in the diagnosis of rupture.[248] The FHR tracing may reveal a sudden prolonged deceleration or repetitive "significant" variable decelerations. It is prudent to proceed more rapidly to cesarean delivery under such circumstances than would be the case in the absence of a prior uterine incision.

Multiple Gestation and Abnormal Fetal Lie

There are no data to contraindicate a VBAC trial in a twin gestation or in a frank breech presentation if the obstetrician is comfortable with selective vaginal breech delivery.

Perinatal Morbidity and Mortality

The perinatal risk for patients considering VBAC is no higher than that for patients delivering by elective repeat cesarean birth.[195,197,208,212,260,271] The overall uncorrected perinatal death rate arising from more than 5,500 women presenting with a prior cesarean birth was 1.4 percent (14/1,000) in a meta-analysis of 10 studies.[212]

Intrapartum fetal deaths arising in the subset of patients who experience dehiscence of a low transverse uterine incision are uncommon. Recent data suggest that maternal and perinatal outcomes are generally good following uterine rupture.

Timing of Elective Repeat Cesarean Delivery

Should the patient refuse a VBAC-TOL or have a recurring indication for cesarean delivery, the clinician has four possible options to determine when elective cesarean delivery should occur. According to the ACOG, fetal maturity may be assumed and amniocentesis need not be performed if the criteria of one of the six options listed in Table 11-2 are met.[237,273] Options 3 and 4 do not preclude use of menstrual dating, particularly if one of these options confirms menstrual dates in a patient with normal menstrual cycles and no immediately recent use of oral contraceptives. Ultrasound is considered confirmatory if there is agreement between menstrual gestational age and crown–rump age at 6 to 12 weeks (option 3) or by the average gestational age de-

Table 11-2 Fetal Maturity Assessment Prior to Elective Repeat Cesarean Delivery

Option 1 (FHR)	One or more of the following is present for the stated duration: For 20 weeks: FHR by nonelectronic fetoscope For 30 weeks: FHR by Doppler
Option 2 (hCG)	For 36 weeks: positive serum or urine pregnancy test
Option 3[a] (Ultrasound)	At 6–12 week's gestation: Ultrasound crown-rump length supports gestational age of ≥39 weeks
Option 4[a] (Ultrasound)	At 12–20 weeks multiple ultrasound measures confirm gestational age of ≥39 weeks as determined by clinical history and physical examination
Option 5	Await spontaneous onset of labor
Option 6	Fetal pulmonary maturity documented by amniotic fluid surfactant assessment

[a]Does not preclude use of menstrual age with agreement within 7 days (option 3) or 10 days (option 4).

termined by multiple measurements at 12 to 20 weeks (option 4).

Peripartum Hysterectomy

Peripartum or obstetric hysterectomy is the surgical removal of the uterus at the time of a planned or unplanned cesarean delivery or in the immediate postpartum period.

Unplanned Emergency Indications

Most peripartum hysterectomies are unplanned and follow cesarean delivery.[120] Most are performed after more conservative efforts to control bleeding have been unsuccessful. Although hysterectomy may be the ultimate remedy for control of obstetric hemorrhage, conservative measures remain the primary approach; hysterectomy is reserved for circumstances in which conservative measures either fail or are not applicable, as would often be the case with abnormal placentation.[284]

Prior cesarean delivery increases the risk for subsequent placenta previa, placenta accreta, and symptomatic uterine rupture, each of which increases the likelihood of need for an emergency hysterectomy.[284,285] The adverse impact of placenta previa as a risk factor for unplanned hysterectomy in patients with a prior cesarean is well established.[86,286] Placenta accreta has been reported in 25 percent of cases of placenta previa and a single prior cesarean delivery and 50 percent of cases with two prior cesarean deliveries.

Maternal morbidity and mortality associated with peripartum hysterectomy is not simply the product of the procedure itself. Maternal mortality and morbidity will in large part depend on whether (1) the procedure is a planned/scheduled or an unplanned/emergency procedure, (2) the patient was previously in labor and had significant risk factors for infection, or (3) the patient had coincidental pregnancy-related complications. Unplanned hysterectomies have a greater risk for maternal mortality than planned procedures, since they are commonly performed in response to life-threatening hemorrhage with independent morbidity and mortality consequences.

Postpartum Sterilization

Tubal ligation in the postpartum period offers several major advantages. The patient is often subjected to only one anesthesia (epidural) for labor and delivery and the ligation process. Should that not be possible, there is still the benefit of an abbreviated hospitalization at a time when maternal responsibilities are less than they will be just weeks later. Furthermore, additional preoperative work-up is not necessary for a second procedure. Increased tissue vascularity and edema pose a theoretical risk of more difficult hemostasis and could contribute to a higher failure rate compared with interval procedures. However, a recent multicenter study of more than 10,000 women who had tubal sterilizations and were followed for 8 to 14 years revealed that postpartum partial salpingectomy and interval unipolar coagulation had the lowest rates of sterilization failure (7.5/1,000 procedures).

A variety of methods of sterilization are available either at the time of cesarean delivery or during the postpartum period. The tubes can be occluded by banding, clipping, resection, or fulguration. In selecting a method for tubal sterilization, consideration should be given to two factors, should the patient later desire reversal: effectiveness relative to later sterility and reversibility. A rational decision for tubal occlusion may later be proven wrong, particularly should sterilization be performed at a young age. Patients are also more likely to regret sterilization procedures performed in association with the stress of pregnancy than considered interval procedures.

From the point of view of later reversibility, the use of clips is probably the best method of sterilization, because clips produce the least damage. Occlusion within the tubal isthmus is desirable should later reanastomosis be attempted, because an isthmic–isthmic reapproximation is most likely to succeed. Salpingectomy, cornual resection, extensive fulguration, and fimbriectomy limit the choices for those patients who later seek restoration of fertility. The timing of the operation relative to the time of birth has little impact. In some instances when there is some concern regarding potential newborn outcome, the procedure may be best postponed.

Postoperative complications are infrequent. Hemorrhage is the most commonly encountered problem. Although patient discomfort associated with the procedure may increase the length of hospitalization by 1 day or more, significant discomfort is seldom encountered after 1 or 2 weeks.

Abdominal Incision

In the early puerperium the tubes are easily isolated through a small abdominal incision, since the uterus is enlarged and the abdominal wall is lax. A small, periumbilical incision offers the most cosmetic result and least postpartum discomfort. However, a small 3- to 4-cm midline vertical or transverse incision at the level of the fundus is often used. The only disadvantage to such a small incision is one of limited exposure that may increase the risk of inadvertent ligation of a round ligament rather than a tube. If the operation is delayed, or if the patient has had previous adnexal surgery and adhesions are anticipated, a transverse or midline vertical incision may be desirable.

Techniques

Pomeroy Technique

The Pomeroy technique is the most popular means of postpartum sterilization (Fig. 11-6) because of its simplicity and effectiveness. As originally described, a small

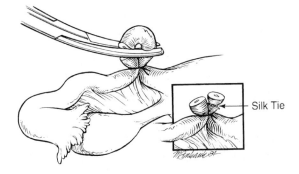

Silk Tie

Fig. 11-6 Pomeroy sterilization. A knuckle of tube is ligated with absorbable suture, and a small segment is being excised. Note that the ligation is performed at a site that will favor reanastomosis, should that become desirable. Some surgeons place an extra tie of nonabsorbable suture around the proximal stump as added protection against recanalization.

knuckle of each tube is picked up approximately 1 inch from its cornual insertion and ligated with a single loop of absorbable suture (plain catgut). A small section of the isolated tubal segment is then resected and submitted to the pathologist to document that the tubal lumina have been interrupted. Presumably the remaining segments of tube will separate when the suture is absorbed, leaving a gap between the proximal and distal ends. A modification wherein the proximal ends of each resected tube are also ligated with a nonabsorbable suture is employed by some in an attempt to reduce the likelihood of recanalization of the proximal tubal lumen. The modified operation has a failure rate of approximately 1/500.

Uchida Technique

Some clinicians advocate the Uchida technique because of its low failure rate and the theoretically reduced risk of associated disturbance of ovarian blood supply. This technique is more complicated than the Pomeroy technique and requires the surgeon to separate the muscular portion of the tube from its serosal cover, which is then cut and ligated. The proximal segment is then buried in the leaves of the broad ligament, leaving the distal segment exteriorized (Fig. 11-7).

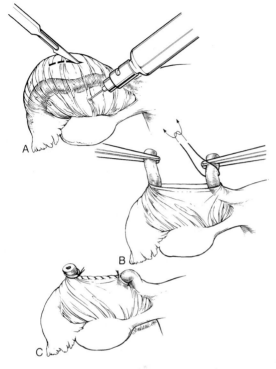

Fig. 11-7 Uchida sterilization. The leaves of the broad ligament and peritubal peritoneum are infiltrated with saline so that the tube can be easily isolated from these structures, divided, and ligated. The broad ligament is then closed, burying the proximal stump between the leaves and including the distal stump in the line of closure.

Irving Technique

Although the Irving operation is slightly more complicated than other techniques, it may have the lowest failure rate. After transecting and ligating the cut ends of the tubes, a tunnel is created by blunt dissection into the adjacent uterine wall at the insertion of the round ligament, a less vascular area. The proximal segment of each tube is carried into the depth of the tunnel by means of a traction suture and transfixed there by an interrupted suture (Fig. 11-8). The cut end of each distal segment is then buried between the leaves of the broad ligament or may be left exposed in the modified Irving procedure.

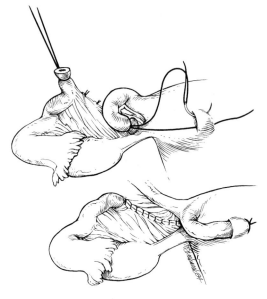

Fig. 11-8 Irving sterilization. The tube is transected 3 to 4 cm from its insertion, and a short tunnel is created by means of a sharp-nosed hemostat in either the anterior or posterior uterine wall. The cut end of the tube can then be buried in the tunnel and, if necessary, further secured by an interrupted suture at the opening of the tunnel. The distal cut end is buried between the leaves of the broad ligament.

Counseling for Tubal Ligation

Patient counseling may include a discussion of the risk of failure, alternative methods of contraception including male sterilization, and procedural complications. Some clinicians include a review of the variety of tubal techniques available, as well as the possibility of adverse long-term effects on ovarian function and sexual interest. A sufficient interval should be allowed following the provision of consent to satisfy the legal requirements of various jurisdictions and, of equal importance, to permit the patient and her family to reconsider their decision. Despite attempts to provide detailed information, a number of patients will later desire reversal of the procedure. Because reversal is not always possible, tubal sterilization should only be recommended as a permanent procedure.

Acute Abdomen in Pregnancy

Appendicitis

Appendicitis is the most common acute surgical condition of pregnancy, with an incidence of 1/2,000 births. It is encountered with relatively the same frequency in every trimester as well as the puerperium. The diagnosis is reputed to be more difficult and likely to be delayed because the clinical picture tends to be masked by the symptoms and physical changes of pregnancy.[302] Some of the factors confusing the diagnosis are the nausea, vomiting, and abdominal discomfort of early pregnancy, upward displacement of the appendix by the expanding uterus, laxity of the abdominal wall, round ligament spasm, physiologic leukocytosis, and elevated sedimentation rate.

Diagnosis

Despite these confusing factors, the signs and symptoms of appendicitis in pregnancy are similar to those in the nonpregnant patient. The initial visceral pain is typically gradual in onset, often colicky (denoting an element of obstruction), and usually referred to the epigastrium or periumbilical area. During the first trimester, the pain localizes in the right lower quadrant as the overlying parietal peritoneum becomes involved. Past the fourth month, the appendix has been displaced upward and laterally. At 6 months, the point of maximal thickness is above the iliac crest, and at 8 months it rises to the level of the right costal margin.[303] Usually, anorexia accompanied by nausea and vomiting begin 1 to 2 hours after the onset of pain. Right lateral rectal tenderness is commonly found, and about one-half of the patients will have abdominal muscle spasm or guarding. Moving the uterus tends to intensify pain in the appendiceal area. By placing the patient on her left side, the clinician can sometimes differentiate pain of uterine origin. If the uterus is the source of the pain, abdominal wall tenderness will diminish as the uterus falls away from the examining fingers.

The patient's temperature can be normal but is usually moderately elevated, up to 101°F. Because of the physiologic leukocytosis of pregnancy, significant alterations of the white blood cell count depend on finding either a rising count over a period of observation or an increasing left shift. Urinalysis is usually negative unless the inflamed appendix is retroperitoneal and lying in close proximity to the right ureter. X-ray studies are rarely helpful, but ultrasound or a computed tomography scan may be valuable.

If the appendix ruptures, either peritonitis follows or the uterus forms the median wall of a localized abscess. In either case, abortion or labor is the usual consequence. As the uterus is emptied, a walled-off abscess tends to rupture, producing generalized peritonitis. For these reasons, early diagnosis and operation in all suspicious cases is particularly important. Diagnostic laparoscopy in doubtful cases encountered during early pregnancy may help to avoid an unnecessary laparotomy.

The differential diagnosis includes pyelonephritis, round ligament pain, a placental accident, torsion of an ovarian cyst, degenerating myomata, pancreatitis, and cholecystitis. Appendicitis can also be confused with early labor and postpartum endomyometritis.

Management

A transverse muscle-splitting incision over the point of maximum tenderness is usually adequate and can easily be extended if necessary. If the appendix is unruptured, the incision is closed without drainage. Neither antibiotics nor tocolytic agents are necessary, and abortion and premature labor are unlikely.

When the appendix is ruptured, the patient should receive multiple antibiotic therapy, including an agent effective against anaerobic organisms. Suction drainage through a flank incision will be needed for an abscess or generalized peritonitis. A cesarean section should be avoided unless a compelling obstetric indication exists. The incision should be separately drained, or the skin should be left open for secondary closure.

Trauma

Trauma is the most common nonobstetric cause of maternal death as well as the leading cause of death into the mid-40s age range.[305] Most reported trauma in pregnancy is blunt trauma secondary to automobile accidents, falls, or penetrating injuries. Uterine injury as a result of external trauma is highly unlikely in early pregnancy; however, vulnerability increases as the uterus becomes an abdominal organ in later pregnancy. The fetus is relatively well protected by its amniotic fluid cushion, but placental separation can occur as a result of a direct blow or hypovolemic shock. Uterine rupture is a less likely consequence of a direct blow or seat belt compression. Distortion of the uterus produced by the sudden compression of a waist-type seat belt can produce placental separation. Adverse fetal outcome is closely linked to placental abruption or direct fetal injury. Abruption may occur in up to 50 percent of patients presenting with major injuries.[306] In the absence of uteroplacental insufficiency the reported newborn outcome is not adversely affected.[307]

Fetal assessment with continuous FHR and uterine contraction monitoring is employed for at least 4 hours after maternal stabilization. If uterine contractions or vaginal bleeding are observed, monitoring should be continued for 24 hours.

Consideration should be given to administration of Rh-negative blood until the Rh type is known. If the patient is later determined to be Rh negative, mini-dose Rh immunoglobulin is appropriate up to 12 to 13 weeks' gestation, whereas 300 μg or more are necessary at more than 13 weeks. Should Kleihauer-Betke testing support a large fetal–maternal blood, a larger dose of Rh immunoglobulin may be required based on the estimated volume of the bleed.[311]

Key Points

- Even when morbidity and mortality arising from the indications leading to cesarean delivery are excluded, maternal morbidity and mortality remain many times higher for cesarean delivery than for vaginal delivery.
- As the percentage of laboring patients presenting with prior cesarean births has increased, there have been associated increases in more difficult repeat cesarean deliveries and complications, including a higher incidence of placenta previa, placenta accreta, symptomatic uterine rupture, hemorrhage, requirement for transfusion, and need for unplanned hysterectomy.
- The reported incidence of maternal mortality following cesarean delivery is estimated to range from 6.1 to 22/100,000 live births. Approximately one-third to one-half of maternal deaths can be attributed directly to the cesarean procedure itself.
- If the patient is massively obese, it may be better to use an incision directly over the lower uterine segment that does not involve the underside of the panniculus, an area that is more heavily colonized with bacteria and that is difficult to prepare surgically, to keep dry, and to inspect in the postoperative period.
- The physician contemplating a cesarean delivery for placenta previa, particularly a repeat procedure, should consider the possibility of hysterectomy. The reported incidence of placenta accreta (1/2,500 deliv-

eries) increases to approximately 4 percent in patients with a placenta previa and may approach 25 percent in patients with a prior cesarean birth.

- Although cesarean delivery is often elected to minimize trauma to the preterm breech fetus, the actual delivery mechanism via the cesarean incision is essentially identical to that of the vaginal route. Should head entrapment be encountered, the first action should be to extend the abdominal incision and to enlarge the uterine incision.

- Most patients with a prior cesarean birth are candidates for VBAC. The only established contraindication is a prior classic incision. VBAC reduces the incidence of postpartum infection, the need for postpartum transfusion, and maternal length of stay and, as a result, offers the potential to generate significant cost savings.

- VBAC trial candidates are no more likely to require a cesarean delivery than a population of women with no prior cesarean deliveries. VBAC-TOL is successful in 60 to 80 percent of acceptable candidates.

SECTION 3
Postpartum Care

The Neonate

Adam A. Rosenberg

The first 4 weeks of an infant's life, the neonatal period, are marked by the highest mortality rate in all of childhood. The greatest risk occurs during the first several days after birth. Critical to survival during this period is the infant's ability to adapt successfully to extrauterine life. During the early hours after birth, the newborn must assume responsibility for thermoregulation, metabolic homeostasis, and respiratory gas exchange, as well as undergo the conversion from fetal to postnatal circulatory pathways. Successful accomplishment of this process starts with proper management in the delivery room.

Delivery Room Management of the Newborn

When an asphyxiated infant is expected, a resuscitation team should be in the delivery room. The team should have at least two persons, one to manage the airway and one to monitor heart rate and provide whatever assistance is needed. Table 12-1 lists equipment necessary.

Steps in the resuscitation process[88] are as follows (Fig. 12-1):

1. Dry the infant well and place under the radiant heat source.
2. Gently suction the oropharynx and nose.
3. Assess the infant's condition (Table 12-2). The best criteria to assess are the infant's respiratory effort (apneic, gasping, regular) and heart rate (more or less than 100). A depressed heart rate indicative of hypoxic myocardial depression is the single most reliable indicator of the need for resuscitation.[87,89]

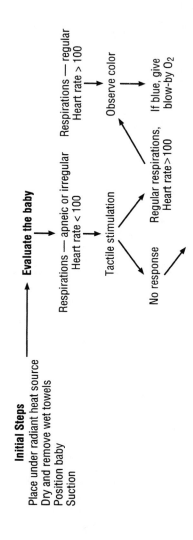

Initial Steps
Place under radiant heat source
Dry and remove wet towels
Position baby
Suction

Evaluate the baby

Respirations — apneic or irregular
Heart rate < 100

Respirations — regular
Heart rate > 100

Tactile stimulation

Observe color

If blue, give
blow-by O₂

Regular respirations,
Heart rate > 100

No response

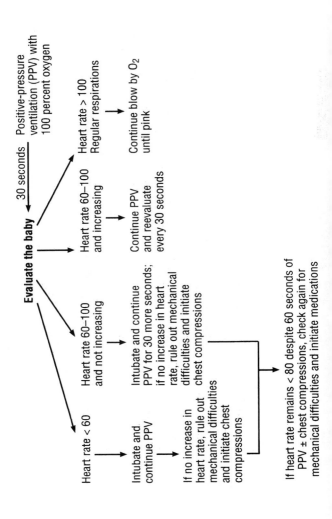

Positive-pressure ventilation (PPV) with 100 percent oxygen

Evaluate the baby — 30 seconds

Heart rate > 100
Regular respirations
→ Continue blow by O₂ until pink

Heart rate 60–100 and increasing
→ Continue PPV and reevaluate every 30 seconds

Heart rate 60–100 and not increasing
→ Intubate and continue PPV for 30 more seconds; if no increase in heart rate, rule out mechanical difficulties and initiate chest compressions

Heart rate < 60
→ Intubate and continue PPV
If no increase in heart rate, rule out mechanical difficulties and initiate chest compressions

If heart rate remains < 80 despite 60 seconds of PPV ± chest compressions, check again for mechanical difficulties and initiate medications

Table 12-1 Equipment for Neonatal Resuscitation

Clinical Needs	Equipment
Thermoregulation	Radiant heat source with platform, mattress covered with warm sterile blankets, servo control heating; temperature probe
Airway management	*Suction:* bulb suction, DeLee suction apparatus, wall vacuum suction with sterile catheters *Ventilation:* manual infant resuscitation bag connected to pressure manometer capable of delivering 100% oxygen, appropriate masks for term and preterm infants *Intubation:* neonatal laryngoscope with #0 and #1 blades; endotracheal tubes 2.5, 3.0, and 3.5 mm outer diameter with stylet
Gastric decompression	Nasogastric tubes 5.0 and 8.0 Fr
Administration of drugs/volume	Sterile umbilical catheterization tray, umbilical catheters (3.5 and 5.0 Fr), volume expanders (Normal saline, 5% albumin), drug box with appropriate neonatal vials and dilutions (Table 12–4), sterile syringes, and needles
Transport	Warmed transport isolette with oxygen source

Table 12-2 The Apgar Scoring System

Sign	0	1	2
Heart rate	Absent	<100/min	>100/min
Respiratory effort	Apneic	Weak, irregular, gasping	Regular
Reflex irritability[a]			

[a] Elicited by suctioning the oropharynx and nose.

Modified from Apgar V: A proposal for a new method of evaluation of the newborn infant. Anesth Analg 32:260, 1953, with permission.

4. Generally, infants with heart rates over 100 bpm will require no further intervention. Infants with heart rates less than 100 bpm with apnea or irregular respiratory efforts should be vigorously stimulated by rubbing the baby's back with a towel while blowing oxygen over the face.

5. If the baby fails to respond rapidly to tactile stimulation, proceed to bag and face mask ventilation, using a soft mask that seals well around the mouth and nose. For the initial inflations, pressures of 30 to 40 cm H_2O may be necessary to overcome surface active forces in the lungs. A 1- to 2-second inspiratory time may be helpful as well.[90] In the premature infant even higher pressures (40 to 60 cm H_2O) may be needed. Adequacy of ventilation is assessed by observing expansion of the infant's chest with bagging and a gradual improvement in color, perfusion, and heart rate. After the first few breaths, attempts should be made to lower the peak pressure. Rate of bagging should not exceed 40 to 60 breaths/min.

6. Most neonates can be effectively resuscitated with a bag and face mask. However, if there is not favorable response in 30 to 40 seconds, one must proceed to intubation:

   a. The head should be stable, with the nose in the sniffing position (pointing straight upward).

   b. Insert the laryngoscope blade, and sweep the tongue to the left.

   c. Advance the blade to the base of the tongue, and identify the epiglottis.

   d. Pick up the endotracheal tube with the right hand.

   e. Slide the laryngoscope anterior to the epiglottis, and gently lift along the angle of the handle of the laryngoscope.

   f. Identify the vocal cords.

   g. Insert the tube in the right side of the mouth, and visualize the tube passing through the vocal cords.

   h. Ventilate as described above.

   i. Failure to respond to intubation and ventilation can result from (i) mechanical difficulties (Table 12-3), (ii) profound asphyxia with myocardial depression, and (iii) inadequate circulating blood volume.

   j. Mechanical causes should be quickly ruled out. Check to be sure the endotracheal tube passes through the vocal cords. Occlusion of the tube should be suspected when there is resistance

Table 12-3 Mechanical Causes of Failed Resuscitation

Category	Examples
Equipment failure	Malfunctioning bag, oxygen not connected or running
Endotracheal tube malposition	Esophagus, right mainstem bronchus
Occluded endotracheal tube	
Insufficient inflation pressure to expand lungs	
Space-occupying lesions in the thorax	Pneumothorax, pleural effusions, diaphragmatic hernia
Pulmonary hypoplasia	Extreme prematurity, oligohydramnios

to bagging and no chest wall movement. If the endotracheal tube is in place and not occluded, and equipment is functioning, a trial of bagging with higher pressures is indicated. A pneumothorax is characterized by asymmetric breath sounds not corrected by repositioning the tube above the carina. Pleural effusions usually occur with fetal hydrops, while a diaphragmatic hernia should be ruled out in the setting of asymmetric breath sounds and a scaphoid abdomen. Pulmonary hypoplasia should be considered if the pregnancy has been complicated by oligohydramnios. It is very unusual for a neonatal resuscitation to require either cardiac massage or drugs. Almost all newborns respond to ventilation with 100 percent oxygen.

7. If mechanical causes are ruled out, external cardiac massage should be performed for persistent heart rate at less than 100 bpm. Compression of 1 to 1.5 cm should be performed, interposed with ventilation at a 3/1 ratio (90 compressions: 30 breaths/min).

8. If drugs are needed (Table 12-4), the drug of choice is 0.1 to 0.3 ml/kg of 1:10,000 epinephrine through the endotracheal tube or preferably an umbilical venous line. Sodium bicarbonate 1 to 2 mEq/kg of the neonatal dilution can be used for a *documented* metabolic acidosis. If volume loss is suspected (e.g., documented blood loss with clinical evidence of hypovolemia), 10 ml/kg of a volume expander (5 percent albumin, normal saline) should be administered through an umbilical venous line. The appropriateness of continued resuscitative efforts should always be reevaluated in an infant who fails to respond to all of the above efforts. Today resuscitative efforts are made even in "apparent stillbirths," that is, infants whose 1-minute Apgar scores are 0 to 1. However, efforts should not be sustained in the face of little or no improvement over a reasonable period of time (i.e., 10 to 15 minutes).[91]

Infants in whom respiratory depression secondary to narcotic administration is suspected may be given naloxone (Narcan). However, this should not be done until the airway has been managed and the infant resuscitated in the usual fashion. A special group are preterm infants. Minimizing heat loss improves survival,

Table 12-4 Neonatal Drug Doses

Drug	Dose	Route[a]	How Supplied
Epinephrine	0.1–0.3 ml/kg	IV or ET	1:10,000 dilution
Sodium bicarbonate[b]	1–2 mEq/kg	IV	0.5 mEq/ml (4.2% solution)
Volume[c]	10 ml/kg	IV	Whole blood, 5 percent albumin, Ringer lactate, normal saline
Naloxone (Narcan)[d]	0.1 mg/kg	IV, ET, IM, or SQ	0.4 mg/ml or 1 mg/ml

[a] IV, intravenous; ET, endotracheal; IM, intramuscular; SQ, subcutaneous.

[b] For correction of metabolic acidosis only after adequate ventilation has been achieved; give slowly over several minutes.

[c] Infuse slowly over several minutes.

[d] After proceeding with proper airway management and other resuscitative techniques.

Modified from American Heart Association and American Academy of Pediatrics: Textbook of Neonatal Resuscitation. Washington, DC, American Heart Association, 1994, p 6–51, with permission.

so prewarmed towels should be available and the environmental temperature of the delivery suite should be raised. In the extremely low-birth-weight infant (less than 1,000 g), proceed quickly to intubation. Volume expanders and sodium bicarbonate should be infused slowly to avoid rapid swings in blood pressure.

Chapter 13

Postpartum Care

Watson A. Bowes, Jr.

Postpartum Involution

The Uterus

Within 2 weeks after birth the uterus has usually returned to the pelvis, and by 6 weeks it is usually normal sized. Hemostasis immediately after birth is accomplished by arterial smooth muscle contraction and compression of vessels by the involuting uterine muscle.

The postpartum uterine discharge or lochia begins as a flow of blood, rapidly diminishing to a reddish-brown discharge through the third or fourth day postpartum. This is followed by a transition to a mucopurulent discharge, lochia serosa, for about 3 weeks. In the majority of patients the lochia serosa is followed by a yellow-white discharge, lochia alba. Sometimes a sudden but transient increase in uterine bleeding occurs between 7 and 14 days postpartum. This corresponds to the slough of the eschar over the site of placental attachment. Although it can be profuse, this bleeding episode is usually self-limited, requiring nothing more than reassurance of the patient. If it does not subside within 1 or 2 hours, the patient should be evaluated for possible retained placental tissue with ultrasound. Those who have an empty uterine cavity will respond to therapy with oxytocin or methylergonovine.[7]

Ovarian Function

Women who breast-feed their infants may be amenorrheic for long periods of time, often until the infant is weaned. Ovulation occurs as early as 27 days after delivery, with the mean time being approximately 70 to 75 days in nonlactating women.[12–14] Among those women who are breast-feeding their infants, the mean time to ovulation is about 190 days.

Menstruation resumes by 12 weeks' postpartum in 70 percent of women who are not lactating, and the mean time to the first menstruation is 7 to 9 weeks. The duration of anovulation depends on the frequency of breast-feeding, the duration of each feed, and the proportion of supplementary feeds.[15] The risk of ovulation within the first 6 months postpartum in a woman exclusively breast-feeding is 1 to 5 percent.

Weight Loss

By six weeks postpartum, 28 percent of women will have returned to their prepregnant weight. The remainder of the weight loss occurs from 6 weeks postpartum until 6 months after delivery. Women with weight gain in pregnancy >35 lb are likely to have a net gain.

Thyroid Function

The postpartum period is a time when women are at increased risk of developing autoimmune thyroiditis followed by hypothyroidism.[20]

Cardiovascular System and Coagulation

By the third postpartum day, plasma volume has increased by 900 to 1,200 ml because of a shift of extracellular fluid into the vascular space.[22] Patients who deliver vaginally have a 5 percent increase in hematocrit, whereas those who have a cesarean delivery have on average, a 6 percent decrease in hematocrit.

The Urinary Tract and Renal Function

The urinary tract becomes dilated during pregnancy, especially the renal pelvis and the ureters above the pelvic brim, the right kidney more than the left. These changes are due predominantly to compression of the ureters by adjacent vasculature and, to a lesser extent, by compression from the enlarged uterus. Ureteral tone above the pelvic brim returns to nonpregnant levels immediately after delivery.[30]

Management of the Puerperium

If a patient has adequate support at home, there is little value in an extended hospital stay, provided the mother is adequately educated about infant care and feeding. Extending the hospital stay will provide time for insecure mothers to gain adequate education and some measure of self-confidence.

Physical activity, including walking up and down stairs, lifting heavy objects, riding in or driving a car, and performing muscle-toning exercises, can be resumed without delay if the delivery has been uncomplicated. Mothers whose lethargy persists beyond several weeks must be evaluated, especially as regards thyroid dysfunction and depression.

Sexual activity may be resumed when the perineum is comfortable. The desire and willingness to resume sexual activity in the puerperium varies greatly among women, depending on the site and state of healing of perineal or vaginal incisions and lacerations, the amount of vaginal atrophy secondary to breast-feeding, and the return of libido.[42]

Six weeks is regarded as the normal period of "disability" following delivery,[44] for employed mothers.

Perineal Care

Analgesia can be accomplished in most patients with nonsteroidal anti-inflammatory drugs such as ibuprofen. These drugs have been shown to be superior to acetaminophen or propoxyphene for episiotomy pain and uterine cramping,[45] and are safe for nursing mothers.

When a patient complains of inordinate perineal pain, the first step is to reexamine the perineum, vagina, and rectum to detect and drain a hematoma or to identify a perineal infection. Perineal pain may be the first symptom of the very rare but potentially fatal complications of angioedema, necrotizing fasciitis, or perineal cellulitis.[46–48]

Sitz baths also provide pain relief. Although hot sitz baths have long been customary therapy for perineal pain, cold or "iced" sitz baths provide immediate pain relief as a result of decreased excitability of free nerve endings and decreased nerve conduction. Further pain relief comes from local vasoconstriction, which reduces edema, inhibits hematoma formation, and decreases muscle irritability and spasm.

The technique for administering a cold sitz bath is first to have the patient sit in a tub of water at room temperature to which ice cubes are then added. The patient remains in the ice water for 20 to 30 minutes.

Frequently what appears to be severe perineal pain is, in fact, the pain of prolapsed hemorrhoids. Witch hazel compresses, suppositories containing corticosteroids, or local anesthetic sprays or emollients may be helpful. Occasionally a thrombus will occur in a prolapsed hemorrhoid. It is a simple task to remove the thrombus through a small scalpel incision using local anesthesia. Dramatic relief of pain usually follows this procedure.

Postpartum Infection

The standard definition of postpartum febrile morbidity is a temperature of 38.0°C (100.4°F) or higher on any 2 of the first 10 days postpartum, exclusive of the first 24 hours. The most common cause of postpartum fever is endometritis, but differential diagnosis includes urinary tract infection, lower genital tract infection, wound infections, pulmonary infections, thrombophlebitis, and mastitis.

Endometritis is an ascending infection from pathogens in the lower genital tract, including a variety of aerobic and anaerobic organisms.[52] Endometritis that presents within 1 or 2 days after delivery is often group A streptococcus. When the symptoms begin on the third or fourth day postpartum, the organism is likely to be an enteric pathogen, most commonly *Escherichia coli* or anaerobic organisms. Late-onset endometritis (after 7 days) is frequently caused by *Chlamydia trachomatis*. Patients predisposed to puerperal endometritis are those with prolonged rupture of membranes, long labors, multiple vaginal examinations during labor, cesarean delivery especially following a long labor, and anemia.

The symptoms of puerperal endometritis, in addition to fever and chills, are lower abdominal pain, anorexia, malaise, and malodorous vaginal discharge. The signs of endometritis are elevated temperature, abdominal tenderness, mucopurulent vaginal discharge, and uterine and parametrial tenderness on bimanual pelvic examination. Lower abdominal rebound tenderness may be present in some cases because of the associated pelvic cellulitis and peritonitis that occur in many of these infections.

Laboratory studies include a complete blood count, urine culture, and anaerobic and aerobic blood cultures in some instances. Transvaginal endometrial cultures are of limited value, because it is difficult to avoid contamination from vaginal flora.

Treatment of suspected puerperal endometritis is prompt, adequate intravenous antibiotic therapy. The most commonly employed regimen is the combination of clindamycin–gentamicin, which provides coverage of most aerobic and anaerobic organisms involved in these infections. Treatment may also be accomplished with single-drug therapy using either a cephalosporin such as cefotetan or cefoxitin, an extended-spectrum penicillin such as piperacillin or mezlocillin, or ampicillin combined with a β-lactaminase inhibitor. When the symptoms and signs of endometritis, including fever, have resolved for 24 hours, parenteral antibiotic therapy can be discontinued. Oral antibiotic therapy thereafter is unnecessary.

If signs and symptoms of infection have not subsided within 48 to 72 hours of intravenous antibiotic therapy, other sources of infection and complications of the original infection must be considered along with the possibility that the offending organism(s) are not adequately covered with the primary antibiotic therapy. Other diagnoses include pelvic abscess, wound infection, septic pelvic thrombophlebitis, urinary tract infection, and mastitis. Pelvic imaging studies, including ultrasound, computed tomography scanning, and magnetic resonance imaging, will often be helpful in detecting retained placental tissue, pelvic abscesses, or ovarian vein thrombosis in patients with persistent puerperal febrile morbidity. In patients with persistent fever in whom these studies have failed to detect other sources of infection, a course of intravenous heparin therapy is often recommended. A response to such therapy within 72 hours suggests the diagnosis of septic thrombophlebitis, for which there is no definitive clinical, laboratory, or imaging test.

Maternal–Infant Attachment

It is now recognized that there should be opportunities for parents to be with their newborns even from the first few moments after birth and as frequently as possible during the first days thereafter. Separation of mother and infant in the first hours after birth has been shown to diminish or delay the development of characteristic mothering behaviors,[54] or "bonding."

The modern hospital maternity ward should enhance and encourage parent–infant attachment by such policies as flexible visiting hours for the father, encouragement of the infant rooming with the mother, and supportive attitudes about breast-feeding.

Lactation and Breast-Feeding

Benefits of breast-feeding include improved infant nutrition, increased resistance to infection, decreased expense, and increased convenience.[62]

Successful breast-feeding depends to a great extent on the motivation of the mother and on the support she receives from family, friends, and health-care providers. A variety of hospital practices, including the use of audiovisual aids, telephone hotlines, and training for personnel, have been shown to increase the incidence of successful breast-feeding.[63]

The Term Infant

Allowing the infant to nurse in its wakeful period immediately after birth when the mouthing movements and rooting reflex are active will give the mother confidence and promote milk production and letdown. Early suckling provides the infant with the important immunologic and anti-infective properties of colostrum, and also has been shown to enhance successful breast-feeding.

Rooming-in allows the parents to become accustomed to demand feeding and provides the mother with opportunities to seek help from the nursing staff while she enhances her breast-feeding skills. Although the rooting and suckling reflexes are intact in a healthy newborn, successful breast-feeding is a learned talent for mother and infant. The infant should be allowed to suckle for 5 minutes per breast per feeding the first day, 10 minutes the second day, and 15 minutes or more per breast per feeding thereafter. If suckling is interrupted before initiation of the letdown reflex, breast engorgement is encouraged and nipple soreness will increase. The initial breast engorgement that occurs on the second to fourth postpartum days is best managed with 24-hour demand feedings.

Nipple soreness, another common complaint during the immediate puerperium, can be relieved by rotating breasts and the infant's position every 5 minutes while nursing; using frequent, shorter feedings rather than prolonged feeding times; avoiding irritating soaps or wet nursing pads; and exposing the nipples for air drying followed by the application of lanolin. In cases of persistent nipple soreness or of sudden appearance of nipple soreness after lactation has been established, *Monilia* infection of the nipple must be considered.[64]

Breast Milk for the Premature Infant

There are substantial data confirming the psychological, nutritional, and immunologic advantages to using a mother's breast milk to feed her premature infant. Furthermore, the immunologically active constituents of breast milk account for the lower incidence of infectious complications found in premature infants fed breast milk.

Most intensive care nurseries and many postpartum wards provide written instructions about milk expression and collection techniques.[78] Electric pumps, which simulate the physiologic suckling action of the infant, are available in many nurseries and can be leased from surgical supply companies.

Optimal milk production is associated with five or more milk expressions per day and pumping durations that exceed 100 min/day. Also, nasal oxytocin (Syntocinon) can be helpful in augmenting milk letdown. Breast milk can be refrigerated for 24 hours at 1° to 5°C or frozen at $-18°$ to $-23°C$ for up to 3 months.

Complications of Breast-Feeding

The most common complication of breast-feeding is puerperal mastitis. This condition is characterized by fever, myalgias, and an area of pain and redness in either breast, and the organism is often staphylococcus. Breast-feeding should not be discontinued, as engorgement may predispose to abscess formation. The combination of a penicillinase-resistant penicillin and continued breast-feeding will result in prompt resolution of the infection in the majority of cases.

Inadequate milk production can usually be corrected by decreasing the interval between feedings and by enhancing milk letdown with oxytocin nasal spray. Metoclopramide[83] (Reglan) has been shown to enhance milk production, presumably by stimulating prolactin secretion, and should be given in doses of 10 mg three or four times a day.

Lactation Suppression

For those patients who will not breast-feed, breast support, ice packs, and analgesic medications are helpful in ameliorating the symptoms of breast engorgement, which will last 24 to 72 hours.

Pregnancy Prevention and Birth Control

Natural Methods

The natural family planning methods, which depend on predicting the time of ovulation by use of basal body temperature or assessment of cervical mucus, cannot be used until regular menstrual cycles have resumed.[94]

Barrier Methods

The proper size of the diaphragm should be determined at the 6-week postpartum visit. The use of condoms alone or in combination with spermicides is often advised for women who are lactating.

Steroid Contraceptive Medications

In patients who are not breast-feeding, oral contraceptive agents are started 3 weeks after delivery. Combined-type oral contraceptive agents have a suppressive effect on lactation, whereas progestin-only medications do not diminish lactation performance,[102] so progestin-only preparations should be offered to women who are breast-feeding.

Depot medroxyprogesterone acetate (DMPA), 150 mg IM every 3 months, has a contraceptive efficacy exceeding 99 percent.[104] The most annoying side effect is unpredictable spotting and bleeding.

Pregnancy rates in women using the levonorgestrel subdermal implants are lower than with any other reversible contraception.[105] Implants inserted after delivery have no effect on lactation or growth of an infant who is nursing, even though small amounts of levonorgestrel are excreted in the milk. Irregular uterine bleeding, expense, and difficulty in removing the implants are the major drawbacks.

Intrauterine Devices

The copper-containing T-shaped device (ParaGard) and the progesterone-releasing device (Progestasert) are highly effective in preventing pregnancy (two to three pregnancies per 100 women-years).[106–108] The advantage of the copper-containing intrauterine device (IUD) is that it is effective for 10 years; its disadvantage is an increase in irregular uterine bleeding. The device that releases progesterone reduces uterine bleeding, but it must be replaced annually.

The major side effects and complications are uterine perforation, abnormal uterine bleeding, uterine and pelvic infection, and ectopic pregnancy.[107]

Sterilization

The Pomeroy or Parkland procedures are as effective as the more complicated procedures. In either case, a portion of the middle third of the fallopian tube is removed, leaving the cut ends ligated together in a single structure, as in the Pomeroy procedure, or separately, as in the Parkland operation.[116] The Irving procedure involves removing a segment from the middle third of the tube and then burying the proximal stump in a small tunnel created in the anterior surface of the uterus under the peritoneum.[119]

Puerperal sterilization compared with interval sterilization is associated with increased incidence of guilt and regret.[121,122] With increasing frequency, couples are postponing tubal ligation procedures until 6 to 8 weeks after delivery.[115] This provides time to ensure that the infant is healthy and to review all the implications of the decision.

Obstetricians must remember that vasectomy is often a more advisable and desirable alternative for a couple considering sterilization.[126] It can be performed as an outpatient procedure under local anesthesia with insignificant loss of time from work. Furthermore, almost all the failures can be detected by a postoperative semen analysis. This is a decided advantage over the tubal ligation, in which failures are discovered only when a pregnancy occurs. Furthermore, vasectomy is less expensive and overall is associated with fewer complications.

Tubal ligation can be reversed, but a patient should not undergo sterilization if she is contemplating reversal. Success as measured by the occurrence of pregnancy following tubal reanastomosis varies from 40 to 85 percent, depending on the type of tubal ligation performed and on the length of functioning tube that remains.[115]

Postpartum Psychological Reactions

The psychological reactions experienced by women following childbirth include the common, relatively mild, and transient "postpartum blues" (50 to 70 percent incidence), more prolonged affective disorders regarded as true postpartum depression (PPD; 10 to 15 percent incidence), and frank puerperal psychosis (0.14 to 0.26 percent incidence).

Postpartum Blues

The most common of the psychological manifestations of the puerperium is the transient state of tearfulness, anxiety, irritation, and restlessness, described as "postpartum blues." The symptoms may appear on any day within the first week after delivery and usually have resolved by postpartum day 10.

Because the syndrome is transient and of short duration, no therapy is indicated. Some of the symptoms may be from sleep deprivation, and increased rest may be helpful.

Postpartum Depression

The signs and symptoms of postpartum depression are not different from those in nonpregnant patients, but they may be difficult to differentiate from normal involutional phenomena (e.g., weight loss, sleeplessness) or from the transient "postpartum blues."[138] However, in addition to the more common symptoms of depression, the postpartum patient may manifest a sense of incapability of loving her family and manifest ambivalence toward her infant.

There is a high risk of recurrence (50 to 100 percent) of PPD in subsequent pregnancies and a 20 to 30 percent risk of PPD in women who have had a previous depressive reaction not associated with pregnancy.

Puerperal hypothyroidism often presents with symptoms including mild dysphoria. Consequently thyroid function studies may be useful in patients presenting with suspected PPD.

If there is not prompt response to general supportive measures and initial use of antidepressant medication, psychiatric consultation is advisable. The prognosis for PPD is good, although symptoms may persist for up to a year.

Postpartum Psychosis

Schizophrenia and manic–depressive reactions are seen with increased frequency in the puerperium, suggesting that there is a psychosis specific to the postpartum condition. Most patients with puerperal psychosis are manic–depressive, with confusion and disorientation prominent features of the clinical presentation. If suicidal thoughts or attempts occur, or if frankly delusional thoughts are expressed, the diagnosis of postpartum psychosis can be made.[141] Clearly, all patients with puerperal psychosis require hospitalization for at least initial evaluation and institution of therapy. Psychotic reactions occurring in the puerperium appear to have a more favorable prognosis, frequently lasting only 2 or 3 months.

Managing Perinatal Grieving

When a patient and her family experience a loss associated with a pregnancy, special attention must be given to the grieving patient and her family. Grief will occur with any significant loss, whether it is the actual death of an infant[145] or the loss of an idealized child in the case of the birth of a handicapped infant.[146]

There are five manifestations of normal grieving. These include somatic symptoms of sleeplessness, fatigue, digestive symptoms, and sighing respirations; preoccupation with the image of the deceased; feelings of guilt; feelings of hostility and anger toward others; and disruption of the normal pattern of daily life. Pathologic grief may occur if acute mourning is suppressed or interrupted. Some of the manifestations of this so-called morbid grief reaction are overactivity without a sense of loss; appearance or exacerbations of psychosomatic illness; alterations in relationships with friends and relatives; furious hostility toward specific persons; lasting loss of patterns of social interaction; activities detrimental to personal, social, and economic existence; and agitated depression.

It is important that the characteristics of the grieving patient be recognized and understood by health professionals caring for such patients. What is actually beneficial at such a time is a sympathetic listener and an opportunity to express and discuss feelings of guilt, anger, and hopelessness and the other symptoms of mourning.

The following are guidelines for managing perinatal loss:

1. Keep the mother informed; be honest and forthright.
2. Recognize and facilitate anticipatory grieving.
3. Encourage the mother's major support person to remain with her throughout labor and delivery.
4. Support the couple in seeing or touching the infant.
5. Describe the infant in detail, particularly for couples who choose not to see.
6. Encourage the mother to make as many choices about her care as possible.
7. Teach the couple about the grieving process.
8. Show infants during postpartum hospitalization on request.
9. Allow photographs of the infant.
10. Prepare the couple for hospital paperwork, such as autopsy requests.
11. Discuss funeral or memorial services.
12. Help the couple to think about informing siblings.

13. Assist the couple in deciding how to tell friends of the death and in packing away the baby's things.
14. Discuss subsequent pregnancy.
15. Use public health nurse referral or schedule additional office visits.

It is also important to realize that the fathers of infants who die have somewhat different grief responses than do the mothers. Their grief is characterized by the necessity to keep busy with increased work, feelings of diminished self-worth, self-blame, and limited ability to ask for help. Stoic responses are typical of men and may obstruct the normal resolution of grief.

Key Points

- By six weeks postpartum, 28 percent of women will have returned to their prepregnant weight.
- Late-onset endometritis (after 7 days) is frequently caused by *Chlamydia trachomatis.*
- *Monilia* infection is a common cause of persistent nipple soreness in women who are breast-feeding.
- Most women with puerperal mastitis can be adequately treated with penicillin V, ampicillin, or dicloxacillin while they continue to breast-feed their infants.
- Breast-feeding will result in 98 percent contraceptive protection for up to 6 months following delivery provided there is little or no supplemental feeding of the infant.
- Progestin-only contraceptive medication does not diminish lactation performance.
- Postpartum, major depression occurs in 8 to 15 percent of parturients.
- Puerperal hypothyroidism often presents with symptoms that include mild dysphoria; consequently, thyroid function studies are suggested in the evaluation of patients with suspected postpartum depression.

Fetal Wastage

Joe Leigh Simpson

Not all conceptions result in a liveborn infant. Of clinically recognized pregnancies, 10 to 15 percent are lost. Of married women in the United States, 4 percent have experienced two fetal losses and 3 percent have experienced three or more.[1] It is accepted that a subset of women genuinely manifest repetitive spontaneous abortions as opposed to merely representing random untoward events. This chapter considers the causes of fetal wastage, the management of couples experiencing repetitive losses, and the topic of ectopic gestations.

Frequency and Timing of Pregnancy Losses

Pregnancy is not generally recognized clinically until 5 to 6 weeks after the last menstrual period, but before this time β-human chorionic gonadotropin (β-hCG) assays can detect preclinical pregnancies. Of pregnancies detected by β-hCG assays at 20 weeks' gestation, about one-third are lost.

Of surviving pregnancies, clinically recognized first-trimester fetal loss rates of 10 to 12 percent overall are well documented. Maternal age greatly increases risk, a 40-year-old woman carrying twice the risk of a 20-year-old woman. Prior pregnancy history is also pivotal. Loss rates are lowest (6 percent) among nulliparous women who have never experienced a loss,[5] rising to 25 to 30 percent after three or more losses.

Studies utilizing ultrasonography have now made it clear that fetal demise occurs before overt clinical signs are manifested. This conclusion is based on cohort studies showing that only 3 percent of viable pregnancies are lost after 8 weeks' gestation.[7] Given an accepted clinical loss rate of 10 to 12 percent, fetal viability must cease weeks before maternal symptoms appear; thus, most fetuses aborting clinically at 9 to 12 weeks must have died weeks previously.

Establishing an etiology for preclinical losses is not easy, but the one proven explanation is morphologic and genetic abnormalities in the early embryo. Consistent with this are studies showing that chromosomal abnormalities exist in approximately 25 percent of pre-implantation embryos that are fertilized in vitro.[11,12] In turn, chromosomal abnormalities exist in 10 percent of sperm of ostensibly normal males and in perhaps 20 percent of oocytes.[13,14] One can conclude that chromosomal abnormalities are not only frequent in morphologically *normal* embryos but even more frequent in morphologically *abnormal* embryos.

Cytogenetic Etiology in Clinically Recognized Losses

The major cause of clinically recognized pregnancy losses is chromosomal abnormalities. At least 50 percent of clinically recognized pregnancy losses result from a chromosomal abnormality.[16–18] The frequency is probably even higher. Among third-trimester losses (stillborn infants) the frequency of chromosomal abnormalities is approximately 5 percent.[21] This frequency is less than that observed in earlier abortuses but still higher than found among liveborns (0.6 percent).

Autosomal Trisomy

Autosomal trisomies comprise the largest (approximately 50 percent) single class of chromosomal complements in cytogenetically abnormal spontaneous abortions. Frequencies of these trisomies are listed in Table 14-1. The most common trisomy is number 16. Most trisomies show a maternal age effect, but the effect is variably marked among certain chromosomes. The maternal age effect is especially impressive for double trisomies.

Autosomal trisomies are more likely to arise cytologically in maternal meiosis than in paternal meiosis. Most trisomies (90 percent) arise during maternal meiosis, usually maternal meiosis I.[25] Trisomy 18 is an exception in arising during meiosis II.

Polyploidy

In polyploidy more than two haploid chromosomal complements exist. Triploidy ($3n = 69$) and tetraploidy ($4n = 92$) occur often in abortuses. Triploid

Table 14-1   Chromosomal Complements in
Spontaneous Abortions: Recognized
Clinically in the
First Trimester[a]

Complement	Frequency	(%)
Normal 46,XX or 46,XY		54.1
Triploidy		7.7
69,XXX	2.7	
69,XYX	0.2	
69,XXY	4.0	
Other	0.8	
Tetraploidy		2.6
92,XXX	1.5	
92,XXYY	0.55	
Not stated	0.55	
Monosomy X		8.6
Structural abnormalities		1.5
Sex chromosomal polysomy		0.2
47,XXX	0.05	
47,XXY	0.15	
Autosomal monosomy (G)		0.1
Autosomal trisomy for chromosomes		22.3
1	0	
2	1.11	
3	0.25	
4	0.64	
5	0.04	
6	0.14	
7	0.89	
8	0.79	
9	0.72	
10	0.36	
11	0.04	
12	0.18	
13	1.07	
14	0.82	
15	1.68	
16	7.27	
17	0.18	
18	1.15	
19	0.01	
20	0.61	
21	2.11	
22	2.26	
Double trisomy		0.7
Mosaic trisomy		1.3
Other abnormalities or not specified		0.9
		100.0

[a] Pooled data from several series, as referenced elsewhere by
Simpson JL, Bombard AT: Chromosomal abnormalities in spontaneous abortion: frequency, pathology and genetic counseling. p.
51. In Edmonds K, Bennett MJ (eds): Spontaneous Abortion,
Blackwell, London, 1987, with permission.

abortuses are usually 69,XXY or 69,XXX, resulting from dispermy.[26,27] Pathologic findings in triploid placentas include a disproportionately large gestational sac, cystic degeneration of placental villi, intrachorial hemorrhage, and hydropic trophoblasts (pseudomolar degeneration).[23,24] Tetraploidy is uncommon, rarely progressing beyond 2 to 3 weeks of embryonic life.

Monosomy X

Monosomy X is the single most common chromosomal abnormality among spontaneous abortions, accounting for 15 to 20 percent of abnormal specimens. Monosomy X embryos usually consist of only an umbilical cord stump. Later in gestation, anomalies characteristic of the Turner syndrome may be seen, specifically cystic hygromas and generalized edema. Although liveborn 45,X individuals usually lack germ cells, 45,X abortuses show germ cells; however, these germ cells rarely develop beyond the primordial germ cell stage. The pathogenesis of 45,X germ cell failure thus involves not so much failure of germ cell development as more rapid attrition in 45,X than in 46,XX embryos.[28,29]

Structural Chromosomal Rearrangement

Structural chromosomal rearrangement accounts for 1.5 percent of all abortuses (Table 14-1). Rearrangements (e.g., translocation) either may arise de novo during gametogenesis or be inherited from a parent carrying a "balanced" translocation or inversion. Phenotypic consequences depend on the specific duplicated or deficient chromosomal segments. Although not a common cause of sporadic losses, inherited translocations are an important cause of *repeated* fetal wastage.

Sex Chromosomal Polysomy (X or Y)

The complements 47,XXY and 47,XYY each occur in about 1/800 liveborn male births; 47,XXX occurs in 1/800 female births. X or Y polysomies are only slightly more common in abortuses than in liveborns.

Mendelian and Polygenic/Multifactorial Etiology

The 30 to 50 percent of first-trimester abortuses that show no chromosomal abnormalities could still have undergone fetal demise as a result of other genetic etiologies. Neither mendelian nor polygenic/multifactorial disorders show chromosomal abnormalities. Many excellent anatomic studies of abortuses have demonstrated structural abnormalities, but lack of cytogenetic data on the dissected specimens makes it nearly impossible to determine the precise role of noncytogenetic mechanisms in early embryonic maldevelopment. Doubtless pivotal to early development are many mendelian genes, mutation of which would be expected to result in embryonic death and pregnancy loss.

Genetic Counseling and Recurrence Risks

The obstetrician faced with a couple experiencing spontaneous abortion has several immediate obligations: (1) inform the couple concerning the frequency of fetal wastage (10 to 12 percent clinically recognized pregnancies) and its likely etiology (at least 50 percent cytogenetic), (2) provide recurrence risk rates, and (3) determine the necessity of a formal clinical evaluation.

Recurrence Risks

Loss rates are definitely increased among women who have experienced previous losses, but not nearly to the extent once thought (Table 14-2). For decades, obstetricians fervently believed in the concept of "habitual abortion." After three losses, the risk of subsequent

Table 14-2 Approximate Recurrence Risk Figures Useful for Counseling Women with Repeated Spontaneous Abortions[a]

	Prior Abortions	Risk (%)
Women with liveborn infants	0	5–10
	1	20–25
	2	25
	3	30
	4	30
Women without liveborn infants	3	30–40

[a] Recurrence risks are slightly higher for older women, for those who smoke cigarettes or drink alcohol, and for those exposed to high levels of selected chemical toxins.

Based on data from Warburton D, Fraser FC: Spontaneous abortion risks in man: data from reproductive histories collected in a medical genetics units. Am J Human Genet 16: 1, 1964, Poland BJ, Miller JR, Jones DC et al: Reproductive counseling in patients who have had a spontaneous abortion. Am J Obstet Gynecol 127:685, 1977, and others.

losses was thought to rise sharply. Such beliefs were based on calculations made in 1938 by Malpas,[33] who concluded that, following three abortions, the likelihood of a subsequent one was 80 to 90 percent. Occurrence of three consecutive spontaneous abortions was thus said for decades to confer upon a women the designation of "habitual aborter." These risk figures not only proved incorrect but also were and unfortunately still seem subconsciously to be used as "controls" for clinical studies evaluating various treatment plans. This practice led to unwarranted acceptance of certain interventions, the most famous of which was diethylstilbestrol (DES) treatment.

In 1964, Warburton and Fraser[34] showed that the likelihood of recurrent abortion rose only to 25 to 30 percent, irrespective of whether a woman had previously experienced one, two, three, or even four spontaneous abortions. This concept has been confirmed in many subsequent studies, although if no previous liveborns have occurred the likelihood of fetal loss is somewhat higher.[35] Lowest risks (5 percent) are observed in nulliparous women with no prior losses.[5] Women who smoke cigarettes or drink alcohol moderately are probably at slightly higher risk.[36] Recurrence risks are higher if the abortus is cytogenetically normal than cytogenetically abnormal.[37]

Taking all the above into account, the prognosis is reasonably good even without therapy, the predicted success rate being 70 percent. Indeed, Vlaanderen and Treffers[38] reported successful pregnancies in each of 21 women having unexplained prior repetitive losses but subjected to no intervention. Other groups have reached similar conclusions.[39,40] To be judged efficacious, therapeutic regimens must achieve successes greater than 70 percent.

Etiology and Clinical Evaluation or Repetitive Abortions

Structural Chromosomal Rearrangements

Structural chromosomal abnormalities are generally accepted as one explanation for repetitive abortions. The most common structural rearrangement encountered is a translocation, found in about 5 percent of couples experiencing repeated losses.[41-43] Individuals with balanced translocations are phenotypically normal, but abortuses or abnormal liveborns may show chromosomal duplications or deficiencies as a result of normal meiotic segregation. About 60 percent of the translocations detected are reciprocal, and 40 percent are Robertsonian. Females are about twice as likely as males to show a balanced translocation.[41]

If a child has Down syndrome as result of a Robertsonian translocation, the rearrangement will prove to have originated de novo in 50 to 75 percent of cases. That is, a balanced translocation will not exist in either parent. The likelihood of Down syndrome recurring in subsequent offspring is minimal. Conversely, the risk is significant in the 25 to 50 percent of families in which individuals have Down syndrome as the result of a balanced parental translocation (e.g., parental complement 45,XX,−14,−21,+[14q;21q]). The theoretical risk of having a child with Down syndrome is 33 percent, but empirical risks are considerably less. The likelihood is only 2 percent if the father carries the translocation and 10 percent if the mother carries the translocation.[44,45] If Robertsonian (centric-fusion) translocations involve other chromosomes, empirical risks are lower. In t(13q;14q), the risk for liveborn trisomy 13 is 1 percent or less.

Reciprocal translocations are those that do not involve centromeric fusion. Empirical data for specific translocations are usually not available, but useful generalizations can be made on the basis of pooled data derived from many different translocations.

Theoretical risks for abnormal offspring (unbalanced reciprocal translocations) are far greater than empirical risks. Overall, the risk is 12 percent for offspring of either female heterozygotes or male heterozygotes.[44,45] Detecting a parental chromosomal rearrangement thus profoundly affects subsequent pregnancy management. Antenatal cytogenetic studies should be offered in subsequent pregnancies. The frequency of unbalanced fetuses is lower if parental balanced translocations are ascertained through repetitive abortions (3 percent) than through anomalous liveborns (nearly 20 percent).[44]

Recurrent Aneuploidy

Already discussed at length as the most common overall cause for sporadic abortions, numerical chromosomal abnormalities (aneuploidy) may be responsible for recurrent losses as well. This reasoning is based on observations that the complements of successive abortuses in a given family are more likely to be either recurrently normal or recurrently abnormal. If the complement of the first abortus is abnormal, the likelihood is 80 percent that the complement of the second abortus also will be abnormal.[50] The recurrent abnormality usually is trisomy.

If couples are predisposed to recurrent aneuploidy, they might logically be at increased risk not only for aneuploid abortuses but also for aneuploid liveborns. The trisomic autosome in a subsequent pregnancy might not always confer lethality, but rather might be compatible with life (e.g., trisomy 21). Indeed, the risk of liveborn trisomy 21 following an aneuploid abortus is about 1 percent.[51]

Luteal Phase Defects

The term *luteal phase defects* (LPDs) is used to describe an endometrium manifesting an inadequate progesterone effect. Progesterone secreted by the corpus luteum is necessary to support the endometrium until the trophoblast produces sufficient progesterone to maintain pregnancy, an event occurring around 7 gestational (menstrual) weeks or 5 weeks after conception. Once almost universally accepted as a common cause for fetal wastage, LPDs now seem to be considered an uncommon cause. Although plausible clinically, there are no randomized studies verifying efficacy of treatment.

LPDs are far less common than once believed. The consensus is that LPDs are either an arguable entity or cannot be proved to be treated successfully with progesterone therapy. Indeed, a meta-analysis by Karamardian and Grimes[65] showed no beneficial effect (pregnancy rate) of treatment. Treatment should be initiated only if the diagnosis is firmly established and only if couples are apprised of the unfounded claims of progesterone teratogenicity. Patients should probably be informed that therapeutic efficacy is unproved. If instituted, treatment usually consists of vaginal progesterone suppositories 25 mg twice daily beginning with the basal body temperature elevation and continuing at least 6 to 8 weeks.

Thyroid Abnormalities

Decreased conception rates and increased fetal losses are associated with overt hypothyroidism or hyperthyroidism. However, subclinical thyroid dysfunction is probably not an explanation for repeated losses.[66]

Diabetes Mellitus

Women whose diabetes mellitus is poorly controlled are at increased risk for fetal loss.[3] In one study, women whose glycosylated hemoglobin level was greater than four standard deviations above the mean showed higher pregnancy loss rates than women with lower glycosylated hemoglobin levels. Poorly controlled diabetes mellitus should be considered one cause for early pregnancy loss, but well-controlled or subclinical diabetes is probably not a cause of early miscarriage.

Intrauterine Adhesions (Synechiae)

Intrauterine adhesions could interfere with implantation or early embryonic development. Adhesions may follow overzealous uterine curettage during the postpartum period, intrauterine surgery (e.g., myomectomy), or endometritis. Curettage is the usual explanation, with adhesions most likely to develop if curettage is performed 3 or 4 weeks postpartum. Individuals with uterine synechiae usually manifest hypomenorrhea or amenorrhea, but 15 to 30 percent show repeated abortions. If adhesions are detected in a woman experiencing repetitive losses, lysis under direct hyperoscopic visualization should be performed. Estrogen administration should also be initiated. Approximately 50 percent of patients conceive after surgery, but the frequency of abortions remains high.

Incomplete Müllerian Fusion

Müllerian fusion defects (Fig. 14-1) are an accepted cause of *second*-trimester losses and pregnancy compli-

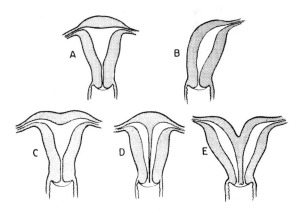

Fig. 14-1 Diagrammatic representation of some müllerian fusion anomalies: (A) normal uterus, fallopian tubes, and cervix; (B) uterus unicornis (absence of one uterine horn); (C) uterus arcuatus (broadening and medial depression of a portion of the uterine septum); (D) uterus septus (persistence of a complete uterine septum); and (E) uterus bicornis unicollis (two hemiuteri, each leading to same cervix). (From Simpson JL: Disorders of Sexual Differentiation: Etiology and Clinical Delineation. San Diego, Academic Press, 1976, with permission.)

cations. Low birth weight, breech presentation, and uterine bleeding are other abnormalities associated with müllerian fusion defects. The major problem in attributing cause and effect for second-trimester complications and uterine anomalies is that the latter are so frequent that adverse outcomes could often be coincidental. Treatment has traditionally involved surgical correction, such as metroplasty.

First-trimester abortions might also be due to müllerian fusion defects. Septate uteri might raise the risk of poor implantation on a poorly vascularized and inhospitable surface. Abortions occurring after ultrasonographic confirmation of a viable pregnancy at 8 or 9 weeks may properly be attributed to uterine fusion defects if the latter are present; however, losses having no confirmation of fetal viability at that time are statistically more likely to represent missed abortions in which fetal demise occurred prior to 8 weeks. Women experiencing second-trimester abortions can be assumed to benefit from uterine reconstruction, but reconstructive surgery is not necessarily advisable if losses are restricted to the first trimester.

Incompetent Internal Cervical Os

A functionally intact cervix and lower uterine cavity are obvious prerequisites for a successful intrauterine pregnancy. Characterized by painless dilatation and effacement, cervical incompetence usually occurs during the middle second or early third trimester. This condition frequently follows traumatic events like cervical amputation, cervical lacerations, forceful cervical dilatation, or conization. A relationship to various connective tissue disorders is plausible but yet unproved. The various surgical techniques to correct cervical incompetence are discussed in Chapter 15.

Infections

Infections are accepted causes of late fetal wastage and logically could be responsible for early fetal loss as well. Microorganisms reported to be associated with spontaneous abortion include *Variola, Vaccinia, Salmonella typhi, Vibrio fetus, Plasmodium, Cytomegalovirus, Brucella, Toxoplasma, Mycoplasma hominis, Chlamydia trachomatis,* and *Ureaplasma urealyticum.* Transplacental infection doubtless occurs with each of these microorganisms, and sporadic losses could logically be caused by any. Unanswered is whether the infectious agents were causative in the fetal losses or merely arose secondarily after demise due to a noninfectious etiology. Confounding variables (e.g., maternal age, prior pregnancy history) are also rarely taken into account. Overall, a purported association between a common microorganism and pregnancy loss could easily reflect chance findings or be explained by other factors. Of all the organisms mentioned, *Ureaplasma* and *Chlamydia* are the most commonly implicated in *repetitive* abortion.

What evaluation and management is recommended? Culturing the endometrium for *U. urealyticum* seems reasonable, with culture-positive women having such infections receiving treatment. Alternatively, tetracycline therapy can be reasoned to be so innocuous that empirical treatment with doxycycline (100 mg orally twice times a day for 10 days, both husband and non-pregnant wife) could be recommended.

Anti-Fetal Antibodies

Perturbations of the immune system can be responsible for fetal wastage. However, the nature of the immunologic process responsible for maintaining pregnancy is complex.

An otherwise normal mother may produce antibodies against her fetus on the basis of genetic dissimilarities. Fetal loss is well documented in Rh-negative (D-negative) women having anti-D antibodies. More apropos for early pregnancy loss is the presence of anti-P antibodies. Most individuals are genotype Pp or PP, but one may be homozygous for p (pp). If a woman of genotype pp has a Pp or PP mate, resulting offspring may or must be Pp. If the mother develops anti-P antibodies, Pp fetuses will be rejected (aborted) early in gestation. Plasmapheresis and other modalities may be therapeutically efficacious.[93,94]

Autoimmune Disease

An association between pregnancy loss and certain autoimmune diseases is generally accepted.[95,96] Individuals having anti-phospholipid antibodies, including lupus anticoagulant (LAC) antibodies and anti-cardiolipin antibodies (aCL) constitute the group most often associated with fetal wastage. Almost all[97] agree that the frequency of midtrimester fetal death in women who show LAC or aCL is increased, perhaps dramatically so. Other pregnancy complications (e.g., growth retardation, preeclampsia) are also more common. These antibodies have closely related specificities and could be members of the same family of autoantibodies. LAC in particular has been associated with subplacental clotting and fetal losses in all trimesters.[98] The abortifacient mechanism is thus presumably decidual. Although a relationship between aCL and *second*/third-trimester losses seems reasonably well established, data do not support a major role for ACL in *first*-trimester pregnancy losses. Treatment with heparin and low-dose aspirin is best restricted to couples with second- or third-trimester losses.

Alloimmune Disease (Shared Parental Antigens)

That parental histo*in*compatibility could be beneficial in pregnancy maintenance continues to be the source of considerable investigation, although any relationship may or may not be related to blocking antibodies. Considerable experimental support for a beneficial effect of fetomaternal incompatibility in animals can be cited. Whether increased human leukocyte antigen (HLA) sharing per se constitutes the mechanism underlying lack of parental differences in humans is less certain.

An alternative interpretation that could explain how some but not all couples sharing HLA antigens experience deleterious effects would be for the normal pregnancy to require fetal–maternal histo*in*compatibility but not at the HLA locus. Another possibility is that the deleterious effect of parental antigen sharing may not be immunologic at all. All observations could be explained entirely on a nonimmunologic basis by postulating existence of a lethal recessive gene closely linked to HLA.

If fetal rejection truly occurs as the result of diminished fetal–maternal immunologic interaction (alloimmune factors), immunotherapy to enhance interaction at the few potentially differing loci would not be unreasonable. However, efficacy of immunotherapy remains highly controversial.

Drugs, Chemicals, and Noxious Agents

Various exogenous agents have been implicated in fetal losses. Indeed, women are exposed frequently to relatively low doses of ubiquitous agents. However, few agents can be implicated with confidence. Rarely are data adequate to determine the true role of these exogenous factors in early pregnancy losses.

Outcomes following exposures to exogenous agents are usually deduced on the basis of case–control studies. In such studies, women who aborted claimed exposure to the agent in question more often than controls. However, case–control studies suffer certain inherent biases, as reviewed in Chapter 2. The primary bias is that controls have less incentive to recall antecedent events than subjects experiencing an abnormal outcome (recall bias). Employers attempt to limit exposure of women in the reproductive age group; thus, exposures to potentially dangerous chemicals are usually unwitting and, hence, poorly documented. Moreover, pregnant women usually are exposed to many agents concurrently, making it nearly impossible to attribute adverse effects to a single agent. Given these caveats, physicians should be cautious about attributing pregnancy loss to exogenous agents. However, common sense dictates that exposure to potentially noxious agents be minimized.

X-Irradiation

Irradiation and antineoplastic agents in high doses are accepted abortifacients. However, pelvic x-ray exposure of up to perhaps 10 rad places a woman at little to no increased risk. Exposure doses are usually far less (1 to 2 rad). Still, it is prudent for pregnant hospital workers to avoid handling chemotherapeutic agents and minimize potential exposures during diagnostic x-ray procedures.

Intrauterine Devices

Conception with an intrauterine device in place clearly increases the risk of fetal loss. However, if the device is removed prior to pregnancy, there is no increased risk of spontaneous abortions. Use of oral contraceptives before or during pregnancy is not associated with fetal loss, nor is spermicide exposure either prior to or after conception (see Ch. 2).

Environmental Chemicals

Among the many chemical agents variously claimed to be associated with fetal losses,[130,131] consensus seems to be evolving around a selected few.[132] These include anesthetic gases, arsenic, aniline dyes, benzene, solvents, ethylene oxide, formaldehyde, pesticides, and certain divalent cations (lead, mercury, cadmium). Workers in rubber industries, battery factories, and chemical production plants are among those at potential risk. The difficulty lies in defining the precise effect of lower exposures and attributing a specific risk. False alarms concerning potential toxins are frequent.

Trauma

Women commonly attribute pregnancy losses to trauma, such as a fall or blow to the abdomen. However, fetuses are actually well protected from external trauma by intervening maternal structures and amniotic fluid. The temptation to attribute a loss to minor traumatic events should be avoided.

Psychologic Factors

That impaired psychologic well-being predisposes to early fetal losses has been claimed but never proved. Certainly neurotic or mentally ill women experience losses just like normal women. Whether the frequency of losses is higher in the former is less certain because potential confounding variables have not been taken into account. Some studies can be cited as consistent with a beneficial effect of psychological well-being,[39,40] but any ostensible positive effect of psychological well-being is probably either more apparent than real or secondary to other factors.

Recommended Evaluation for Recurrent Pregnancy Losses

1. Couples experiencing only one first-trimester abortion should receive pertinent information, but not necessarily be evaluated formally. Mention the relatively high (10 to 15 percent) pregnancy loss rate in the general population and the beneficial effects of abortion in eliminating abnormal conceptuses. Provide the relevant recurrence risks, usually 20 to 25 percent subsequent loss in the presence of a prior liveborn and somewhat higher in the absence of a prior liveborn. Risks are higher for older women and those who smoke. Occurrence of an anomalous stillborn or liveborn warrants genetic evaluation irrespective of the number of pregnancy losses.

2. Investigation may or may not be necessary after two spontaneous abortions, depending upon the patient's age and personal desires. After three spontaneous abortions, evaluation is usually indicated. One should then (a) obtain a detailed family history, (b) perform a complete physical examination, (c) discuss recurrence risks, and (d) order the selected tests needed.

3. Parental chromosomal studies should be performed on all couples having repetitive losses. Antenatal chromosomal studies should be offered if a balanced chromosomal rearrangement is detected in either parent or if autosomal trisomy occurred in any previous abortus.

4. Although it is impractical to karyotype all abortuses, cytogenetic information on abortuses may exist. Detection of a trisomic abortus suggests the phenomenon of recurrent aneuploidy, justifying prenatal cytogenetic studies in future pregnancies.

5. The validity of luteal phase deficiency as a discrete entity is arguable. Progesterone therapy has been proposed, but its efficacy has not been proved.

6. Other endocrine causes for repeated fetal losses seem unlikely except for poorly controlled diabetes mellitus (hyperglycemia). Subclinical thyroid dysfunction and carbohydrate intolerance are rare causes of pregnancy losses.

7. To determine the role of infectious agents, the endometrium may be cultured for *U. urealyticum*. Alternatively, a couple could be treated empirically with doxycycline (100 mg two times per day for 10 days) before pregnancy. Of other infectious agents, only *C. trachomatis* seems genuinely possible.

8. If an abortion occurs after 8 to 10 weeks' gestation, a uterine anomaly or submucous leiomyoma should be considered. The uterine cavity should be explored by hysteroscopy or hysterosalpingography. If a müllerian fusion defect (septate or bicornuate uterus) is detected in a woman experiencing one or more second-trimester spontaneous abortions, surgical correction may be warranted. However, the same statements do not necessarily apply following *first*-trimester losses. Cervical incompetence should be managed by surgical cerclage during the next pregnancy.

9. To exclude autoimmune disease involving antiphospholipid antibodies, assessment should include LAC and aCL. Women with antibodies who experience midtrimester losses may benefit from treatment with heparin and aspirin, but the same does not necessarily hold when these antibodies are detected in asymptomatic women having first-trimester pregnancy losses.

10. Controversy persists concerning the propriety of immunologic evaluations and especially the role of immunotherapy for couples sharing HLA antigens or otherwise having blunted maternal response to paternal antigens.

11. One should discourage exposure to cigarettes and alcohol, yet remain cautious in ascribing cause and effect in individual cases. Similar

counsel should apply for exposures to other potential toxins.

Ectopic Pregnancy

In ectopic pregnancy, implantation occurs at a site other than the endometrium. Ectopic pregnancies are responsible for approximately 10 percent of all maternal mortality.[139] Moreover, the prognosis for future reproduction is poor. Only one-half of women having an ectopic pregnancy are eventually delivered of a liveborn infant. Most of these never become pregnant, and up to 25 percent of those who do suffer a repeat ectopic pregnancy.[140] Various factors contribute to ectopic pregnancies, the most common being infection.

Most ectopic pregnancies (96 percent) are tubal. The remainder are interstitial uterine ectopic pregnancies and, rarely, cervical, abdominal, or ovarian pregnancies.[142] Most tubal pregnancies are located in the distal (ampullary) two-thirds of the tube. A few ectopic pregnancies are isthmic, located in the proximal portion of the extrauterine part of the tube. On rare occasions both intrauterine and extrauterine gestations can coexist (heterotopic pregnancy).

Signs and Symptoms

Abdominal pain and irregular vaginal bleeding are the most common presenting symptoms in ectopic pregnancy.[143,144] Of 328 patients presenting with ectopic pregnancy, 94 percent have pain, 89 percent had a missed menstrual period, 80 percent have vaginal bleeding, and 20 percent have hypotension.[145] An abdominal mass is palpable in only one-half of patients with an ectopic pregnancy. Of course, passage of a decidual cast in association with vaginal bleeding nearly unequivocally indicates ectopic pregnancy, but this is uncommon. The Arias-Stella phenomenon is frequently found in the endometrium in association with ectopic pregnancies; however, this phenomenon is also seen in 70 to 80 percent of therapeutic and spontaneous abortions,[146] and thus it is not specific for ectopic gestation.

Ectopic pregnancies should now be diagnosed before the onset of hypotension, bleeding, pain, and overt rupture. Ectopic pregnancy can be detected by 6 weeks' gestation, often as early as at 4 1/2 gestational weeks.

Diagnosis

Direct vision by laparoscopy was once the diagnostic standard for ectopic pregnancy. However, if the pregnancy is early and the gestational sac small, the gestation may not be visualized. Thus algorithms incorporating a single measurement of serum progesterone, serial measurement of the β-subunit of hCG, pelvic ultrasonography, and uterine curettage are accepted.[146] Figure 14-2 shows a useful approach.

Single Measurement of Serum Progesterone

Ectopic pregnancy can be excluded and viable intrauterine pregnancy diagnosed with 97.5 percent sensitivity if serum progesterone (P) levels are 25 ng/ml or higher (≥79.5 nmol/L), obviating the need for further testing. Conversely, serum P can identify nonviable pregnancies with 100 percent sensitivity if P levels are 5 ng/ml or lower (≤15.9 nmol/L).[147–150] If a single P level is 5 ng/ml or lower, diagnostic uterine evacuation can be performed even if ectopic pregnancy cannot otherwise be distinguished from a spontaneous intrauterine abortion. P values above 5 but below 25 ng/ml necessitate establishing viability by ultrasonography.

Serial Serum β-hCG Measurements

β-hCG is produced by trophoblastic cells. In normal pregnancies, β-hCG concentration increases 67 percent over a 2-day interval.[151] Abnormal intrauterine or ectopic pregnancies have impaired β-hCG production and, hence, a prolonged hCG doubling time.

Transvaginal Ultrasound

If β-hCG is greater than 1,500 mIU/ml and the pregnancy is intrauterine, a gestational sac should be visualized by transvaginal ultrasound. By transabdominal ultrasound the gestational sac may not be identified until β-hCG reaches 6,000 mIU/ml. If β-hCG is greater than these levels but the gestational sac cannot be visualized, an ectopic location should be assumed.

Uterine Curettage

Villi float in saline, a characteristic permitting identification of tissue obtained by curettage. If no villi are recognized and a decrease in the β-hCG level of 15 percent or more 8 to 12 hours occurs after curettage, a completed abortion can be assumed to exist. If villi are not visualized and β-hCG titers plateau or rise, trophoblasts can be assumed *not* to have been removed by

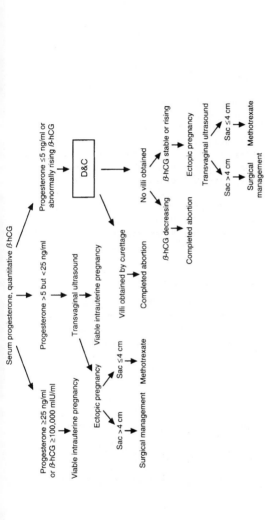

Fig. 14-2 Algorithm for the diagnosis of unruptured ectopic pregnancy without laparoscopy. Progesterone measurements increase the sensitivity of the algorithm by inexpensively screening large numbers of patients during the first trimester of pregnancy. The definitive diagnosis is made by transvaginal ultrasound or uterine curettage and does not depend on the serum progesterone concentrations obtained during screening. (From Carson SA, Buster JE: The ectopic pregnancy: new advances in diagnosis and treatment. N Engl J Med 329:1174, 1993, with permission.)

the uterine curettage; thus an ectopic pregnancy can be presumed to be present.

Surgical Treatment

Salpingectomy by laparotomy has long offered almost a 100 percent cure. However, current emphasis is not just to prevent death but also to facilitate rapid recovery, preserve fertility, and reduce costs. Laparoscopic salpingostomy and partial salpingectomy are thus rapidly replacing laparotomy. Laparotomy should be performed only when a laparoscopic approach is too difficult, the surgeon is not trained in operative laparoscopy, or the patient is hemodynamically unstable.

Linear salpingostomy is the standard laparoscopic operation when an ectopic mass is unruptured yet more than 4 cm in length by ultrasound.[147,153–157] Over the bulging antimesenteric border of the implantation site, a longitudinal incision is made by electrocautery, scissors, or laser. The products of conception are removed by forceps or suction. After hemostasis is achieved, the incision is allowed to heal by secondary intention. Alternatively, sutures can be placed. Approximately 95 percent of laparoscopic salpingostomies are successful (i.e., no additional procedures are needed).[147]

Segmental resection is necessary if ectopic pregnancies are located in the isthmus (the midportion of the oviduct). Subsequent laparotomy is then necessary for reanastomosis of the surgically divided oviduct. Laparoscopic salpingectomy is also desirable for patients who do not wish to become pregnant again.

Medical Treatment

Although operative laparoscopy has substantially fewer complications than laparotomy, there remains irreducible morbidity intrinsic to surgery and anesthesia. Medical treatments can greatly reduce this morbidity. The agent used is the folic acid antagonist methotrexate, which inhibits synthesis of purines and pyrimidines and thus interferes with DNA synthesis and cell multiplication. Actively proliferating trophoblasts have long been known to be vulnerable to methotrexate, as illustrated by its successful use in the treatment of gestational trophoblastic disease.

Hemodynamically stable patients with ectopic pregnancies are eligible for treatment with methotrexate if the mass is unruptured and measures 4 cm or less in diameter by ultrasound.[147] Patients with larger ectopic masses, embryonic cardiac activity, or evidence of acute intra-abdominal bleeding (acute abdomen, hypotension, or falling hematocrit) are not eligible for methotrexate therapy.[147] Outcome of treatment with systemic methotrexate[147,161] compares favorably with that of laparoscopic salpingostomy.

High doses of methotrexate can cause bone marrow suppression, acute and chronic hepatotoxicity, stomatitis, pulmonary fibrosis, alopecia, and photosensitivity. Fortunately, these side effects are not only infrequent with the shorter treatment schedules used for an ectopic pregnancy but can be mitigated against by the administration of leucovorin (citrovorum factor). Experience with methotrexate in gestational trophoblastic disease provides little reason for concern about the risks of subsequent neoplasia or congenital anomalies in later pregnancies.[162]

Safeguards are necessary to enhance the success and minimize the toxicity of systemic methotrexate. First, the patient should undergo a pelvic examination by only a single examiner and then only once. Self-control concerning this part of management should be similar to that employed with placenta previa. Second, both physician and patient must recognize that transient pain is common, usually occurring 3 to 7 days after initiation of methotrexate therapy. The pain, presumably caused by tubal abortion, normally lasts 4 to 12 hours. Perhaps the most difficult aspect of methotrexate therapy is distinguishing the transient abdominal pain associated with successful therapy from that of rupturing ectopic pregnancy. Surgical intervention becomes necessary only when pain is accompanied by orthostatic tachycardia, hypotension, or a falling hematocrit. Because colicky abdominal pain is common during the first 2 or 3 days of methotrexate therapy, patients should be warned to avoid gas-producing foods such as leeks and cabbage. Patients should also avoid exposure to the sun because of the photosensitivity methotrexate produces.

Key Points

- Approximately 22 percent of all pregnancies detected on the basis of urinary hCG assays are lost, usually before clinical recognition.
- The clinical loss rate is 10 to 12 percent. Most of these pregnancies are lost before 8 weeks' gestation. Only 3 percent of pregnancies are lost after an ultrasonographically viable pregnancy at 8 to 9 weeks, and only 1 percent are lost after 16 weeks' gestation.
- Pregnancy losses may be recurrent; 4 percent of U.S. women experience two losses and 3 percent three or more losses. Although increasing after one loss, the

recurrence risk generally reaches no more than 25 percent after three or four losses. Loss rates for 40-year-old women are approximately twice those of 20-year-old women.

- By far the most common causes of pregnancy losses are chromosomal abnormalities. At least 50 percent of clinically recognized pregnancy losses show a chromosomal abnormality. The types of chromosomal abnormalities differ from those found in liveborns, but autosomal trisomy still accounts for 50 percent of abnormalities. A balanced translocation is present in about 5 percent of couples having repeated spontaneous abortions.

- Many other causes of repetitive abortions have been proposed, but few are proved. These include luteal phase defects and infectious processes (e.g., *Ureaplasma*). It is reasonable to evaluate couples for these conditions, but efficacy of treatment remains uncertain.

- Uterine anomalies are accepted causes of second-trimester pregnancies. Couples experiencing such losses may benefit from metroplasty or hysteroscopic resection of a uterine septum. Uterine anomalies are less common causes of first-trimester losses.

- Drugs, toxins, and physical agents are associated with spontaneous abortion, but usually not in repetitive pregnancies. Avoiding potential toxins is obviously desirable, but one should not assume that such exposures explain repetitive losses.

- LAC antibodies and aCL are clearly associated with second-trimester losses, but their role in first-trimester losses is more arguable. Controversy persists concerning the propriety of immunologic evaluations and immunotherapy for couples sharing HLA antigens or otherwise showing blunted maternal response to paternal antigens (alloimmune disease).

- The diagnosis of ectopic pregnancy can be made by ultrasound and sensitive β-hCG assays. Treatment may be surgical (linear salpingostomy performed through the laparoscope) or medical (methotrexate).

- The earlier detection of an unruptured ectopic pregnancy has greatly modified treatment. Laparotomy is now rarely necessary. Laparoscopic procedures are commonly employed, with an increase in subsequent pregnancy rates and a decrease in repeat ectopic gestations. About one-third of women with ectopic pregnancies prove eligible for medical treatment (methotrexate).

Preterm Birth

Jay D. Iams

Premature birth is the single largest cause of perinatal mortality and morbidity in nonanomalous infants in developed nations. In the United States, complications of prematurity account for more than 70 percent of fetal and neonatal deaths annually in babies without anomalies.[1] Long-term sequelae of prematurity disproportionately contribute to developmental delay, visual and hearing impairment, chronic lung disease, and cerebral palsy.[2] Advances in neonatal care during the last 30 years have led to increased survival and reduced short- and long-term morbidity for infants born before 37 weeks of pregnancy, but the rate of preterm birth has actually increased since 1970.

Efforts to identify and treat the conditions leading to prematurity have been largely disappointing, fulfilling the prophetic words of Nicholson Eastman in 1947: "Only when the factors underlying prematurity are completely understood can any intelligent attempt at prevention be made."[4]

The Problem of Prematurity

Definitions

Infants born before 37 weeks' gestation (259 days from the first day of the mother's last menstrual period, or 245 days after conception) are *premature*. *Low-birth-weight* (LBW) infants weigh less than 2,500 g at birth, regardless of gestational age. *Very-low-birth-weight* (VLBW) infants weigh less than 1,500 g at birth. Extremely low-birth-weight (ELBW) infants weigh less than 1,000 g at birth. Because gestational age and birth weight are directly correlated throughout most of gestation, birth weight has been used as an indirect indicator of gestational age in many studies, especially those in which data are obtained from poorly dated pregnancies. Interchanging the two measures has led to significant misinterpretation of data at every level of analysis, because the problems of LBW infants may be the result of prematurity in some instances, of poor intrauterine growth in others, and of both in still others. Similarly, problems due to prematurity in infants whose birth weight exceeds 2,500 g may go unrecognized because of their apparently "full-term" appearance.

The incidences of LBW and VLBW deliveries have changed little since 1975.[6] Rates of LBW and VLBW in newborn blacks are consistently about twice as high as corresponding rates for nonblacks. Even when corrected for age and educational level, black women continue to deliver more LBW infants than do white women.

Perinatal Mortality and Morbidity

Analysis of perinatal mortality and morbidity statistics has long been confounded by the various definitions of fetal, perinatal, neonatal, and infant time periods that have been used across the United States and around the world.[8] The definitions endorsed by the American College of Obstetricians and Gynecologists are used here.[9]

Significant improvements in survival rates for extremely preterm infants (26 weeks or younger) weighing less than 1,000 g have been observed in several studies. From 1988 to 1991, after the introduction of neonatal surfactant therapy, survival increased to 15 percent at 23 weeks, 56 percent at 24 weeks, and 80 percent at 25 weeks. The survival figures cited include all liveborn infants born at the reporting institutions, even those not successfully transferred from the delivery room to the nursery. Higher survival rates are reported when only neonatal unit admissions are analyzed.

Despite the marked improvement in neonatal survival over the past 40 years, the United States still compares relatively unfavorably with other developed countries with respect to neonatal mortality. This is due entirely to a small excess of preterm births in the United States. For example, reduction in preterm delivery in the United States to the rate observed in Norway would produce a perinatal mortality rate equivalent to that in Norway. The prevention of excess perinatal mortality in the United States depends more on prevention of prematurity, especially extreme prematurity, than on prevention of low birth weight.

Perinatal Morbidity

Common complications in premature infants include respiratory distress syndrome, intraventricular hemorrhage, bronchopulmonary dysplasia, patent ductus arteriosus, necrotizing enterocolitis, sepsis, apnea, and retinopathy of prematurity. Extremely preterm infants are at greatest risk.

Preterm infants are at increased risk for neurodevelopmental handicaps such as severe mental retardation, cerebral palsy, seizure disorders, blindness, and deafness. The rate of intact survival has steadily increased for VLBW and ELBW infants.

The proportion of survivors within each birth weight group who have serious handicaps has not increased since the introduction of neonatal intensive care. For infants born between 1975 and 1985, 26 percent of surviving infants with birth weights below 800 g, 17 percent of survivors with birth weights between 750 and 1,000 g, and 11 percent of survivors with birth weights between 1,000 and 1,500 g have major handicaps at 1 or 2 years of age. More moderate impairment, defined as an IQ between 70 and 80, was reported in an additional 41 percent of neonates born at less than 800 g, 31 percent born between 750 and 1,000 g, and 16 percent between 1,000 and 1,500 g birth weight.[14] These children were all born before the introduction of surfactant and aggressive use of antenatal corticosteroids.

Overview of the Pathogenesis of Prematurity

The Epidemiology of Preterm Birth

The list of maternal and fetal diagnoses antecedent to preterm deliveries is indeed long and broad: preterm labor, preterm ruptured membranes, preeclampsia, abruptio placenta, multiple gestation, placenta previa, fetal growth retardation, excessive or inadequate amniotic fluid volume, fetal anomalies, amnionitis, and incompetent cervix. Maternal medical problems such as diabetes, asthma, drug abuse, and pyelonephritis may all lead to preterm delivery. Maternal characteristics that have been associated with an increased risk of preterm delivery are also diverse: maternal black race, low socioeconomic status, poor nutrition, low pre-pregnancy weight, a history of previous preterm birth, inadequate prenatal care, age less than 18 or more than 40, strenuous work, high personal stress, anemia, cigarette smoking, bacteriuria, cervical injury or abnormality, uterine anomaly or fibroids, excessive uterine contractility, and premature cervical dilation.

Spontaneous Versus Indicated Preterm Delivery

The multitude of clinical disorders and risk factors has been organized into two broad categories called *spontaneous* and *indicated* preterm birth. Approximately 75 percent of preterm births occur spontaneously after preterm labor (PTL) or preterm premature rupture of membranes (preterm PROM). The *spontaneous preterm delivery* category also includes deliveries after amnionitis and patients with incompetent cervix. *Indicated preterm births* follow medical or obstetric disorders that place the fetus at risk (e.g., acute or chronic maternal hypertension, diabetes, placenta previa or abruption, and intrauterine growth restriction).

The Epidemiology of Spontaneous Preterm Birth

More than one-half of spontaneous preterm births (SPTBs) occur in women who have no *apparent* risk factors. The recurrence risk rises as the number of prior preterm births increases and increases still further as the gestational age of the prior preterm birth decreases.

It is helpful to look at risk factors as either unique to the affected pregnancy and therefore nonrecurrent or as potentially operative in successive pregnancies. Risk factors such as placenta previa and abruption, polyhydramnios and oligohydramnios, second-trimester bleeding, and multiple gestation typically are not recurrent. Risk factors that may be expected to influence successive pregnancies may be immutable (e.g., a history of preterm delivery, black race) or recurrent but potentially amenable to intervention (e.g., maternal genital tract colonization, reduced cervical competence, uterine malformations, poor nutritional status, or maternal work).

A history of prior preterm birth predicts recurrent SPTB in 15 to 80 percent of subsequent pregnancies and the most recent birth is the most predictive (Table 15-1). The likelihood of recurrent preterm birth also increases as the number of prior preterm births increases. Nevertheless, most women with a prior preterm birth do not deliver another preterm baby.

Infection and Prematurity

There have been numerous reports of an association between preterm birth and infection.[37,38] Positive amniotic fluid cultures have been reported in 20 to 30 percent of women with preterm labor[39-41] and espe-

Table 15-1   Risk of Preterm Birth According to Obstetric History

| First Birth | Second Birth | Number | Subsequent/Preterm Birth | |
			Percent	Relative Risk
Term	—	25,817	4.4	1.0
Preterm	—	1,860	17.2	3.9
Term	Term	24,689	2.6	0.6
Preterm	Term	1,540	5.7	1.3
Term	Preterm	1,128	11.1	2.5
Preterm	Preterm	320	28.4	6.5

From Bakketeig LS, Hoffman HJ: Epidemiology of preterm birth: results from a longitudinal study of births in Norway. *In* Elder LS, Hendricks CH (eds): Preterm Labor. Boston, Butterworths, 1981, p 17, with permission.

cially in women whose preterm labor was refractory to tocolytic drugs.[42] The incidences of maternal and neonatal infections following preterm birth is higher than for term birth.

Microbiologic studies have observed an association between preterm birth and maternal vaginal colonization with bacterial vaginosis. Treatment of bacterial vaginosis with metronidazole has reduced the rate of preterm birth in one controlled trial.

Infections, Contractions, and the Cervix

The National Institute of Child Health and Human Development (NICHD) Preterm Birth Prediction Study, a prospective observational study of risk factors for SPTB, collected demographic and medical–obstetric information about nearly 3,000 subjects who were representative of the population at 10 participating university centers. Serial cervical and vaginal cultures,[49] digital and transvaginal ultrasound examinations of the cervix,[56] and an assay for the presence of oncofetal fibronectin (fFN) in cervical and vaginal secretions[61] were obtained at regular intervals between 24 and 34 weeks of pregnancy. Fibronectin is an extracellular matrix protein that is best described as the "glue" that attaches the fetal membranes to the underlying uterine decidua.[62] Fibronectin is normally found in the cervicovaginal secretions before 20 to 22 weeks of pregnancy and again at the end of normal pregnancy as labor approaches. It is not normally present in cervicovaginal secretions between 22 and 37 weeks.

The strongest predictors of SPTB were, in decreasing order, cervicovaginal fFN,[59] transvaginal sonographic cervical length,[56] an obstetric history of previous preterm birth,[25] and presence of bacterial vaginosis.[49] fFN was strongly correlated with the presence of bacterial vaginosis, almost completely predicting which subjects with bacterial vaginosis were at risk for SPTB.

Sonographic cervical length and obstetric history were also strongly and continuously correlated with each other and with the risk of SPTB in a *continuous* manner.[58] That is, for subjects with a history of prior SPTB, the risk of recurrent SPTB increased as the gestational age at the time of the prior PTB decreased. The length of the cervix as measured by transvaginal sonography was inversely and continuously related to the likelihood of SPTB in the current pregnancy and to a history of SPTB, especially for SPTB before 32 weeks' gestation. Cervical length is a marker for the functional ability of the cervix to resist delivery and that cervical competence operates as a continuum. If the cervix is a structure with degrees of "competence," then cervical incompetence may not be a distinct disorder but instead may be viewed as the end of a spectrum.

Diagnosis and Treatment of Spontaneous Preterm Birth

Clinical decision-making for patients with impending preterm delivery is based on a careful assessment of the risks for both mother and infant of continuing the pregnancy versus delivery.

Diagnosis of Preterm Labor

The diagnosis of PTL is traditionally made by the combination of persistent uterine contractions and change in the dilatation and/or effacement of the cervix by digital examination.[74] Randomized trials of drugs to arrest PTL have found that approximately 40 percent of subjects diagnosed by these criteria and treated with placebo will deliver at term.[75] False-negative diagnosis is also a significant problem. One study found an 18 percent rate of preterm birth in women who were sent home without treatment after evaluation for possible PTL.[76]

Difficulty in accurate diagnosis is the product of the high prevalence of the symptoms and signs of early PTL among normal healthy women and the imprecision of the digital examination of the cervix. Symptoms of PTL are nonspecific and *are not necessarily those of labor at term*. Women treated for PTL may report symptoms of pelvic pressure, an increase in vaginal discharge, backache, and menstrual-like cramps, all of which may occur in normal pregnancy. Contractions may be painful or painless and may be distinguished from the normal contractions of pregnancy (Braxton-Hicks contractions) only by their persistence.

Contraction frequency can also be misleading. A prospective study[78] of uterine contractions in normal pregnancies in 109 low-risk subjects, who all delivered at term and who were monitored for 24 hours twice weekly from 20 weeks until delivery, found a wide variation in contraction frequency according to gestational age and time of day. A strong clustering of contractions occurred at night and became more pronounced after 24 weeks. Uterine contraction frequency was decreased following maternal rest and increased after coitus in this study. Prior to 37 weeks' gestation, as many as seven contractions per hour fell within two standard deviations above the 95th percentile, depending on the time of day. Therefore, contraction frequency alone can be seen to be insufficient to establish the diagnosis of PTL.

Although digital assessment of cervical dilation of at least 3 cm is relatively straightforward, assessment of dilation of less than 3 cm, effacement, and cervical consistency (soft or firm) are highly subjective. Softening of the lower segment and effacement are more predictive of impending labor than are other features of the cervical examination, including dilatation.

A number of studies have reported that failed tocolysis, defined as delivery within 24 to 48 hours despite tocolysis, was associated with cervical dilatation above 3 cm at presentation. Thus patients with persistent contractions whose cervix is effaced at least 80 percent and dilated more than 2 cm should be treated without waiting for additional information. A retrospective study of 209 patients with PTL[81] suggested that, for patients whose initial digital examination was 2 cm or less, there was no change in perinatal outcome if treatment was initiated only after obvious change in dilatation.

Two new methods of improving the accuracy of diagnosis in symptomatic women have been reported: transvaginal sonography to measure cervical length, and the presence of fetal fibronectin in cervicovaginal fluid.

Cervical Sonography

Transabdominal sonographic measurement of cervical length is affected variably by maternal body habitus and bladder filling and is not possible in many patients. Transvaginal sonography performed with an empty maternal bladder is unaffected by maternal habitus and provides satisfactory images in more than 95 percent of subjects. Cervical sonography appears to be useful in excluding preterm labor in some patients and in making a positive diagnosis in others. A cervical length of 30 mm or more by transvaginal sonography is good evidence that significant effacement has not occurred (30 mm is approximately the 25th percentile of length).

Fibronectin

A clinical assay for fetal fibronectin was approved by the FDA in 1995 as an aid in the diagnosis of preterm labor. The presence of fFN in the cervix or vagina after the 20th week is abnormal and may indicate disruption of the attachment of the membranes to the decidua. Fibronectin reappears in cervicovaginal secretions as labor approaches at term.

Fibronectin is superior to the traditional methods of diagnosis of PTL in predicting SPTB within 7 days of presentation. Fibronectin has superior sensitivity, specificity, and predictive values compared with contraction frequency, cervical dilation more than 1 cm, and vaginal bleeding.

The clinical utility of the fibronectin assay lies primarily in the negative predictive value as a test to avoid overdiagnosis and unnecessary treatment. It may also improve sensitivity by identifying additional women who may benefit from further observation and/or treatment.

Experience with combined use of the fibronectin assay and cervical sonography in clinical practice is limited but suggests that the two tests are complementary. A positive fibronectin assay indicates the presence of an acute process that may lead to SPTB within 7 to 14 days in 15 to 30 percent of symptomatic women, while sonographic cervical length measurement correlates best with risk of SPTB at less than 35 weeks. Fibronectin appears to be the better test for acute risk. The likelihood that this process will in fact progress to preterm birth may in part be a function of the sonographic cervical length. A positive fibronectin assay is more likely to be associated with preterm delivery in women with a short cervix. Both a long cervix (more than 30 mm by transvaginal ultrasound) and a negative fibronectin assay have excellent negative predictive value for preterm delivery in symptomatic women. A short cervix with a negative fibronectin assay suggests that labor is not currently present but would be difficult to arrest if it did occur.

Treatment of Preterm Labor

Goals of Treatment

Once diagnosed, the ultimate goal of therapy for PTL is delivery at term of an infant who suffers none of the sequelae of prematurity. Treatment with tocolytic drugs has not been shown to reduce premature delivery for treated subjects. However, tocolytics can delay delivery for at least 48 hours. The immediate goals of tocolytic therapy are sufficient delay in delivery to allow antepartum transfer of the mother to the most appropriate hospital, treatment of underlying causes of PTL (e.g., maternal pyelonephritis), and corticosteroid treatment. Both antepartum maternal transport and steroid therapy have been shown to reduce neonatal morbidity and mortality.

The following sections describe the parenteral ad-

Clinical Evaluation of Patients With Possible Preterm Labor

1. Patient presents with signs/symptoms suggesting preterm labor:
   - Persistent contractions (painful or painless)
   - Intermittent abdominal cramping, pelvic pressure, or backache
   - Increase or change in vaginal discharge
   - Vaginal spotting or bleeding

2. Sterile speculum examination for pH, fern, pooled fluid, cultures for group B Streptococcus (outer one-third of vagina and perineum), *Chlamydia* (cervix), and *N. gonorrhoeae* (cervix), and fibronectin swab (external cervical os and posterior fornix, avoiding areas with bleeding)

3. Transabdominal ultrasound examination for placental location, amniotic fluid volume, estimated fetal weight and presentation, and fetal well-being

4. Digital examination (if preterm PROM ruled out by above):
   - Cervix ≥ 3 cm dilatation: The diagnosis of PTL confirmed. Candidate for tocolysis.
   Cervix 2–3 cm dilatation: The diagnosis of PTL likely but not established. Assay fibronectin and monitor contraction frequency. Repeat digital examination 30–60 minutes. Candidate for tocolysis if any cervical change, contractions increase in frequency, or fibronectin is positive.
   - Cervix < 2 cm dilatation: The diagnosis of PTL uncertain. Monitor contraction frequency, assay fibronectin, and repeat digital examination in 1–2 hours. Candidate for tocolysis if there is a 1-cm change in cervical dilatation or if fibronectin is positive.

5. Treatments for symptomatic fibronectin-positive results:
   - Parenteral tocolysis
   - Maternal transfer
   - Steroids
   - Hospitalize × 3–7 days
   - Group B Streptococcus prophylaxis

6. Treatments for symptomatic fibronectin-negative
   results:
   - Parenteral tocolysis begun (cx ≥2 cm)
     Risk of delivery ≤7 days = 1.7%–3.5%
     Conclude course of tocolysis
     Reduce hospital stay
   - Tocolysis not begun
     Risk of delivery ≤7 days = 0%–1.8%
     Observe in outpatient setting
   - Cervical sonography should be considered in
     these patients to assess risk of SPTB.

ministration of current tocolytic drugs. The use of these agents in oral form following the acute care of an episode of PTL is not advised because of the absence of evidence of effectiveness in prolonging pregnancy.

The β-Mimetic Tocolytics

Ritodrine is the only agent approved by the FDA for use as a tocolytic. Terbutaline is marketed in the United

Contraindications to Tocolysis

Maternal contraindications to tocolysis
    Significant hypertension (eclampsia, severe pre-
        eclampsia, chronic hypertension)
    Antepartum hemorrhage
    Cardiac disease

Fetal contraindications to tocolysis
    Gestational age ≥ 37 weeks
    Advanced dilatation/effacement
    Birth weight ≥ 2,500 g
    Demise or lethal anomaly
    Chorioamnionitis
    In utero fetal compromise
    - Acute: fetal distress
    - Chronic: intrauterine growth retardation, or
      substance abuse

States only as a drug for asthma but is widely used as a tocolytic.

Efficacy of β-Mimetics

There is good evidence that β-mimetic agents are successful in prolonging pregnancy for at least 48 hours. The trials were conducted prior to the introduction of neonatal surfactant therapy and at a time when antepartum use of corticosteroids was infrequent. A large multicenter Canadian prospective randomized trial of ritodrine reported a reduction in deliveries within 2 to 7 days of diagnosis, but there was no significant difference in births before 37 weeks or before 32 weeks.

There is a consensus that short-term tocolysis with these agents is effective in delaying delivery long enough to allow maternal transport and to administer steroids and antibiotics for group B streptococcal prophylaxis.

Pharmacokinetics of Ritodrine

The therapeutic blood level of ritodrine varies according to the degree of uterine activity rather than to cervical dilatation or status of the membranes.[93] Actual serum ritodrine levels vary greatly at a given infusion rate. Serum ritodrine levels reach 75 percent of maximum levels within 20 minutes of a constant intravenous infusion.[94] The manufacturer's recommended protocol for intravenous therapy starts at 0.1 mg (100 μg) per minute and is increased by 0.05 mg (50 μg) every 10 minutes until contractions cease, side effects occur, or the maximum rate (0.35 mg [350 μg]/min) is reached. The infusion is then maintained at the effective level for 12 hours after contractions cease.[95] Side effects occur most often when the infusion rate and concentration of ritodrine are increasing, and the rate of change in the infusion rate or drug concentration was more important than absolute drug level.[94] An alternate protocol uses as little drug as necessary, starting at 50 μg/min and increasing by 50 μg/min every 20 minutes only if contractions are more frequent than every 10 minutes. The dose may exceed 350 μg/min in some patients if the maternal pulse remains below 110 bpm, as some of these individuals are exhibiting rapid clearance of the drug. Once labor is stopped, the infusion rate is maintained for 1 hour and then reduced every 20 minutes to the lowest rate that inhibits contractions adequately. This rate is then maintained for 12 hours.

A single intramuscular injection of 5 to 10 mg of ritodrine results in labor-inhibiting concentrations with clinically insignificant cardiovascular effects. The intramuscular route is preferable for women who are being transferred to another hospital.

Terbutaline

Pharmacokinetics. At infusion rates above 5 µg/min, this drug can be accumulated with raised serum levels and increased symptoms,[94] probably reflecting the longer half-life of terbutaline over ritodrine. The onset of action is rapid with both intravenous bolus (1 to 2 minutes) and subcutaneous (3 to 5 minutes) administration.

Dosage. Currently published protocols often employ subcutaneous administration, with the usual dose being 0.25 mg (250 µg) every 3 hours.[97] Intravenous administration is begun at 2.5 µg/min and increased by 2.5 µg/min every 20 minutes until a maximum of 17.5 to 20 µg/min is reached.[98]

Tachyphylaxis with β-Mimetic Drugs

Tachyphylaxis, or desensitization, of the adrenergic receptor occurs throughout the body after prolonged exposure to β-agonists. Animal studies suggest that contractions resume after only several hours of *continuous* intravenous therapy with high-dose β-mimetic therapy; the myometrium remains quiescent longer with *pulsatile* administration of lower doses of the same tocolytic agent.[99]

Side Effects and Complications of Parenteral β-Mimetic Tocolysis

Maternal side effects of the β-adrenergic agonists are common and diverse, as shown in Table 15-2. Serious maternal cardiopulmonary and metabolic complications have been reported, including maternal death when β-adrenergic agents were given to mothers with unrecognized cardiac disease. A thorough history and review of possible cardiac symptoms before initiating treatment and prompt attention to any patient with persistent symptoms during treatment are important in preventing these complications.

Pulmonary Edema. Pulmonary edema is the most serious complication of tocolytic therapy and can often be prevented. Evaluation of cardiac function with Swan-Ganz catheters or echocardiography has failed to demonstrate left ventricular failure in cases of pulmonary edema.[106] Noncardiogenic causes that may be important are decreased colloid oncotic pressure and in-

Table 15-2   Side Effects and Complications of β-Mimetic Tocolysis

Maternal	Fetal and Neonatal
Physiologic	Fetal
Apprehension	Tachycardia
Jitteriness	Cardiac arrhythmia
Headache	Myocardial and septal
Nausea and vomiting	hypertrophy
Fever	Myocardial ischemia
Hallucinations	Heart failure
Metabolic	Hyperglycemia
Hyperglycemia	Hyperinsulinemia
Hyperinsulinemia	Death
Hyperlactic acidemia	Neonatal
Hypokalemia	Tachycardia
Hypocalcemia	Hypoglycemia
Antidiuresis, water retention	Hypocalcemia
Altered thyroid function	Hyperbilirubinemia
Elevated transaminases	Tachycardia
Cardiac	Myocardial ischemia
Tachycardia	Hypotension
Pulmonary edema	Intraventricular
Hypotension	hemorrhage
Arrhythmias/palpitations	Decreased myocardial
Heart failure	contractility
Myocardial ischemia, altered	
ECG and chest pain	
Shortness of breath	
Other	
Skin rash	
Pruritis	
Ileus	
Death (cardiac)	

Data from Hill WC: Risks and complications of tocolysis. Clin Obstet Gynecol 38:725, 1995, with permission.

creased pulmonary vascular permeability, especially when premature labor is associated with amnionitis. In one study, tocolysis for PTL was associated with a higher incidence of pulmonary edema in the presence of maternal infection (21 percent) than when it was absent (1 percent).[107]

It is uncommon for pulmonary edema to develop in the first 24 hours of β-mimetic therapy; 90 percent of reported cases of pulmonary edema occur after 24 hours of therapy. Recommendations to avoid pulmonary edema related to tocolytic treatment are outlined in the box.

Myocardial Ischemia and Cardiac Dysrhythmias. Symptomatic cardiac dysrhythmias and symptomatic

Recommendations To Avoid Tocolytic-Related Pulmonary Edema

1. Restrict fluid intake to 2.5 liters/day (total IV and PO)

2. Limit salt content of fluids (avoid saline or Ringer's lactated solution)

3. Restrict total dose and length of intravenous β-mimetic therapy

4. Respect contraindications to β-mimetic use

myocardial ischemia and infarction have occurred during β-agonist tocolytic therapy. If a patient develops chest pain during therapy, one should discontinue the β-mimetic and administer oxygen.

Hypotension. The β-mimetics in current use produce a mild (5 to 10 mm Hg) fall in diastolic blood pressure. However, the extensive peripheral vasodilatation makes it difficult for the patient to mount a normal, vasoconstrictive response to hypovolemia and so β-mimetics are dangerous in the face of antepartum hemorrhage. Another is that the important early signs of excessive blood loss, such as maternal and fetal tachycardia, are masked by these drugs.[104]

Hyperglycemia and Hypokalemia. β-Mimetic agents compound the problems of patients with overt or gestational diabetes mellitus. Increased glycogenolysis with resultant hyperglycemia markedly increases the risk of ketoacidosis.[110] These drugs should in general be avoided in women with diabetes. If it is absolutely necessary to use β-mimetics, a simultaneous intravenous insulin infusion should be employed. In the nondiabetic woman, β-mimetics will cause a significant increase in serum glucose level, although rarely over 180 mg/dl.[98] β-Mimetics also lead to potassium flux from plasma into cells, thereby causing a fall in serum measurements without a change in excretion. Hence there is no change in total body potassium. After 24 hours of therapy, both the serum glucose and potassium levels will have begun to return to baseline even without specific therapy.[111] No potassium replacement is needed unless the serum potassium level falls below 2.5 mEq/L.

Neonatal Side Effects of β-Mimetics. β-Mimetic tocolysis has been linked to an increased risk of neonatal intraventricular hemorrhage. Neonatal hypoglycemia, hypocalcemia, and ileus have also been reported with β-mimetics and can be clinically significant if the maternal infusion is not discontinued more than 2 hours before delivery.[113] With all tocolytic drugs, adverse neonatal effects are greatest when the fetus is born close to a period of high-dose parenteral therapy.[114] These drugs should be discontinued when there is advanced cervical dilatation and delivery appears inevitable.

Magnesium Sulfate

Efficacy

The efficacy of magnesium as a tocolytic agent has been studied in relatively few trials that enrolled relatively few subjects. Randomized studies of magnesium compared with β-mimetics[118,119] found no differences in tocolytic effect.

Dosage

Magnesium sulfate must be administered parenterally in order to elevate serum levels above the normal range. Therapeutic dosage is similar to that used for intravenous treatment of preeclampsia: a 4- to 6-g loading dose given over 20 minutes, followed by an infusion of 2 to 4 g/hr, until contractions cease.[117] Serum magnesium levels alone should not serve as the endpoint of therapy. The drug should be titrated on the basis of clinical efficacy or maternal toxicity. Deep tendon reflexes should be checked regularly. One study suggested that stopping the drug was more effective than weaning in preventing recurrences of PTL. Excess magnesium is rapidly excreted by the kidney, provided there is normal renal function. Should there be any evidence of renal impairment, the patient should be followed with serum levels and doses adjusted accordingly. Magnesium sulfate should not be used in patients with myasthenia gravis.

Maternal Side Effects

Flushing, nausea, vomiting, headache, generalized muscle weakness including especially complaints of diplopia and shortness of breath, and pulmonary edema have all been reported. Magnesium sulfate, however, is tolerated better than ritodrine. It has therefore become the tocolytic agent of choice in a number of major medical centers. There can be, however, major and life-threatening complications with magnesium therapy, including chest pain and pulmonary edema (1 percent).

Neonatal Side Effects

Although magnesium crosses the placenta and achieves serum levels comparable to maternal levels, serious neonatal complications are uncommon. Lethargy, hypotonia, and even respiratory depression may occur.

Indomethacin

Prostaglandins are important mediators of the final pathways of uterine muscle contraction. Inhibition of cyclooxygenase by nonsteroidal anti-inflammatory drugs (NSAIDs) leads to reduced synthesis of prostaglandins. Indomethacin is the most widely used agent in this class.

Efficacy. Indomethacin has been reported to be effective in two small randomized, placebo-controlled trials. Indomethacin has significantly fewer maternal side effects when compared with ritodrine.

Dosage

Indomethacin is well absorbed orally or per rectum. The usual dose is a 50-mg loading dose by mouth or 50 to 100 mg per rectum if the patient cannot tolerate the oral dose. Subsequently, 25 mg is administered orally every 6 hours. Therapy is usually limited to 2 days because of concern about fetal side effects.

Maternal Side Effects

The principal advantage of this agent is the relative infrequency of serious maternal side effects when the agent is used in a brief course of tocolysis. Gastrointestinal side effects such as nausea and heartburn are the most common but are usually mild. More serious complications include gastrointestinal bleeding, alterations in coagulation, thrombocytopenia, and asthma in aspirin-sensitive patients. Hypertensive women may experience acute increased blood pressure after indomethacin treatment. Drugs of this class are antipyretic agents and may obscure a clinically significant fever. Maternal contraindications to indomethacin tocolysis include renal or hepatic disease, active peptic ulcer disease, poorly controlled hypertension, asthma, and coagulation disorders.

Fetal and Neonatal Side Effects

The potential for fetal and neonatal complications of indomethacin tocolysis is worrisome. In actual practice, serious complications have been rare. Three principal side effects of indomethacin have been of concern: constriction of the ductus arteriosus, oligohydramnios, and neonatal pulmonary hypertension. Tricuspid regurgitation occurs in some fetuses but all ductal abnormalities resolve within 24 hours after the medication is discontinued. The likelihood of ductal constriction increases after 32 weeks of pregnancy.[134] Ductal constriction is usually transient and responds to discontinuation of the drug. However, persistent ductal constriction and right heart failure have been reported after prolonged therapy.

Oligohydramnios associated with indomethacin tocolysis is dose related and reversible. The oligohydramnios is a consequence of reduced fetal urine production due to reduction by indomethacin of the normal prostaglandin inhibition of antidiuretic hormone.

Primary pulmonary hypertension in the neonate is a potentially fatal illness that has also been associated with prolonged (more than 48 hours) indomethacin therapy.[138,139] Primary neonatal pulmonary hypertension has not been reported with 24 to 48 hours of therapy, but the incidence may be as high as 5 to 10 percent with long-term therapy.[132]

Other complications, including necrotizing enterocolitis, small bowel perforation, patent ductus arteriosus, jaundice, and intraventricular hemorrhage, have been observed when indomethacin was used outside of standardized protocols that did not limit the duration of treatment and/or employed the drug after 32 weeks,[140] and employed multiple tocolytics. Several follow-up studies of children treated in utero with indomethacin have not found significant long-term effects.

Because of the effect on fetal urine production and amniotic fluid volume, indomethacin may be an appropriate tocolytic when PTL is associated with polyhydramnios. Several studies report successful treatment of PTL with indomethacin for patients with polyhydramnios and for polyhydramnios without labor.[146–150]

Calcium Channel Blockers

Nifedipine and nicardipine more selectively inhibit uterine contractions than verapamil. These drugs are rapidly absorbed via oral or sublingual administration, and the duration of action of a single dose can be as long as 6 hours.

Several reports have compared nifedipine with either ritodrine or terbutaline. In each trial, nifedipine was equal or superior to the β-mimetic agents in delaying delivery with fewer side effects.

Dosage

Nifedipine is usually given as a 10- to 20-mg dose every 6 hours orally. Patients in active PTL may be given a loading dose of 10 mg sublingually every 20 minutes for up to three doses, followed by oral administration every 6 hours.

Side Effects. Maternal cardiovascular side effects of the calcium channel blockers are similar to but milder than those with the β-mimetics. A mild decrease in blood pressure and a rise in pulse have been noted by most authors, with occasional cases of significant hypotension.[155] Nifedipine is not associated with a decrease in serum potassium, although modest increases in glucose have been noted. Maternal symptoms are infrequent but include headache, flushing, dizziness, and nausea.

Treatment with Multiple Tocolytics

Sustained treatment with the combination of magnesium and a β-mimetic has been found to increase the risk of significant side effects and should be avoided. Patients who fail the first agent can be switched to the other. Initial success rates are comparable at approximately 70 percent for either ritodrine or magnesium sulfate, and most women who fail the initial agent respond favorably to the alternative. The combination of magnesium and calcium channel blockers may lead to skeletal muscle blockade.

Ancillary Treatment for Women with Preterm Labor

The initial goal of treatment of women with PTL is to delay delivery long enough to allow three interventions that have been shown to reduce the neonatal morbidity and mortality:

1. Transfer of mother and fetus to a hospital equipped to care for a premature infant
2. Administration of glucocorticoids to reduce neonatal respiratory distress syndrome and intraventricular hemorrhage
3. Administration of antibiotic prophylaxis to prevent neonatal group B Streptococcus infection

Maternal and Neonatal Transfer

Regionalization of neonatal intensive care and maternal perinatal care has been shown to improve the rates of morbidity and mortality for LBW and especially for VLBW infants. Transfer of the mother with fetus in utero is the preferred alternative whenever possible.

Antenatal Glucocorticoids

Numerous studies have confirmed the beneficial effects of maternal steroid treatment in reducing newborn respiratory distress syndrome, intraventricular hemorrhage and necrotizing enterocolitis, and, most importantly, in decreasing perinatal mortality. Antenatal steroids enhance cell differentiation and maturation rather than cell growth. Two essentially identical glucocorticoid regimens are equally effective; betamethasone 12 mg IM qd for two doses or dexamethasone 6 mg IM q12h for four doses. Prednisone may not be effective because of poor placental transfer and should not be considered effective for this indication.

A 50 percent reduction in respiratory distress syndrome occurs in steroid-treated neonates. Some questions remain about the efficacy of steroids in reducing respiratory distress syndrome in patients with preterm PROM, but the magnitude and the consistency of the benefit across multiple trials have eliminated any doubt of efficacy of antenatal steroids in reducing respiratory distress syndrome in patients with intact membranes. Steroids are effective in infants across a wide range of gestational ages from 24 through 34 weeks, and may still have some benefit up till the 37th week. Maternal steroid treatment has been shown to ameliorate the severity of RDS when it does occur. The effects of steroids and surfactant have been found to be additive for infants who receive both treatments. Antenatal steroid treatment is associated with a 50 percent reduction in the incidence of intraventricular hemorrhage.

Other Effects. Antenatal steroid treatment has been associated with other favorable effects on neonatal outcome, including a 65 percent reduction in the incidence of necrotizing enterocolitis, patent ductus arteriosus, and a 40 percent reduction in early neonatal mortality.

Risks. The major short-term concern is the risk of reduced resistance to infection for both the mother and infant. Neither of the two largest studies[172,186] noted any increased incidence of neonatal or maternal infections. Another short-term result of prenatal glucocorticoid therapy is impairment of maternal glucose tolerance, particularly in a woman with insulin-dependent diabetes. To prevent ketoacidosis, these patients may require management with insulin infusions for several days. In most patients without diabetes, the hyperglycemic effect of glucocorticoids is limited to 2 to 3 days.

There is no evidence of delayed adverse effects after in utero therapy. The original cohort of fetuses treated before 1972 have displayed no differences when compared with gestational age-matched controls in physical or mental function.

Questions regarding the need for and risk of repeated weekly courses of steroids remain unanswered. A weekly reassessment of the need for steroids, rather than a policy of routinely administering steroids each week to high-risk patients, is probably the wisest course.

Antibiotics for Women with Preterm Labor

The indication for antibiotics in women with PTL is prophylaxis of neonatal group B streptococcal infection, an intervention that is clearly effective. Administration of antibiotics to women being treated for PTL has not improved efficacy of tocolysis.

Problems and Controversies with Tocolytic Therapy

Persistent Contractions Despite Maximum Dose Therapy

Persistent contractions despite aggressive and prolonged tocolysis may occur at the opposite ends of the spectrum of PTL. The most common reason is an inaccurate diagnosis of PTL, in which contractions persist but the cervix does not change. The availability of fibronectin and cervical sonography has provided methods to reassure these patients that their contractions do not indicate the presence of PTL. Persistent contractions may also indicate an underlying stimulus such as chorioamnionitis or abruption.

Who Needs an Amniocentesis?

Evaluation of amniotic fluid for fetal pulmonary maturity studies is especially helpful when the gestational age is in doubt or when the size of the fetus suggests poor or excessive intrauterine growth. Amniotic fluid glucose, Gram stain, and culture may be indicated when infection is suspected because of maternal fever, leukocytosis, or persistent contractions. Amniocentesis should also be considered prior to corticosteroid treatment of patients after 34 weeks.

What Is the Role of Home Uterine Activity Monitoring After Preterm Labor?

Several trials of home uterine activity monitoring (HUAM) after preterm labor found no advantage to monitored contraction data compared with self-palpation and frequent nursing contact.[210,211] In these studies, the monitored contraction data were typically used to adjust the dose of oral β-mimetic drugs to suppress contractions. The inability to demonstrate an advantage for patients who used the home monitor in these studies may be explained in part by the ineffectiveness of oral tocolysis, as described in the following section.

Oral Tocolytic Treatment: Is There a Role for Oral Tocolytic Medications After Parenteral Therapy?

Use of oral tocolytic medication after suppression of an acute episode of PTL is not supported by existing literature. Two meta-analyses[213,214] of randomized controlled trials of oral β-mimetics, the drugs most frequently prescribed, found no reduction in preterm birth, no prolongation of pregnancy, and no reduction in recurrent PTL associated with this treatment. The FDA has withdrawn its approval for oral ritodrine. Also, studies[111,216] have documented a clear deterioration in glucose tolerance with more than 5 days of oral terbutaline.

The dosages of oral β-mimetics and magnesium do not achieve levels in the blood comparable to levels produced by parenteral therapy.[217] Treatment with oral β-mimetic agents for more than 2 to 3 weeks is associated with tachyphylaxis, a decreased pharmacologic effect caused by down-regulation of the β-receptor after prolonged use.

Abnormal Cervical Competence

The diagnosis of incompetent cervix has traditionally been made and is still most confidently established by an obstetric history of passive and painless dilatation of the cervix in the second trimester. A history of the amniotic sac found bulging through a well-effaced and partially dilated cervix in the absence of contractions, bleeding, infection, or amniorrhexis is classic but is not common. There are many other women who present for care in the second trimester with uterine cramps, leaking amniotic fluid, chorioamnionitis, or even bleeding, and whose cervical dilatation and effacement seem out of proportion to the duration and/or severity of the presenting complaints.

The same cervical changes (shortened cervix, funneled internal os) that are associated with increased risk of SPTB have also been described in women who present with typical cervical incompetence.[224] The only difference is duration of pregnancy at the time of examination.

The cervix is of *variable* competence, and cervical function is described by a bell-shaped curve that roughly corresponds to length. Women with cervical lengths below the 5th or 10th percentile clearly have the greatest risk for SPTB, but the clinical presentation is not uniform. Some will present with PTL, others with preterm PROM, and still others with the classic picture of incompetent cervix. The importance of reduced cervical "competence" as a contributing factor in the pathogenesis of preterm delivery increases as the gestational age at the time of delivery decreases. Cervical resistance to delivery is a continuous variable, but so also are the factors favoring delivery, such as uterine volume and contractile activity and infectious insults. For example, a cervix at the 10th to 25th percentiles of length may be adequate for a singleton pregnancy in a woman who does not perform manual labor but inadequate to resist delivery in a twin pregnancy in a woman who works 60 hours per week as a house officer.

Length Versus Competence

Cervical length alone is not sufficient to determine the function of the cervix in pregnancy. The ratio of muscle to collagen has been shown to be increased in women with a history of incompetent cervix.[225] Women with a history of cervical cone biopsy may have significant cervical shortening without increased risk of preterm birth.

Etiology

Reduced cervical competence may be congenital and/or acquired. Some women have typical histories of painless dilatation in the first and every subsequent pregnancy, while others experience progressively earlier delivery with each pregnancy until a typical "incompetent" history occurs.

Cervical trauma may occur in the course of either vaginal or cesarean delivery. Obstetric trauma may accompany dilatation and curettage for completion of spontaneous or induced abortion. The current practice of pretreating nulliparous patients with *Laminaria*, using local anesthesia, and using tapered cervical dilators before dilatation and curettage has greatly reduced cervical trauma. Depending on the amount of tissue removed, cervical cone biopsy may lead to reduced cervical competence.

Congenital structural changes in the cervix can occur in association with müllerian uterine malformations or after diethylstilbestrol exposure. We have followed women with prior conization, müllerian anomalies, and in utero diethylstilbestrol exposure with serial transvaginal sonography and have had success in selecting candidates for cerclage when funneling or shortening below 20 mm occurs, thus limiting cerclage to relatively few patients with these risk factors.

Diagnosis

Reduced cervical competence is a clinical diagnosis marked by gradual, painless dilatation and effacement of the cervix with membranes visible through the cervix. This history establishes the diagnosis but is probably a fortuitous presentation; eventually, women with this cervical status may develop membrane rupture, labor, or even amnionitis with intact membranes. Short labors with the delivery of an immature fetus or loss of the pregnancy at progressively earlier gestational ages in successive pregnancies is characteristic of reduced competence. The use of dilators or balloons to determine cervical resistance and/or hysterosalpingograms to measure the width of the cervical canal between pregnancies have not been sensitive or specific, and digital examination of the cervix is highly subjective.

The sonographic characteristics of reduced competence are a short cervix, with a length of less than 20 mm, often but not always accompanied by funneling of the internal os. Funneling may be thought of as "effacement in progress": the process proceeds from the inside out, beginning at the internal os and moving caudad. Local or coordinated uterine activity may accompany the funneling of the internal os, but more commonly there is no palpable or measurable uterine contraction.

A diagnosis of reduced cervical competence may be made prior to pregnancy if a typical history of painless dilatation and effacement of the cervix in a prior pregnancy can be documented. Women with a history of a previous second-trimester loss in which cervical sonography documented the classic picture of funneling and shortened cervical length are also candidates for prophylactic cerclage sutures. However, when the history is atypical or uncertain, it is more appropriate to follow the patient closely with frequent transvaginal ultrasound examinations beginning at 16 weeks' gestation, looking for the criteria noted above and for funneling in response to fundal pressure. Transfundal pressure may be useful in eliciting cervical funneling as an aid in making a diagnosis of incompetent cervix, as funneling does not occur in normal early pregnancies but can be seen in about half of women with a history suggestive of abnormal competence. The positive predictive value of funneling for preterm birth before 35 weeks was only 17.3 percent when funneling was noted at 24 weeks and just 11.6 percent at 28 weeks.

Cerclage Technique

Prophylactic Cerclage

In 1955, Shirodkar[233] reported successful management of cervical incompetence with the use of a submucosal band, first of fascia lata and later of mersilene, placed at the level of the internal os. This procedure, which could be performed during pregnancy, required anterior displacement of the bladder and submucosal dissection. Several years later, McDonald[234] described the use of a pursestring technique that could easily be performed during pregnancy. This approach involves either four or five "bites" as high on the cervix as possible. The knot is placed anteriorly to facilitate removal and a permanent suture is used. This operative technique is illustrated in Figure 15-1. The McDonald procedure has proved to be as effective as the Shirodkar technique[235] and requires considerably less dissection. Prophylactic cerclage sutures may be placed at 10 to 14 weeks' gestation.

After prophylactic cerclage, intercourse, prolonged standing (more than 90 minutes), and heavy lifting are not permitted. We follow these patients with periodic vaginal sonography to assess stitch location and funneling.[236-238] No additional restrictions are recommended as long as the stitches remain within the middle or upper third of the cervix without the development of a funnel, and the length of the cervix is 25 mm or longer.

Emergency Cerclage

In the setting of advanced dilatation with bulging membranes, several techniques may be helpful. Amniocentesis to remove sufficient fluid to reduce the bulging membranes (and obtain cultures) has been helpful in the most advanced cases. Overfilling the bladder with

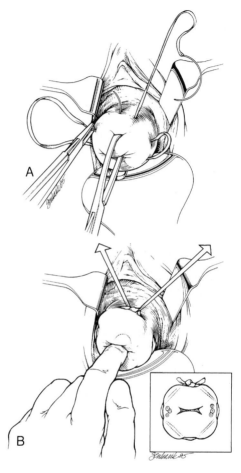

Fig. 15-1. Placement of sutures for McDonald cervical cerclage. (A), I use a double-headed Mersilene band with four "bites" in the cervix, avoiding the vessels. (B) The suture is placed high upon the cervix close to the cervical–vaginal junction, approximately the level of the internal os.

1,000 ml of saline may help by elevating the membranes out of the operative field, but may also obstruct the surgeon's view.[241] We often place a Foley catheter balloon inside the cervix and overfill it with 50 ml of saline or more to push the membranes gently out of the lower segment. The cerclage can then be placed and tied as the balloon fluid is evacuated. For patients who have a very short or amputated cervix or who have failed a vaginal suture, a transabdominal cerclage may be necessary.

Cerclage is uncommonly performed after 26 weeks' gestation. The great risk of inducing PROM or PTL and the ability to prolong gestation with bedrest and suppressive medications argue against surgical intervention in such cases.

Risks of Cerclage

Cervical injury at the time of delivery is the most commonly reported morbidity from a McDonald cerclage. While fibrous scar tissue may form at the site of the stitch, producing an abnormal labor curve, most patients will labor normally after cerclage removal.[243] A fibrous "band" may rupture, leading to a cervical laceration (1 to 13 percent), or never dilate (cervical dystocia, 2 to 5 percent), requiring cesarean birth.[227] Rarely, a laceration may extend to the broad ligament or corpus of the uterus, requiring extensive repair or even hysterectomy.

Later in the pregnancy, displacement of the suture also can occur (3 to 12 percent). A second cerclage has a much lower success rate.[227] When fluid leakage occurs in a patient with a cerclage, the suture(s) should be removed immediately[244] to reduce the risk of infection. The patient may then be managed according to protocols for preterm PROM.

Efficacy of Cervical Cerclage

The practice of cerclage was established in the era before randomized trials became standard. There has never been a randomized prospective study documenting the benefit of cerclage for women with a "classic" history of cervical incompetence. Success, defined as fetal survival, has occurred in 80 to 90 percent of the pregnancies.

Three prospective randomized trials of cerclage[220,245,246] have been conducted in patients with increased risk of preterm birth, *excluding* women with classic indications for cerclage. Two trials[245,246] found no benefit from cervical cerclage in this patient population. The third, a prospective and randomized study[220] limited to women ($n = 905$) in whom the obstetrician was uncertain about the need for cerclage, found a decrease in the occurrence of preterm births before 33 weeks in women treated with a cerclage compared with controls (13 vs. 18 percent, $p = 0.03$).

Preterm Premature Rupture of the Membranes

PROM is defined as leakage of amniotic fluid beginning at least 1 hour prior to the onset of labor at any gestational age. The following discussion is limited to the diagnosis and management of preterm PROM, defined as PROM that occurs before 37 weeks' gestation.

Etiology

Epidemiologic studies have identified several risk factors associated with a higher risk of preterm PROM. Genital tract infection or colonization with various microorganisms, coitus, low socioeconomic status, poor nutrition, smoking, and bleeding in pregnancy have all been linked to an increased chance of preterm PROM. These risk factors are consistent with a syndrome of spontaneous premature delivery in which preterm PROM is just one of several possible clinical presentations. Most evidence points to a pathway in which various genital microorganisms gain access to the decidua–membrane interface. Organisms may ascend through a short or dilated cervix that poorly defends the intrauterine contents during pregnancy, may reach this space via hematogenous spread, or may even have colonized the endometrium *before* conception.[57] According to this paradigm, it is the inflammatory interaction between host defenses and microorganisms that initiates a process that may ultimately result in several clinical presentations, including both preterm PROM and PTL.

Preterm PROM is the predominant clinical presentation in indigent patients, whereas PTL is more common than PROM among women who receive private obstetric care. Smokers are three times more likely than nonsmokers to experience PROM before 34 weeks' gestation, with a dose-dependent effect. A history of previous preterm PROM and second-trimester bleeding are also significant risk factors.

Evidence of the association of infection with preterm PROM is abundant and diverse.[255] Histologic studies of membranes after preterm PROM often demonstrate significant bacterial contamination diffusely along the choriodecidual interface with minimal involvement of the amnion.

Specific genital tract pathogens have also been correlated with the occurrence of PROM. The strongest association has been found for bacterial vaginosis and SPTB due to both preterm PROM and preterm labor. The NICHD Preterm Prediction Study[49] found a significant relationship between maternal acquisition of bacterial vaginosis between 24 and 28 weeks of pregnancy and SPTB due to both preterm PROM and PTL. However, a significant relationship between bacterial vaginosis and SPTB was not observed for women who were colonized with bacterial vaginosis at both 24 and 28 weeks, suggesting that it was the acquisition of bacterial vaginosis during pregnancy that was important in this study.

Diagnosis

The most common presentation is a gush of fluid from the vagina followed by persistent, uncontrolled leakage, but some patients report only small, intermittent leakage or perineal wetness. Any history of passing fluid through the vagina should be evaluated by a sterile speculum examination to collect fluid for confirmatory tests. Digital examination of the cervix in women with possible PTL or preterm PROM should be avoided until after ruptured membranes have been excluded. Once preterm PROM is diagnosed, digital examination should be avoided until delivery is anticipated because of the risk of introducing bacteria into the endocervix. Even a single digital examination has been found to increase the likelihood of subsequent amnionitis and neonatal infection. A study of women with preterm PROM found that the mean interval from rupture to delivery was 2.1 days in 121 women who had a digital examination compared with 11.3 days in 144 women who had only a sterile speculum examination.[262] A visual estimate at the time of sterile speculum examination can identify women with advanced dilatation.[263] The sterile speculum examination may also reveal a collection or "pool" of fluid that can be tested for pH with nitrazine paper. Since amniotic fluid is slightly alkaline, vaginal secretions containing amniotic fluid will usually result in pH changes in the blue-green range, 6.5 to 7.5. Nitrazine testing is accurate in 90 to 98 percent of cases.[264] False-positive values can result from vaginal infections that raise vaginal pH, especially *T. vaginalis*, as well as the presence of blood or, more rarely, cervical mucus. False-negative reactions are frequent when only a scant amount of fluid is present.

Another helpful test relies on the property of amniotic fluid to "fern." When placed on a clean slide and allowed to air dry, amniotic fluid produces a microscopic crystallization in a "fern" pattern. This phenomenon is due to the interaction of amniotic fluid proteins and salts and accurately confirms PROM in 85 to 98 percent of cases. False-positive tests can result from the collection of cervical mucus, which also "ferns" but usually in a more floral pattern. The fern test is unaffected by meconium, changes in vaginal pH, and blood/amniotic fluid ratios of up to 1/5.[265, 266] The fern pattern in samples heavily contaminated with blood is atypical and appears more "skeletonized."

In patients in whom the diagnosis of membrane rupture is equivocal, the volume of amniotic fluid seen on ultrasound may be helpful in evaluating the patient. Although nonspecific, a finding of decreased or absent fluid supports a diagnosis of ruptured membranes. Another useful step in equivocal cases is to repeat the sterile speculum examination after the patient has rested in a semiupright position for approximately 1 hour to encourage the pooling of secretions in the posterior vagina. Fibronectin is present in amniotic fluid, and the fibronectin assay will be strongly positive in the presence of ruptured membranes. It may prove useful when other tests are equivocal in a patient with reduced fluid. In rare instances, a dilute solution of indigo carmine may be injected via amniocentesis to look for subsequent transcervical leakage onto a tampon, thus making an absolute diagnosis. Methylene blue has been associated with hemolytic anemia and hyperbilirubinemia in the infant and should not be used.

Natural History

Studies that report aggregate outcomes for all women with preterm PROM between 20 and 34 weeks have observed that the duration of pregnancy after PROM is inversely related to the gestational age at time of membrane rupture. When PROM occurs prior to 26 weeks' gestation, 30 to 40 percent of cases will gain at least one additional week before delivery and 20 percent will gain over 4 weeks.[267] In contrast, 70 to 80 percent of patients who experience PROM between 28 to 36 weeks' gestation deliver within the first week after PROM, and more than one-half of these within the first 4 days.[268]

Maternal Risks

Whether a cause or a result of preterm PROM, intrauterine infection is a potentially serious complication to the mother. A clinical diagnosis of chorioamnionitis accompanies preterm PROM in approximately 10 percent of cases.[257] Regardless of clinical signs of infection, as many as 25 to 30 percent of women with preterm PROM will have a positive amniotic fluid culture. Most instances of amnionitis respond well to antibiotic administration and delivery, but infertility may be a late sequela of postpartum infection.

Fetal and Neonatal Risks

Infection is a major potential complication for the fetus and neonate as well as for the mother. The same vaginal organisms that lead to maternal infection can result in congenital pneumonia, sepsis, or meningitis. In published series, the incidence rate of neonatal sepsis in cases of preterm PROM with or without clinical amnionitis has ranged from 2 to 19 percent and the incidence rate of neonatal deaths caused by infection from 1 to 7 percent.

There is a higher risk of frank or occult cord prolapse, particularly if the fetus is not in a cephalic presentation. The risks of fetal distress in labor leading to cesarean delivery are significantly higher with preterm PROM than with isolated preterm labor, usually due to severe variable decelerations.

Placental abruption occurs in 4 to 6 percent of cases of preterm PROM. When abruption occurred after PROM, nearly half of these pregnancies were complicated by acute intrapartum fetal distress.[275]

Pulmonary hypoplasia is a particular concern when fetal membranes are ruptured prior to 26 weeks' gestation. About 25 percent of babies delivered after 26 weeks' gestation following PROM that occurred before 26 weeks' gestation were found to have pulmonary hypoplasia following birth.[267] The duration and degree of oligohydramnios are associated with the chance of pulmonary hypoplasia. Both overall survival and the risk of pulmonary hypoplasia were related to the gestational age at the time of amniorrhexis.

Skeletal deformities related to compression following oligohydramnios may also occur but often resolve in the first year of life. Twenty-seven percent of fetuses with PROM prior to 26 weeks who experienced prolonged rupture before delivery developed skeletal deformations.[278]

Initial Evaluation and Management

Gestational age should be carefully established in order to estimate the relative risks for the fetus of delivery versus expectant management. All clinical and ultrasound dating criteria should be reviewed. Because oligohydramnios may flatten the fetal head, biparietal diameter measurements to estimate fetal weight by ultrasound may be inaccurate in women with preterm PROM.[279, 280]

Before 32 weeks' gestation, the neonatal risks of prematurity will usually outweigh the in utero risks of infection and fetal compromise, while the reverse is usually the case after 35 weeks' gestation.[281] The relative risks of prematurity, infection, and fetal well-being must be repeatedly evaluated for women with preterm PROM.

Amniocentesis for Women with Preterm PROM

Continuing the pregnancy, called *expectant management*, is accompanied by ongoing risks of maternal and fetal infection, cord prolapse, and abruption that must be reassessed. Demonstration of either fetal pulmonary maturity or intra-amniotic bacteria often leads to a decision for delivery, thus obviating the difficulties of fetal and maternal surveillance. Amniotic fluid may be obtained from either free-flowing vaginal fluid or amniocentesis for studies of fetal maturity, but amniocentesis is required to obtain fluid for culture, Gram stain, and glucose tests for infection. Placing the patient in the Trendelenburg position prior to the amniocentesis may facilitate the procedure by favoring intrauterine retention of fluid. Although the amniotic fluid pocket may be small, amniocentesis is reasonably safe when performed with ultrasound guidance.

Tests for Infection in Patients with Preterm PROM

Ultimately, the endpoint for tests of "infection" in this clinical setting should be clinically important maternal or fetal/neonatal infection. Intermediate endpoints, such as amniotic fluid bacteria, white blood cells, glucose, and even culture, while associated with perinatal infection, do not equate uniformly with clinical infectious morbidity or mortality. The incidence of clinical amnionitis approximates 10 percent in women with preterm PROM. Of infants born to mothers with clinical amnionitis, only 1 to 15 percent will have positive cultures, confirming a diagnosis of neonatal sepsis. Finally, the rate of perinatal mortality caused by infection has ranged from 0 to 13 percent in studies of infants born after preterm PROM. The principal causes of perinatal morbidity and mortality after preterm PROM are still related more to prematurity than to infection. However, a two- to fourfold increase in perinatal mortality, intraventricular hemorrhage, and neonatal sepsis has been reported in infants born after amnionitis compared with gestationally matched controls born to noninfected mothers.[289] Most importantly, antepartum treatment of maternal amnionitis clearly decreases the incidence of neonatal sepsis.

Approximately 10^5 organisms per milliliter of amniotic fluid is needed before a Gram stain will be positive. Thus not all culture-positive fluids have positive Gram stains, though virtually all positive Gram stains result from culture-positive fluids. Amniotic fluid culture has a reported sensitivity of 65 to 85 percent and a specificity of 85 percent to predict clinical chorioamnionitis. The presence of white blood cells in amniotic fluid has not proven helpful in predicting infection, but a low amniotic fluid glucose level (16 to 20 mg/dl or less) has been found to correlate well with a positive fluid culture, with sensitivity and specificity of approximately 90 percent. The amniotic fluid glucose is simple, rapid, and available around the clock.

Nonstress testing for patients with preterm PROM is widely and appropriately practiced to look for evidence of cord compression, but it is not a reliable test for incipient or occult infection, as there have been intrauterine fetal deaths due to sepsis within 24 hours of a reactive NST.[272] A more consistent relationship has been reported between a biophysical profile score of 6 or less and subsequent maternal or neonatal infection.

Management Strategies

Three basic management options can be followed. The first is expectant management, in which the patient is hospitalized for intensive surveillance for signs of fetal compromise or infection, at which time labor is allowed or induced if necessary. This approach is associated with a low rate of cesarean delivery but relies on methods of fetal assessment which are not always accurate. An alternate choice is immediate delivery for pregnancies beyond a certain gestational age (e.g., 32 weeks or more) or estimated fetal weight (e.g., 1,500 to 1,800 g or more). This strategy avoids the need for ongoing surveillance for fetal well-being and infection but commits to delivery some women who might have continued the pregnancy longer. This strategy has a high rate of cesarean delivery for failed induction. The third strategy is an attempt to delay delivery in order to influence the relative risks of prematurity and infection, for example, by reducing the risk of infection with antibiotic treatment, administering steroids to accelerate fetal lung maturation, and/or treatment with tocolytic drugs to allow the steroids and antibiotics to have a therapeutic effect. All three strategies are appropriate choices, depending on the individual and population-based assessments of the risk of infection and prematurity.

Use of Corticosteroids

Antenatal corticosteroids have an unequivocal benefit on the risk of intraventricular hemorrhage for infants born at 32 weeks or earlier, regardless of the status of the membranes before delivery. Randomized trials of the effects of corticosteroids on respiratory distress syndrome in the presence of PROM after 32 weeks have revealed conflicting results. The NICHD summary statement[197] encouraged more study of steroids for reduction of respiratory distress syndrome in preterm PROM after 32 weeks.

Use of Antibiotics

Because the risk of perinatal group B streptococcal infection is associated with both premature birth and duration of membrane rupture before delivery, women with preterm PROM should be cultured for group B streptococcal colonization and treated presumptively with an appropriate antibiotic pending culture results. Antibiotic prophylaxis prolongs the interval from rupture to delivery, and decreases neonatal morbidity from respiratory distress syndrome, sepsis, pneumonia, and chronic lung disease.

Erythromycin was used in some studies in addition to ampicillin to treat *Mycoplasma* and *Ureaplasma*. Significant reductions in neonatal morbidity can also be achieved with broad-spectrum antibiotic treatment, especially in populations with a high prevalence of chorioamnionitis.

Use of Tocolytics

There is currently little evidence to support the routine use of tocolytic agents in patients with preterm PROM. Prospective randomized trials of prophylactic tocolysis have revealed no consistent benefit to adjunctive tocolytics for these patients. However, the studies indicating benefit for adjunctive steroids have raised new questions of short-term tocolysis in order to allow a course of steroids and possibly antibiotics.

Identification of Women With Increased Risk of Preterm Birth

Evaluating pregnant women for risk of preterm delivery can be done with a simple obstetric history, placing emphasis on just a few major risk factors:

1. *A prior preterm delivery* between 16 and 36 weeks carries a two- to threefold increase in risk of recurrent preterm birth. The magnitude of risk is related to the outcome of the most recent pregnancy[26] and increases substantially as the gestational age of the previous preterm birth decreases.
2. *Multiple gestation* is an increasingly prevalent risk factor.
3. *Vaginal bleeding* after the first trimester is a significant risk factor.
4. *Low pre-pregnancy weight* (less than 19.8 kg/m^2 [58,63] or approximately 50 kg average) increases the risk of preterm birth.

Biophysical Assessment of Prematurity Risk

There are clear associations of the likelihood of preterm birth with both contractions and cervical examination. However, the clinical value of this information has been disappointing.

Uterine Contractions

Studies of uterine activity in human pregnancy performed in women with risk factors for preterm birth have shown a rise in uterine activity as pregnancy progresses and more frequent contractions in women destined to labor or deliver prematurely. An entire industry has arisen to provide daily monitoring of uterine contractions for women with risk factors such as multiple gestation or a prior preterm delivery. Monitored contraction data are transmitted over telephone lines and read by specially trained nurses in the expectation that an early diagnosis of preterm labor might lead to prompt and therefore more effective use of tocolysis. Numerous studies of the effects of this strategy have been performed, with conflicting conclusions.[212,343–350] There is consensus that the monitoring technique produces accurate data and that frequent supportive nursing contact and education for high-risk women is associated with a small but significant decline in the incidence of preterm birth. The mechanism of this effect is not understood. The independent value of uterine activity monitoring data as an aid to early detection of PTL has not been demonstrated. Meta-analyses of published reports have largely concluded that uterine activity monitoring as currently employed is ineffective in reducing preterm birth in at-risk women.

Digital Cervical Examination

Several studies have observed an association between digital examination showing premature cervical dilatation and effacement and risk of subsequent preterm birth.[52-54] As with uterine contractions, however, the observation of an association has not led to a clinical benefit such as reduced incidence of PTL or delivery.

Cervical Sonography

Digital examination of the cervix is reasonably accurate in active labor but is subject to great interexaminer variation when dilatation is less than 3 cm or effacement is less than 80 percent.[80] Measurement of cervical length using transvaginal sonography[56] has been reported to identify women at risk for preterm birth on the basis of a cervical length less than the 10th percentile, or about 25 mm at 24 to 28 weeks of pregnancy. However, these data have not been tested as part of any program of intervention (e.g., prophylactic use of maternal rest, tocolysis, antibiotics, or cerclage).

Genital Colonization with Microorganisms

The association of maternal colonization with various genital microorganisms and risk of preterm birth has led to investigations of screening tests to identify and treat women at risk. No reduction in preterm birth is associated with screening and treatment for *C. trachomatis, Ureaplasma urealyticum*, or group B Streptococcus. A randomized trial of screening and treatment for bacterial vaginosis, in which treatment with metronidazole and erythromycin was provided after 26 weeks, reported a significantly reduced rate of SPTB, from 49 percent in the placebo group to 31 percent in the antibiotic group.[365] This trial was limited to women with a history of prior preterm birth, and some are now recommending routine screening and treatment for bacterial vaginosis for high-risk women.

Biochemical Markers of Risk for SPTB

Biochemical markers have long been sought to identify women who will deliver premature infants. Increased levels of estriol in maternal saliva have been reported to correlate with the risk of preterm birth.[368]

Fibronectin

Fetal fibronectin in cervicovaginal mucus may predict early PTL in symptomatic subjects. There may be a broader use for the fibronectin assay as a screen for risk of preterm delivery in asymptomatic subjects. The NICHD Preterm Prediction Study indicated that a single positive fibronectin assay performed at 24 to 26 weeks may identify up to 60 percent of women destined to deliver before 28 weeks' gestation. The sensitivity of the 24- to 26-week fibronectin assay for predicting preterm birth declined after 30 weeks. There are as yet no reports describing use of fibronectin as a screening test leading to a successful intervention to reduce prematurity.

Unifactorial Interventions To Prevent Preterm Birth

Social Support and Improved Access to Prenatal Care

Prenatal care has something to do with the rate of SPTB in both black and white women, but the specific contribution of prenatal care to lower rates of SPTB is not clear. Prospective interventions designed to reduce preterm birth through better access to care or reduced stress have been unsuccessful.[374,375]

Prophylactic Medications

Tocolytic agents have been widely used without cervical change (i.e., prophylactically) in this country. However, the large-scale use of ritodrine has not been associated with a reduction in either preterm or LBW deliveries.[376]

Bedrest and Activity Modification

There is consistent evidence of a weak relationship between maternal physical activity and risk of SPTB. Strong relationships between hours worked per week, occupational fatigue score, and risk of SPTB have been observed. However, bedrest offers no benefit that has been documented.

Unifactorial Versus Multifactorial Approaches to Preterm Birth Prevention

The foregoing would appear to indicate that, for every factor associated with spontaneous preterm birth there has been an ineffective intervention trial. Failure of each individual trial to affect the rate of SPTB is understandable, but it remains to be seen whether multifactorial interventions will succeed against SPTB. Identification and simultaneous elimination of multiple factors may be necessary to reduce prematurity, and ultimately a national strategy of *primary* prevention may be required.

Key Points

- Preterm birth is the single greatest cause of perinatal morbidity and mortality in nonanomalous infants, being responsible for 70 percent of fetal, neonatal, and infant deaths.
- Spontaneous preterm birth (that following PTL, preterm PROM, and abnormal cervical competence) is a syndrome in which multiple continuous risk variables operate collaboratively to produce several related clinical disorders.
- The mechanism of injury may be infectious, ischemic, or "allergic," alone or in combination.
- Major risk factors for preterm birth are a prior history of preterm delivery, multifetal gestation, bleeding after the first trimester of pregnancy, and a low maternal body mass index, but these factors precede less than 50 percent of preterm births. Every pregnancy is potentially at risk.
- Cervical "competence" is not an absolute or categorical property of the cervix but rather is a continuum. The risk of SPTB increases as the length of the cervix decreases.
- Accurate early diagnosis of PTL is a major problem. Up to 50 percent of patients diagnosed with PTL do not actually have PTL, yet as many as 20 percent of symptomatic patients diagnosed as not being in labor will deliver prematurely. The addition of fetal fibronectin and cervical sonography to the evaluation should improve the accuracy of diagnosis.
- Tertiary care of the clinical disorders that precede spontaneous preterm birth that can reduce perinatal morbidity and mortality are (1) transfer of the mother and fetus to an appropriate hospital, (2) administration of antibiotics to prevent neonatal group B Streptococcus infection, (3) administration of corticosteroids to reduce neonatal respiratory distress syndrome and intraventricular hemorrhage, and (4) administration of labor-arresting (tocolytic) medications to allow the above to occur.
- There is no truly reliable test for fetal well-being or infection in women with preterm PROM.

Chapter 16

Multiple Gestations

Usha Chitkara and
Richard L. Berkowitz

Obstetricians have long been aware that pregnancies complicated by twinning are at higher risk than those of most singletons. Twins are either monozygotic (MZ) or dizygotic (DZ). In the former case a single fertilized ovum splits into two distinct individuals after a variable number of divisions. Such twins are almost always genetically identical and therefore of the same sex. When two separate ova are fertilized, DZ twins result. These individuals are as genetically distinct as any other children born to the same couple. Sets of DZ twins may have the same or opposite sex. DZ half-siblings have been reported in which two ova were fertilized by different fathers. In most cases, DZ twins are genetically dissimilar true siblings, while MZ twins are genetically identical.

The frequency of MZ twins is fairly constant throughout the world at a rate of approximately 4/1,000 births. This rate does not seem to vary with maternal characteristics such as age or parity. DZ twinning, however, is associated with multiple ovulation, and its frequency varies between races and within countries. In general, the frequency of DZ twins is low in Asians, intermediate in whites, and high in blacks. In the United States, the overall incidence of twins is approximately 12/1,000 births, and two-thirds are DZ.[1]

The frequency of DZ births is affected by maternal age, increasing from a rate of 3/1,000 in women under age 20 to 14/1,000 at ages 35 to 40. Above age 40 the rate declines.

Infertility patients treated with menopausal urinary gonadotropins (Pergonal) or clomiphene citrate are well known to have a dose-dependent increase in multiple births when compared with women who conceive without these agents. The use of in vitro fertilization and embryo transfer has further increased the incidence of multiple pregnancies.

Placentation

Twin placentas are described in terms of their membranes (Fig. 16-1). The sac of a singleton pregnancy consists of an outer chorion and an inner amnion. Each DZ twin develops within a similar sac because both blastocysts generate their own placentas. If implantations of these blastocysts are not proximal to each other, two separate placentas will result, each of which will have a chorion and an amnion. Should they implant side by side, intimate fusion of the placental discs will occur, but these placentas are always diamniotic and dichorionic, and vascular anastomoses rarely occur. While MZ twins may also have placentas with two amnions and two chorions, this generally is not the case. Monochorionic placentas have a single chorion that usually surrounds two amnions, but occasionally there is only a single amnion. Triplets and quadruplets have also been delivered with monochorial placentas and shown to be MZ. Almost all monochorial placentas have blood vessel communications between the fetal circulations.

The type of placenta that develops in an MZ pregnancy is determined by the timing of cleavage of the fertilized ovum. If twinning is accomplished during the first 2 to 3 days, it precedes the setting aside of cells that eventually become the chorion. In that case, two chorions and two amnions will be formed. After approximately 3 days, however, twinning cannot split the chorionic cavity, and from that time on a monochorial placenta must result. If the split occurs between the third and eighth days, a diamniotic monochorial placenta will develop. Between the eighth and thirteenth days, the amnion has already formed, and the placenta will therefore be monoamniotic and monochorionic. Embryonic cleavage between the thirteenth and fifteenth days will result in conjoined twins within a single amnion and chorion; beyond that point, the process of twinning cannot occur.

Because monochorial placentas can only occur in MZ pregnancies, study of the membranes will establish zygosity in 20 percent of cases in the United States. In approximately 35 percent of cases the twins will be of opposite sex and therefore necessarily DZ. This leaves only 45 percent of cases (twins of like sex having dichorionic placentas) in which further studies are necessary in order to determine zygosity. This 45 percent breaks down into 8 percent MZ and 37 percent DZ. The more genotypic markers that are studied, the greater the likelihood of demonstrating dizygosity. At present, the most accurate method for determination of twin zygosity is by analysis of DNA polymorphism.[7,8]

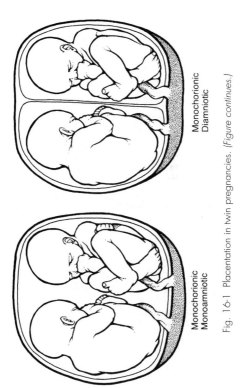

Monochorionic
Diamniotic

Monochorionic
Monoamniotic

Fig. 16-1 Placentation in twin pregnancies. *(Figure continues.)*

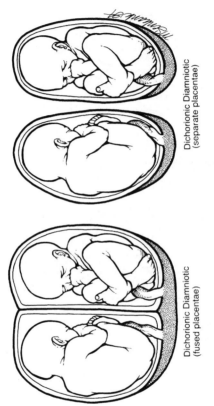

Dichorionic Diamniotic
(separate placentae)

Dichorionic Diamniotic
(fused placentae)

Fig. 16-1 (Continued).

Perinatal Morbidity and Mortality

Perinatal morbidity and mortality are greater in twins, approximately three times greater than that of comparable singletons at the same institutions. Both preterm delivery and intrauterine growth restriction (IUGR) contribute to this problem. Twins also have an increased frequency of congenital anomalies, placenta previa, abruptio placenta, preeclampsia, cord accidents, and malpresentations.

A decline in perinatal mortality has been reported over the past two decades. Most of the improved neonatal outcome is due to increased survival rates in neonates weighing 1,000 to 1,500 g at birth. In one series, more than 70 percent of the deaths occurred before 30 weeks' gestation, either in utero or during the neonatal period. If obstetricians are to have a major impact on the perinatal survival of twins, they must concentrate on the period between 25 and 30 weeks' gestation.

Although perinatal mortality rates have decreased, the risk of prematurity in multifetal gestations has not changed significantly over the past 20 years. The average gestational age at delivery for triplets consistently seems to be about 33 weeks. Approximately 75 percent of these patients deliver prior to 37 weeks, and at least 20 percent deliver prior to 32 weeks.

Among survivors, the incidence of severe handicap is significantly higher among multiple births, 1.7-fold and 2.9-fold higher among twins and triplets compared with singletons.

Diagnosis

Before widespread use of ultrasound, 50 percent of twins remained undiagnosed until the time of delivery.[25] Multiple gestations should be suspected whenever the uterus seems to be larger than dates, or the pregnancy has occurred following ovulation induction or in vitro fertilization.

Separate gestational sacs can be identified ultrasonically as early as 6 weeks from the first day of the last menstrual period. With transabdominal scanning, an embryo within each sac should be visible by 7 weeks, and beating fetal hearts should be seen by 7.5 to 8 weeks.[30] With good equipment the fetal cranial pole is also identifiable during this period, but the intracranial landmarks used for accurate biparietal diameter measurements are usually not seen until 14 to 16 weeks. Increasing sophistication in the development and use of endovaginal scanning has made it possible to visualize these developmental landmarks 1 to 2 weeks earlier than with abdominal scanning techniques, so that the embryonic pole and fetal heart can be seen by 6 weeks and the intracranial landmarks are visible by 10 to 12 weeks' gestation.[31]

It is mandatory to visualize separate fetuses. Retromembranous collections of blood or fluid or a prominent fetal yolk sac should not be confused with a twin gestation. Demonstration of the viability of each fetus at the time of the examination requires visualization of independent cardiac activity.

Early Wastage in Multiple Gestations

The incidence of multiple gestations in humans is higher than is usually appreciated and a significant amount of early wastage occurs. This has led to the concept of the "vanishing twin."

One explanation for the disappearance of a gestational sac is resorption which has been ultrasonically described in human multiple gestations between 7 to 12 weeks. Another explanation is the presence of a blighted ovum or anembryonic pregnancy, a gestational sac having a volume of 2.5 ml more in which no fetus can be identified on ultrasound examination. The only complication of regression of a blighted ovum is slight vaginal bleeding, and a coexisting normal pregnancy has a good prognosis for carrying to term.

Growth and Development

Normal individual twins grow at the same rate as singletons up to 32 weeks' gestation. After that time, they do not gain weight as rapidly as singletons of the same gestational age.[43] Twin birth weights drop below the mean for singletons by 32 weeks but remain within the low-normal range until the thirty-sixth week, after which time they fall progressively below the tenth percentile. Twin birth lengths, head circumferences, and femur lengths, however, remain within the low-normal range for singletons throughout the entire pregnancy. Alterations in twin growth occur primarily in the third trimester, worsen as gestational age progresses, and are usually asymmetric in nature.

Discrepancies in birth weight could be due, in part, to constitutional factors, especially in DZ twins. There are also several pathologic situations in which twins may be born with substantial weight differences. These include the twin-to-twin transfusion syndrome, the combination of an anomalous fetus with a normal co-twin, and growth retardation affecting only one twin because of local placental factors.[33] IUGR, in contrast, can affect both twins relatively equally, in which case they would both be small but not discordant in size. Charts derived from singleton pregnancies may be reliably used to estimate gestational age of twins. As the difference between twin BPDs increases, the likelihood that the smaller fetus will be growth retarded increases.

Crane et al.[54] defined discordance in utero as an intrapair difference in BPD of 5 mm or more and a fall in BPD below two standard deviation (SD) for gestational age on their normal twin curve. They suggested that head circumferences (HCs) be measured if BPD intrapair differences exceed 5 mm. Since HC is less likely to be affected by molding in utero, an intrapair HC difference of less than 5 percent suggests that true discrepancy does not exist.

A survey of multiple parameters on serial ultrasound examinations provides the most accurate assessment of the size of each individual fetus in twin gestations. The highest accuracy for predicting either appropriate or retarded growth is obtained by estimating the fetal weight. Among individual parameters, abdominal circumference is the single most sensitive measurement in predicting both IUGR and growth discordancy.[61,62,66,67] An intrapair difference in abdominal circumference measurement of 2 cm or more can be effectively used as a screening test for discordant fetal growth and IUGR in the smaller twin.[62,66,67] However, individual measurements of BPD, HC, or femur length are relatively poor predictors for either IUGR or growth discordance.[61,66,67] We recommend that women with twins be scanned every 3 to 4 weeks after the 26th week. The incidences of IUGR and fetal death are higher in monochorionic than dichorionic twins, and the twin-to-twin transfusion syndrome (TTS) occurs only in monochorionic twins.

Ultrasonographic Prediction of Amnionicity and Chorionicity

The sonographic prediction of chorionicity and amnionicity should be systematically approached by determining the number of placentas visualized and the sex of each fetus and then by assessing the membranes that divide the sacs. The pregnancy is clearly dichorionic if the twins are of different sex. When a single placenta is present and the twins are of the same sex, careful sonographic examination of the dividing membrane will usually result in a correct diagnosis. Evaluation should be done of three features in the intertwin membrane: (1) thickness of the intertwin membrane, (2) the number of layers visualized in the membrane, and (3) assessment of the junction of the membrane with the placental site for the "twin peak" sign. In dichorionic diamniotic pregnancies, the dividing membrane appears thick[69–71] and has a measured diameter of 2 mm or greater,[72] and either three or four layers can often be identified.[73,74] With a monochorionic diamniotic pregnancy only two layers of membranes will be identified, and the membrane appears to be thin and hairlike.[73] A floating monochorionic diamniotic membrane may fold back upon itself and give a false impression of having four layers; inspection of the membranes near their placental insertion will reduce this artifact. Significant magnification of the image is helpful in counting the number of layers. Determination of membrane thickness allows correct identification of di- or monochorionic gestation in 80 to 90 percent of cases,[68–70] and counting the number of layers can increase the predictive accuracy to almost 100 percent.[73,74]

The *twin peak sign*, which identifies dichorionic pregnancies, is a triangular projection of tissue with the same echogenicity as the placenta extending beyond the chorionic surface of the placenta. This tissue is insinuated between the layers of the intertwin membrane, wider at the chorionic surface and tapering to a point at some distance inward from that surface. This space exists only in a dichorionic pregnancy and is produced by reflection of each chorion away from its placenta at the place where it encounters the chorion and placenta of the co-twin (Fig. 16-2). The absence of the twin peak sign alone does not guarantee that the pregnancy is monochorionic.

In some pregnancies with monochorionic diamniotic placentation, the dividing membranes may not be sonographically visualized because they are very thin. In other cases they may not be seen because severe oligohydramnios causes them to be closely apposed to the fetus in that sac. This results in a "stuck twin" appearance, where the trapped fetus remains firmly held against the uterine wall despite changes in maternal position. Diagnosis of this condition confirms the presence of a diamniotic gestation, which should be distinguished from a monoamniotic gestation where dividing membranes are absent. In the latter situation free movement of both twins, and occasionally entanglement of their umbilical cords, can be demonstrated.[79]

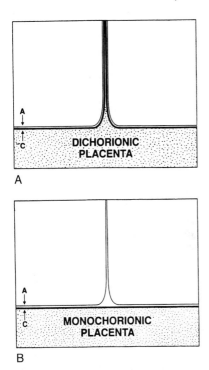

Fig. 16-2 (A) In a dichorionic pregnancy with fused placentas, both the amnions (A) and the chorions (C) reflect away from the placental surface at the point of origin of the septum. This creates a potential space in direct continuity with the chorionic villi and into which they can extend. (B) In a monochorionic twin pregnancy, the septum is formed by reflection of the two amnions away from the placenta. There is a continuous single chorion, which provides an intact barrier, preventing extension of placental villi into the potential interamniotic space.

Doppler Studies in Multiple Gestation

Although some investigators favor continuous wave systems, we think that Doppler studies in multiple gestations are best performed using a pulsed Doppler duplex system to be certain that the vessel being studied belongs to a targeted fetus. Umbilical artery S/D ratios in normal twins decrease with advancing gestation, the same as in singletons.

Abnormal Doppler studies may precede documentation of IUGR by sonographic biometry or abnormalities in other tests of fetal well-being.[83] Abnormal umbilical artery waveforms may reflect vascular lesions in the placenta, which can be presumed to increase resistance to blood flow through the umbilical arteries.[86] An S/D ratio difference of 0.4 or more is a better predictor than ultrasound for birth weight discordancy in the small-for-gestational-age (SGA)/AGA twin pairs but is poor in predicting discordant weight in the SGA/SGA, AGA/AGA, or AGA/large-for-gestational-age (LGA) twin pairs.

While the overall sensitivity of Doppler alone for predicting an SGA fetus is only 58 percent, abnormal Doppler findings precede sonographic diagnosis of SGA by about 3.7 weeks. A combination of sonographic and Doppler parameters improved the sensitivity to 84 percent, suggesting that Doppler velocimetry complements real-time ultrasonography in the early detection of abnormal growth in twin pregnancies.

Our routine for the surveillance of patients with multiple gestations is as follows:

1. Initial ultrasound evaluation is performed at 18 to 20 weeks' gestation. This includes standard assessment of amniotic fluid volume in each sac, and evaluation of each fetus's anatomy and an attempt to determine chorionicity.
2. If the first study is normal, subsequent scans for fetal growth are performed at 24 to 26 weeks and every 3 to 4 weeks thereafter.
3. If there is evidence of IUGR, discordant fetal growth, or discordant fluid volumes, fetal surveillance is intensified and includes frequent nonstress testing along with biophysical profile and Doppler velocimetry studies.

Abnormalities Associated With Multiple Gestation

Twin-to-Twin Transfusion Syndrome

TTS in humans has only been reported in association with monochorionic placentas. The potential for the transfusion syndrome occurs when the arterial circulation of one twin is in communication with the venous circulation of the other through arteriovenous shunts. In this situation, one fetus becomes a donor that transfuses its co-twin. The donor becomes anemic and growth retarded. Although occasionally it may become hydropic as a result of high-output failure, more frequently this twin is significantly smaller than the other. The recipient, conversely, becomes polycythemic and can suffer from congestive heart failure as a result of circulatory overload.

The perinatal mortality associated with TTS is as

high as 70 percent. Three antenatal factors almost invariably predict a fatal outcome in these pregnancies: (1) an early gestational age at diagnosis with delivery before 28 weeks, (2) severe hydramnios requiring therapeutic amniocentesis, and (3) fetal hydrops.

When severe, the syndrome usually manifests itself clinically as a result of hydramnios that is almost always found to exist in the sac of the larger twin. Sonographic criteria that provide an antenatal diagnosis of TTS include (1) the presence of same-sex twins with a single placenta; (2) thin (two-layer) separating membrane between the sacs; (3) significant discordance in fetal growth (although this is not inevitably present); (4) discordant amniotic fluid volume with polyhydramnios in the sac of the larger recipient twin and a "stuck twin" appearance as a result of oligohydramnios in the sac of the donor twin; and (5) signs of hydrops or cardiac failure in either fetus, although this occurs more frequently in the larger twin.

When twins of unequal size are discovered on ultrasound examination, it is important to distinguish the transfusion syndrome from a pregnancy in which one fetus is growth retarded but the other is developing normally. In the latter situation the normal twin is usually surrounded by an appropriate quantity of amniotic fluid, and oligohydramnios may or may not be present in the other sac. In TTS, however, the donor is smaller than it should be and not simply smaller than its larger sibling. This latter point may be useful in ruling out a third uncommon situation, namely, that of a normal fetus and a larger hydropic co-twin that is anomalous or erythroblastotic.

Cordocentesis on both twins is unable to demonstrate consistently a hemoglobin difference of 5 g or more between the recipient and donor twins. The "pancuronium test" involves cordocentesis and intravascular injection of pancuronium bromide into one twin. Paralysis of both twins under these circumstances would confirm transplacental vascular communications.

Various therapeutic maneuvers have been attempted in an effort to improve pregnancy outcome in severe cases of TTS. These approaches include therapeutic amniocentesis, to decrease pressure on the cord insertion site,[112–115] laser ablation of vascular anastomoses,[116] and selective feticide.[117,118] Selective feticide of one twin in the presence of the placental vascular communications expected in TTS can have devastating consequences, including death or survival with permanent damage of the co-twin.[123]

Repeated therapeutic amniocenteses provide the best option for treatment until delivery is possible with survival rates from 37 to 83 percent.[112-114] The total number and frequency of amniocenteses must be individualized since some patients show improvement following one or two procedures whereas others may require that it be performed far more frequently. The volume of fluid aspirated at any one time should again be individualized, with an aim to removing as much fluid as possible from the polyhydramniotic sac and attaining a relatively "normal" fluid volume.

Congenital Anomalies in Multiple Gestations

Anomalies occur more frequently in twins than in singletons. One series reported a rate of anomalies of 1.4 percent for singletons, 2.7 percent for twins, and 6.1 percent for triplets.[124] Among cases of twins in which anomalies were detected, both twins were affected in 14.8 percent.

Anomalies Related to Twinning

Acardia and conjoined twins are directly related to the twinning process. *Acardia* is a malformation that occurs in one fetus of MZ pregnancies with a frequency of approximately 1/30,000 deliveries.[5] These patients always have monochorial placentas and vascular anastomoses that sustain the life of the acardiac twin.

There is also a high incidence of chromosomal abnormalities in these pregnancies. In 6 of the 12 acardiac cases an abnormal karyotype was found in the perfused twin, while the karyotype of the pump twin was normal. By ultrasound the anomalous twin may appear to be an amorphous mass or may show a wide range of abnormalities. The pump twin, although structurally normal, is at increased risk for in utero cardiac failure, and mortality rates of 50 percent or higher have been reported.[132]

Conjoined twins occur with a frequency of about 1/50,000 deliveries and in approximately 1/600 twin births.[142-144] Dystocia may be a frequent and serious complication if vaginal delivery is attempted at term. It is therefore recommended that conjoined twins except craniopagus twins be delivered by cesarean section. If they are considered to have a poor chance of surviving and are small enough to pass through the birth canal without damaging the mother, vaginal delivery might be an option.

Death of One Twin in Utero

The death of one twin in utero occurs in 2.2 to 6.8 percent of twins. When only one twin dies in utero, it may become a fetus papyraceous. In that condition, the fluid is resorbed from the dead twin's body and is compressed into the adjacent membranes by the growth of the living fetus.

When a dead twin remains undelivered, a legitimate concern is the potential for disseminated intravascular coagulation (DIC) in the mother, but this is rare in twins.

In selected situations it may be possible to treat the chronic maternal coagulopathy associated with a retained dead twin with heparin in order to allow a premature living co-twin to continue to develop in utero. When death in utero of one twin is detected before 34 weeks, conservative management is the wisest course. This should include weekly maternal clotting profiles and serial assessments of fetal growth and well-being. No coagulation disorders have been observed after spontaneous or induced first-trimester death of one or more fetuses in a multiple gestation.

Successful reversal of a consumption coagulopathy within the maternal circulation does not ensure that the surviving fetus will be unaffected by the process. If vascular anastomoses exist within a monochorial placenta, the shared circulation may permit volume and blood pressure changes in the other twin. Cortical necrosis,[172] multicystic encephalomalacia,[173] and other structural abnormalities[174,176] have been reported in liveborn MZ twins with stillborn macerated co-twins. Damage to the survivor occurs far less frequently in the case of DZ twins or MZ twins with dichorionic placentas. There is a 17 percent chance that the "surviving twin" in a monochorionic gestation will either die or suffer major morbidity.

Selective Termination of an Anomalous Fetus

Intracardiac injection of potassium chloride is the procedure of choice because of its safety and is currently preferred both for selective termination procedures in the second trimester and for elective reduction of fetal numbers in the first trimester.[36–38,125,171,182] The procedure carries a risk of losing the entire pregnancy of about 5 percent. Procedures done after 20 weeks carry an increased risk of prematurity.

In considering selective termination of an abnormal twin, particular caution must be exercised to exclude the possibility of a monochorionic gestation. Vascular connections between fetal circulations occur in approximately 70 percent of MZ twins. In this situation, a lethal agent injected into the anomalous twin could enter the circulation of its normal sibling and result in death or permanent damage.[123] This has led perinatologists to attempt to occlude completely the circulation of the anomalous monochorionic twin at the time of the procedure by performing cord ligation.

First-Trimester Multifetal Pregnancy Reduction

The increasingly successful use of ovulatory drugs and in vitro fertilization has resulted in a growing incidence of multifetal pregnancies with three or more fetuses. Because of a high risk of perinatal morbidity and mortality from premature delivery in these pregnancies, first-trimester reduction[36-38] of the number of fetuses has been advocated as a method to improve outcome.

The loss rate after multifetal reduction is 8.7 percent. The spontaneous loss rate prior to 24 weeks in a series of 106 triplets following documentation of cardiac activity was reported to be 20.7 percent.[195] Therefore, the losses in the multifetal pregnancy reduction series may, in fact, represent an improvement over natural loss rates in multifetal pregnancies.

Perinatal morbidity and mortality are likely to improve when pregnancies with four or more fetuses are reduced to smaller numbers. The advantages of reducing triplets to twins is far more controversial, which cannot be justified on the basis of improving perinatal mortality. However, a reduction in the morbidity associated with severe prematurity may result from reducing triplets to twins.

Problems Related to Placentation

Prolapse of the cord and rupture of a vasa previa with fetal exsanguination are more common in twins than in singletons. A velamentous cord insertion occurs in 7 percent of twin placentas as opposed to 1 percent in singletons.

Monoamniotic twins have a high risk of fetal mortality, with double survival rates of 40 percent. The high fetal mortality associated with a single amniotic sac is due to prematurity, vascular anastomoses in the placenta, and, most commonly, entanglement of the umbilical cords, which occurs in as many as 70 percent of monoamniotic twins. Inability to visualize a membrane separating two sacs in a twin gestation is suggestive of a monoamniotic pregnancy but is not diagnostic because occasionally the membrane can remain undetected even though it is present. The observation of entangled umbilical cords in the absence of a membrane separating twin fetuses provides a reliable sign for the sonographic diagnosis of monoamniotic twin gestation. It is essential to trace both cords into the entangled mass before making this diagnosis. Another uncommon mishap that can result from this type of placentation is inadvertant clamping of the undelivered twin's cord after delivery of the first twin, such as when a tight cord around the neck of twin A was clamped and divided and then found to belong to twin B. It is suggested that, whenever possible, division of a cord around the first twin's neck should be avoided.

Because of an impression of increasing morbidity and mortality rates in monoamniotic twins with advancing gestations, prophylactic preterm delivery by 32 weeks has been advocated to prevent cord-related deaths late in pregnancy. The potential for a disastrous outcome either from complications of cord entanglement or from fetal interlocking is substantial and makes cesarean delivery recommended in all viable monoamniotic twin pregnancies.

Amniocentesis in Multiple Gestations

When Should Both Sacs Be Tapped?

In some situations it is obviously necessary to perform amniocentesis on each twin sac. Two series have found a close correlation between lecithin/sphingomyelin (L/S) ratios in amniotic fluid samples from twin sets. However, the firstborn of triplets and quadruplets have been found to have higher pharyngeal L/S ratios and less severe respiratory distress than those of their siblings delivered subsequently. In patients not in labor at the time of delivery, no significant intrapair differences in L/S ratio are found. In labor, however, there may be a significant increase in the L/S ratio of the presenting twin when compared with its sibling.

In most cases of nonlaboring patients with twins, an L/S ratio from one sac will accurately reflect the status of both fetuses. If one twin appears to be abnormal for any reason, however, or if the patient is in premature labor, both sacs should be tapped to assess pulmonary maturity. Should the operator elect to tap only one sac in these situations, it should be that of the twin who appears to be normal in the former case and that of the second twin in the latter. The stressed twin, or the presenting twin in these two instances, can be assumed to have an L/S ratio at least as mature as that of its sibling.

The Technique of Tapping Multiple Sacs

An amniocentesis needle is introduced into one sac. After indigo carmine or Evans blue is injected to serve as a marker and the needle is removed, a different needle is then inserted, and the aspiration of untinged fluid indicates that the second sac has been successfully entered.

Several points should be stressed:

1. A thorough ultrasound examination should precede the amniocentesis. It is particularly important to note the position of one fetus relative to the other(s) and to label the aspirated fluids appropriately, as well as placing a drawing in the patient's chart so that at a later date it is possible to correlate a particular fetus with its fluid specimen. This becomes critically important in the case of genetic studies if at a later date selective termination of one fetus is to be considered.

2. Direct ultrasonic visualization of the needle tip during its insertion allows for precision in guiding the needle to an optimal sampling site.

Second-trimester amniocentesis in twin pregnancies has not been associated with excess pregnancy loss.

Management of Multiple Gestations

The Antepartum Period

No benefit of bedrest in the hospital for a patient carrying twins has been confirmed, and in one study preterm delivery was more common among the hospitalized group. These women should only be hospitalized for the same indications that would be used to admit women with singletons. Prophylactic administration of tocolytic agents to women with twins has not been successful in preventing preterm birth.

Prophylactic cervical cerclage in women with multiple gestations has been disappointing.[2] Since this surgical procedure may be associated with adverse sequelae for both the mother and her fetuses, it is recommended that cerclage placement be limited to women with a strong suggestive history of or objectively documented cervical incompetence.

Cervical evaluation clinically or with ultrasound can select a group of patients with twins at increased risk for preterm delivery. Ambulatory home monitoring of uterine contractions with a mobile tocodynamometer has not proven to be of benefit.

Nonstress tests in twins, whether reactive or nonreactive, appear to be prognostically comparable to those in singleton third-trimester pregnancies.

Triplets and Greater

Gonen et al.[18] reported the outcome and follow-up data of 30 multiple gestations (24 triplets, 5 quadruplets, and 1 quintuplet) managed over a 10-year period from 1978 to 1988. In their study, the early neonatal mortality rate was 31.6/1,000, late neonatal mortality was 21/1,000, and perinatal mortality was 51.5/1,000 live births. The incidence of respiratory distress syndrome was 43 percent, bronchopulmonary dysplasia 6 percent, retinopathy of prematurity 3 per cent, intraventricular hemorrhage 4 percent, and cerebral palsy 2 percent. Follow-up of 84 infants for a period of 1 to 10 years showed 75 percent of them to be free from any neurologic or developmental handicap, 22 percent had mild functional delay, one infant was mildly handicapped, and one was moderately handicapped.

Management of multifetal gestations with three or more fetuses can be achieved on an outpatient basis in most cases, but must include intensified surveillance of the mother and fetuses. Our protocol includes (1) modified bedrest at home initiated at 16 weeks' gestation; (2) frequent prenatal visits with cervical assessment for evidence of effacement or dilatation (routine cerclage is not recommended, but is offered to patients with clinical documentation or historical evidence of cervical incompetence); (3) serial ultrasound studies for evaluation of fetal growth; (4) early initiation of weekly nonstress tests at 26 to 28 weeks' gestation; (5) hospitalization for any evidence of preterm labor or other obstetric/medical complications; (6) tocolytic agents and betamethasone restricted to patients with documented preterm labor; and (8) elective cesarean delivery recommended in all cases either at onset of labor near term or at 36 completed weeks' gestation following documentation of lung maturity.

The Intrapartum Period

Intrapartum twin presentations can be classified into three groups: twin A vertex, twin B vertex (43 percent); twin A vertex, twin B nonvertex (38 percent); and twin A nonvertex, twin B either vertex or nonvertex (19 percent). When both twins are in vertex presentation, a cesarean delivery should only be performed for the same indications applied to singletons.

Currently, cesarean delivery is the method of choice when the presenting twin is in a nonvertex position. If the second twin is in a vertex presentation and faces its sibling, the potential for locking exists. The frequency of locking is approximately 1/1,000 twin deliveries, with an associated fetal mortality of 31 percent. This condition occurs most commonly in breech–vertex presentations when the fetal chins overlie each other. It is usually not recognized until the body of the presenting twin is out of the vagina and the aftercoming head cannot be delivered. Eventually it becomes clear that entry of the first twin's head into the pelvis is being obstructed by that of the second twin. Also, it is possible that the second twin could complicate the delivery of the first twin in more subtle ways, such as by deflexing its head.

The management of women whose twins are in vertex–breech or vertex–transverse lies is particularly controversial. Depressed Apgar scores and increased perinatal mortality rates associated with vaginal breech delivery of the second twin have led some investigators to recommend cesarean delivery whenever twin B is in a nonvertex lie. Others have found no perinatal deaths when nonvertex first or second twins weighing more than 1,499 g were delivered by cesarean section or when nonvertex second twins with similar birth weights were delivered vaginally.

In external cephalic versions performed on transverse and breech malpositioned second twins,[246] version to vertex presentation is successful in 46 to 73 percent of cases. External version was associated with a higher failure rate than breech extraction, and also a higher rate of fetal distress, cord prolapse, and compound presentation.

We currently feel that elective cesarean delivery is the safest for triplets or higher order multiple pregnancies.

Time Interval Between Deliveries

There are reports of significant delays in the delivery of twins who were premature to allow more maturation of the second twin. Intervals range from a few days to 12 weeks. A management protocol for these patients includes high ligation of the umbilical cord of the delivered twin with an absorbable suture, bedrest, ongoing monitoring of the patient for evidence of infection and/or coagulation disorders, corticosteroid administration, and serial monitoring for growth and well-being of the viable fetus(es). This type of management, however, should not be considered "standard of care."

At term, another variable that many investigators have considered important in the outcome of twin pregnancies is the time interval between their deliveries. After delivery of the first twin, uterine inertia may develop, the second twin's cord can prolapse, and partial separation of its placenta may render the second twin hypoxic. In addition, the cervix can clamp down, making rapid delivery of the second twin extremely difficult if fetal distress develops. Many reports have suggested that the interval between deliveries should ideally be within 15 minutes and certainly not more than 30 minutes.[5,10,25,254,255] These data were obtained before the advent of intrapartum fetal monitoring.

Rayburn et al.[253] reported the outcome of 115 second twins delivered vaginally at or beyond 34 weeks' gestation after the vertex delivery of their siblings. The second twin was visually monitored ultrasonically on some occasions, and continuous monitoring of the fetal heart was performed in all cases. Oxytocin was used if uterine contractions subsided within 10 minutes after delivery of the first twin. In this series, 70 second twins delivered within 15 minutes of the first twin, 28 within 16 and 30 minutes, and 17 more than 30 minutes later. The longest interdelivery interval was 134 minutes. All these infants survived, and none of them had traumatic deliveries. All 17 of the neonates delivering beyond 30 minutes had 5-minute Apgar scores of 8 and 10.

It therefore seems apparent that, whereas some second twins may require rapid delivery, others can be safely followed with fetal heart rate surveillance and remain undelivered for substantial periods of time.

Ultrasound and the Intrapartum Management of Multiple Gestations

On admission to the delivery floor, the position of each twin can be quickly and accurately assessed. It is also possible to rule out extension of the head when a fetus is in breech presentation.

When a patient with twins is taken to the delivery room, the real-time scanner should accompany her. After delivery of the first infant, real-time examination immediately and precisely establishes the position of the second twin. Visualization of the fetal heart allows twin B to be monitored for evidence of bradycardia until one fetal pole settles into the pelvis, membranes are ruptured, and a scalp electrode is applied.

In addition to monitoring heart rate, visualization of the second twin permits both external and internal manipulations to be performed in a more controlled fashion. Externally, it is often possible to guide the vertex over the inlet by directing pressure from the ultrasound transducer over the fetal head while pushing the buttocks toward the fundus with the other hand.[262] If this is unsuccessful, an internal version can be made less difficult by visualizing the operator's hand within the uterus and directing it toward the fetal feet.

Key Points

- Perinatal/neonatal morbidity and mortality are significantly higher in multiple gestations than singleton pregnancies.
- Any patient with a multiple gestation should be clinically managed as a high-risk pregnancy.
- The incidence of congenital structural malformations is two to three times higher in fetuses of multiple gestations when compared with those of singleton gestations.
- Ultrasound evaluation is the single most important diagnostic test in multiple gestations.
- All patients with multiple gestations should have a thorough second-trimester ultrasound examination to assess for individual fetal growth, congenital malformations, amnionicity, and chorionicity.
- Twin-to-twin transfusion syndrome is a serious potential complication in monozygotic twins.
- Prophylactic cerclage, tocolytics, or hospitalization for bedrest do not have any proven advantage in the management of multiple gestations.
- In twin pregnancies with discordant growth, fetal lung maturity studies obtained from amniotic fluid of the larger twin will usually also represent similar or greater lung maturity of the smaller twin.
- The presentation of each fetus must be sonographically verified as soon as a patient with twin pregnancy comes in labor.
- As a general rule, mode of delivery should be vaginal when both twins are vertex, individualized for vertex–nonvertex twins, and cesarean section when the first twin is nonvertex. For triplets or more, the safest mode of delivery is by cesarean section.

Chapter 17

Intrauterine Growth Restriction

Ira Bernstein and
Steven G. Gabbe

Intrauterine growth restriction (IUGR) is an important cause of antepartum fetal death and a leading contributor to the perinatal mortality rate.[1] The perinatal mortality rate for these infants is 6 to 10 times greater than that for a normally grown population. Approximately 30 percent of all stillborn infants are growth restricted. The incidence of intrapartum asphyxia in cases complicated by IUGR has been reported to be 50 percent.[2] A portion of these perinatal complications are preventable. If the growth-restricted fetus is appropriately identified and managed, the perinatal mortality can be lowered.[3]

Definition

A commonly used classification has developed that reserves the obstetric label of IUGR for the fetus who suffers morbidity and/or mortality associated with the failure to reach growth potential (Fig. 17-1) and the pediatric term "small for gestational age" (SGA) as the more general term for the small fetus for whom no pathology has yet emerged. For the purposes of this chapter, we have chosen the terms *fetal* or *intrauterine growth restriction* and apply the label in the prenatal period based on estimates of fetal size alone. We believe that this term appropriately characterizes the syndrome and eliminates the negative cognitive associations of the term *retardation*.

Neonatal growth restriction is recognized as a syndrome encompassing small size as well as specific metabolic abnormalities, including hypoglycemia, hypothermia, and polycythemia. In contrast, IUGR is currently characterized by failure to reach growth potential.

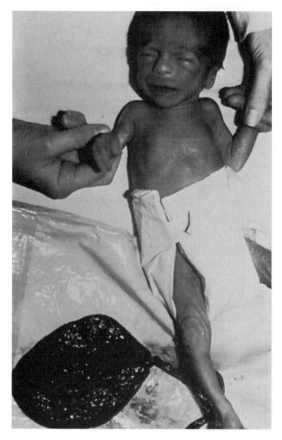

Fig. 17-1 A growth-retarded infant exhibiting subcutaneous wasting.

Ultrasound criteria have emerged as the diagnostic standard employed in the identification of fetal growth restriction. Two patterns of altered head growth were originally described. In "late flattening" IUGR, which represents approximately two-thirds of all cases, the biparietal diameter (BPD) increases normally until late pregnancy and then lags behind. In the "low-profile" type, impaired head growth occurs much earlier in gestation.

As an individual parameter, abdominal circumference (AC) has demonstrated the greatest sensitivity in the identification of IUGR.[15] The use of AC, a directly measurable fetal parameter, in combination with head circumference (HC) has been widely adopted. The most common assessment of fetal size in the United States is the estimation of fetal weight. Investigators have identified distinct fetal parameters identifiable by ultrasound that are useful.[17-20] All of these estimations incorporate an index of abdominal size. These techniques generally have 95 percent confidence limits that deviate approximately 15 percent around the actual value.

An absolute threshold used for the definition of growth restriction can be applied to any of the parameters evaluated (BPD, AC, or estimated fetal weight [EFW]). Birth weight below the population 10th percentile, corrected for gestational age, has been the most widely used criterion for defining growth restriction at birth, and this has been generalized to imply a sonographically estimated fetal weight below the 10th percentile for appropriate population-based cross-sectional growth charts.

Using the birth weight 10th percentile cutoff, approximately 70 percent of the infants thus identified as growth restricted are normally or constitutionally small, so-called SGA.[22] These neonates are *not* at increased risk for poor outcome, but represent one end of the spectrum of normal neonatal size. The remaining 30 percent of this group, does include infants who are truly growth restricted and who are at risk for increased perinatal morbidity and mortality.

Etiology

Etiologies for fetal growth restriction can be crudely separated into fetoplacental and maternal in origin. The fetoplacental origins of growth restriction include chromosomal abnormalities, genetic syndromes, and infectious etiologies, as well as those secondary to placental pathology.

Fetoplacental Origins

Intrauterine infection, although long recognized as a cause of growth restriction, accounts for less than 10 percent of all cases. Herpes, cytomegalovirus, rubella, and toxoplasmosis are well documented, and other intrauterine infections are strongly suspected (see Ch. 22). The infectious process produces early disruption of fetal growth during the stage of cell hyperplasia and is therefore associated with a poor prognosis for normal development. For the agents associated with IUGR, prevention of the infection is the most important therapy.

Fetoplacental Etiologies of Fetal Restriction

Chromosomal abnormalities
  Trisomies (13, 18, 21)
  Trisomy 9 mosaicism
  Trisomy 4P
  4P−, 5P−, 11P−, 13Q− syndromes
  Partial trisomy 10Q

Genetic syndromes
  Cretinism (hypothyroidism)
  Russell-Silver
  Bloom
  Lowe
  De Lange
  Progeria
  Leprechaunism

Congenital malformations
Infectious diseases
  Cytomegalovirus
  Toxoplasmosis
  Rubella

Placental pathology
  Previa
  Abruption
  Circumvallate
  Mosaicism
  Infarction
  Twins

Chromosomal abnormalities, congenital malformations, and genetic syndromes have been associated with less than 10 percent of cases of IUGR. Abnormalities in cell replication and reduced cell number produce a pattern of impaired growth that is early in onset and symmetric. Neonatal prognosis in these cases is determined by the specific abnormality identified.

An absolute or relative decrease in placental mass affects the quantity of substrate the fetus receives and has been recognized ultrasonographically to antedate fetal growth restriction.[27] Thus a circumvallate placenta, partial placental abruption, placenta accreta, or placental infarction may result in growth restriction. Intrinsic placental pathology has been identified in some cases of growth restriction, including the presence of a single umbilical artery. Placental location has also been linked to growth restriction. Placenta previa without bleeding has been suggested as a risk factor, because the low implantation site may not be optimal for nutrient transfer.[34]

Twin gestation represents a relative decrease in placental mass in relation to fetal mass and is therefore often associated with IUGR (see Ch. 16). Next to prematurity, growth restriction represents the second most prevalent cause of morbidity for these infants.

Maternal Origins

Decreased uteroplacental blood flow, with its associated reduction in transfer of nutrients to the fetus, is responsible for the majority of clinically recognized cases of IUGR. Maternal vascular disease, whether chronic hypertension, preeclampsia, or diabetes with vasculopathy, has been associated with impaired fetal growth.[37-39] Preeclampsia is generally marked by asymmetric IUGR with maintenance of normal fetal head growth and reduction in the size of the fetal liver, heart, thymus, spleen, pancreas, and adrenal glands.

Maternal pre-pregnancy weight and weight gain in pregnancy are two of the most important variables contributing to birth weight.[45,46]

Maternal drug ingestion may produce IUGR by a direct effect on fetal growth as well as through inadequate dietary intake. Smoking produces a symmetrically smaller fetus through reduced uterine blood flow and impaired fetal oxygenation.[51] The consumption of alcohol and the use of coumarin or hydantoin derivatives are now well known to produce particular dysmorphic features in association with impaired fetal growth. Maternal use of cocaine has been associated with not only IUGR but also reduced head circumference growth.[53]

A history of poor pregnancy outcome is clearly correlated with the subsequent delivery of a growth-restricted infant.[57] Prior birth of an IUGR infant is the obstetric factor most often associated with the subsequent birth of a growth-restricted infant. Women whose first pregnancy results in a growth-restricted infant have a 1 in 4 risk of delivering a second infant below the 10th percentile. When all indices of risk have been applied, the one-third of the population considered at highest risk accounts for two-thirds of the infants identified as growth restricted. Two-thirds of pregnancies, although not judged to be "at risk" for IUGR, yield one-third of neonates below the 10th percentile.[58] Most of these babies are constitutionally small.

Diagnosis

In the past, clinical parameters such as maternal weight gain and measurement of fundal height were used to reflect fetal growth. Studies have confirmed the lack of sensitivity of fundal height measurements for detecting fetal growth restriction.[63] The presence of risk factors should therefore prompt ultrasound estimation of fetal size independent of maternal weight gain or fundal height growth.

Fetal Measurements

The use of estimated fetal weight has been the most common method for characterizing fetal size and thereby growth abnormalities. An accurate ultrasonographic assessment of fetal weight is essential in detecting and following patients suspected of having growth-restricted infants.[64]

Fetal growth as opposed to fetal size is a dynamic process and requires more than a single evaluation for

---

Risk Factors for Fetal Growth Restriction: Indications for Ultrasound

History of fetal growth restriction
Hypertension
Diabetes mellitus
Elevated maternal serum α-fetoprotein/human chorionic gonadotropin
Antiphospholipid syndrome
Chronic medical illnesses
Low maternal pre-pregnancy weight (<90% ideal body weight)
Poor maternal weight gain
Twin gestation
Substance abuse (tobacco, alcohol, drugs)
Preterm labor
Abnormalities of placentation
Vaginal bleeding
Maternal anemia (hemoglobin < 10 g/dl)
Maternal hypoxia (cyanotic cardiac or pulmonary disease, altitude)
Maternal hemoglobinopathies
Drug ingestion (hydantoin, warfarin)

its estimation. The absence of fetal growth over a sustained period is a concern. The routine clinical evaluation of fetal growth is based on fundal height enlargement during the course of pregnancy. In pregnancies at risk or in those in which fetal size is already estimated to be below the 10th percentile, serial ultrasound estimations of fetal size are performed. The most commonly recommended interval between evaluations is 2 to 3 weeks.[3,74]

In an attempt to increase detection of the fetus with asymmetric growth restriction, HC-to-AC ratios can be assessed (Figs. 17-2 and 17-3).[77,78] In the normally

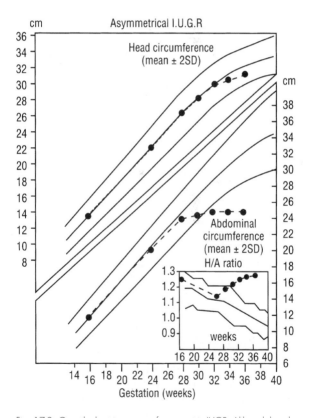

Fig. 17-2 Growth chart in a case of asymmetric IUGR. Although head circumference is preserved, AC growth falls off early in the third trimester. For this reason, the H/A ratio shown in the lower right corner of the graph becomes elevated. IUGR, intrauterine growth retardation. (From Chudleigh P, Pearce JM: Normal and Abnormal Growth. In Obstetric Ultrasound. Edinburgh, Churchill Livingstone, 1986, p 141, with permission.)

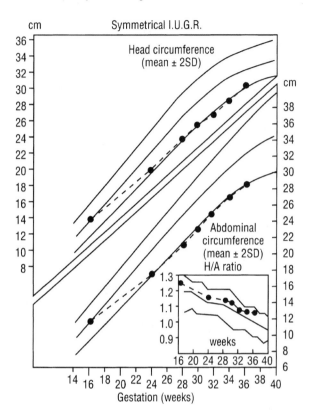

Fig. 17-3 Growth chart in a case of symmetric IUGR. Note the early onset of both HC and AC growth retardation. For this reason, the H/A ratio shown in the lower right corner remains normal. IUGR, intrauterine growth retardation. (From Chudleigh P, Pearce JM: Normal and Abnormal Growth. In Obstetric Ultrasound. Edinburgh, Churchill Livingstone, 1986, p 139, with permission.)

growing fetus, the HC/AC ratio exceeds 1.0 before 32 weeks' gestation, is approximately 1.0 at 32 to 34 weeks' gestation, and falls below 1.0 after 34 weeks' gestation. In fetuses affected by asymmetric growth restriction, the HC remains larger than that of the body (Fig. 17-2). The HC/AC ratio is then elevated. In symmetric IUGR, both the HC and the AC are reduced, and the HC/AC ratio remains normal (Fig. 17-3). Using the HC/AC ratio, 85 percent of growth-restricted fetuses are detected, with a reduction in false-negative diagnoses.

In some cases, measurement of the HC may be difficult as a result of fetal position. One can then compare femur length (FL), which is relatively spared in asymmetric IUGR, to the AC.[79] The FL/AC ratio is 22 at all gestational ages from 21 weeks to term and so can be applied without knowledge of the number of weeks of gestation. An FL/AC ratio greater than 23.5 suggests IUGR.

Oligohydramnios

Decreased amniotic fluid volume has been associated clinically with IUGR and may be the earliest sign detected on ultrasonography, preceding an elevation in HC/AC ratio and lagging fetal growth. Decreased perfusion of the fetal kidneys and reduced urine production explain this observation.[80]

The patient with an uncertain gestational age who presents late in pregnancy poses a difficult diagnostic dilemma because interpretation of BPD and HC/AC ratios must be related to accurate gestational age. Under these conditions, measuring an amniotic fluid pocket, or an FL/AC ratio, may be helpful, as these do not rely on knowledge of the gestational age. A 2-cm vertical pocket is considered normal, 1 to 2 cm is marginal, and less than 1 cm is decreased. One may also use the amniotic fluid index to quantitate amniotic fluid volume (Ch. 4), although this technique requires a knowledge of gestational age.

Summary

The ability to determine appropriate fetal growth using fundal height measurements in a normal population is limited. Fundal height measurements lack both sensitivity and specificity in the identification of the small fetus. It is therefore reasonable to employ a better tool (ultrasound) whenever clinical circumstances point to an increased risk for a growth-restricted fetus. A number of clinical conditions that increase the risk for IUGR were listed earlier. In the absence of routine clinical indications, ultrasound screening of these high-risk pregnancies should be performed at 16 to 18 weeks for dating (if not otherwise established) and again at 32 to 34 weeks.

Management

In developing a plan for the management of suspected growth restriction, it is important to remember the major etiologic groups. Most infants thought to be growth restricted are constitutionally small and require no intervention. Unfortunately, this diagnosis is usually made retrospectively. Approximately 15 percent exhibit symmetric growth restriction due to an early fetal insult for which there is no effective therapy. Here, an accurate diagnosis is essential. Finally, approximately 15 percent have growth restriction or extrinsic growth failure due to placental disease or reduced uteroplacental blood flow. In such cases, antepartum fetal monitoring and carefully timed delivery may be critical.

Once growth restriction is suspected, a well-organized approach to management should be undertaken. The clinician should evaluate and treat problems that may be contributing to growth restriction. Therapy of growth restriction is often nonspecific but should be directed at the underlying cause of poor fetal growth if one can be determined. When a maternal medical problem such as inflammatory bowel disease is contributing to poor growth, specific therapy should be instituted. Alleviation of hypoxia, therapy for high blood pressure and anemia, and hyperalimentation are three examples. Certainly, mothers should be counseled to stop smoking and ingesting alcohol. Nonspecific therapies include bedrest in the left lateral decubitus position to increase placental blood flow. While an inadequate diet has not been clearly established as a cause of growth restriction in this country, dietary supplementation may be helpful in those women with poor weight gain or low pre-pregnancy weight.

Testing

Serial evaluations of fetal growth should be instituted as soon as the diagnosis of growth restriction is confirmed or for patients in whom the suspicion for growth restriction is high. In the clinic setting, special effort should be made to have the same examiner see the patient each visit to measure the fundal height and assess fetal weight. Ultrasound examinations should be scheduled every 3 weeks and should include determinations of the BPD, HC/AC, fetal weight, and amniotic fluid volume. Arrested head growth is of great concern, especially in light of the most recent data available on ultimate developmental potential for the growth-restricted infant.[120] Clear documentation of arrested head growth over a 4-week period is alarming, and the feasibility and safety of delivery should be reviewed.[121]

Ultrasound should be used not only to document abnormal growth but also to detect lethal congenital malformations such as renal agenesis. In cases of severe symmetric growth restriction, amniocentesis, placental biopsy, or cordocentesis should be considered to rule out a chromosomal abnormality such as trisomy 13, 18, or 21.

Fetal well-being should also be assessed regularly once the diagnosis of growth restriction is entertained. These infants have an increased incidence of intrauterine demise, presumably from cord compression as well as placental insufficiency. Monitoring these infants decreases the stillbirth rate by detecting the compromised fetus and allowing timely intervention.[3]

Experience with the nonstress test (NST) in cases of growth restriction has confirmed that a reactive NST correlates highly with a fetus that is not in immediate danger of intrauterine demise. Twice-weekly nonstress testing is an appropriate interval.[122] The appearance of spontaneous decelerations during the NST may reflect oligohydramnios and cord compression and has been associated with a high perinatal mortality rate.[124] The addition of a measure of amniotic fluid volume to the NST has been called a "modified biophysical profile." When compared with a weekly contraction stress test, the twice-weekly modified biophysical profile results in similar perinatal outcome.[125]

Nonreactive NST results are often falsely positive and should be further evaluated before any management decision is made. Contraction stress testing (CST) or a biophysical profile are both options for additional testing. A negative CST result, even when the CST is performed early in the third trimester, is an indication of adequate placental respiratory reserve.[126] Conversely, positive CST results occur in 30 percent of the pregnancies complicated by proven growth restriction. Information from antepartum fetal heart rate testing must always be reviewed in concert with the gestational age of the fetus, as well as other indices of fetal well-being and fetal growth.

The fetal biophysical profile score can provide appropriate follow-up to nonreassuring fetal heart rate testing or can be used as an alternative method for primary antenatal surveillance. As a backup test for nonreassuring fetal heart rate testing, the biophysical profile leads to lower rates of intervention when compared with the CST, with no impact on perinatal outcome.[132]

Maternal monitoring of fetal activity has also been used extensively for the assessment of pregnancies complicated by IUGR. The techniques available for monitoring fetal movement are reviewed in Chapter 6.

The major focus of Doppler studies for the assessment of fetal health has been the umbilical–placental circulation. The small arterial vessel count in the tertiary stem villi of the placenta is significantly lower in patients with high umbilical artery systolic/diastolic (S/D) ratios than in those with normal S/D ratios. These observations suggest that the increased resistance to flow as demonstrated by a high S/D ratio is associated with and may be due to obliteration of the small muscular arteries in the tertiary stem villi.

Doppler flow studies of the umbilical artery may help to assess fetal jeopardy and reduce perinatal mortality in the pregnancy complicated by IUGR. Fetuses with absent end-diastolic flow are significantly more growth restricted and require delivery at an earlier gestational age than those in whom end-diastolic flow is observed. These fetuses are also more likely to suffer perinatal death, necrotizing enterocolitis, and hemorrhage. Absent end-diastolic umbilical flow signals the need for aggressive antenatal surveillance at a level greater than that usually provided.[148] Reversed end-diastolic flow in the umbilical artery reflects severe fetal compromise and is an ominous finding. Perinatal mortality rates were 50 and 64 percent in two studies examining the prognostic significance of this finding. Consideration of delivery should be made when reversed end-diastolic flow is detected.[149,150]

Delivery

Proper timing of delivery is often the critical management issue when dealing with the growth-restricted fetus. The crux of management is to balance the hazards of prematurity with the threat of intrauterine demise. Careful consideration should be given to the reliability of the information on which the gestational age of the fetus has been established, the fetal growth curve, and the results of antepartum fetal monitoring.

Amniocentesis may be an important adjunct to this decision-making process. The lecithin/sphingomyelin (L/S) ratio may also provide information that allows more accurate dating of the pregnancy. A surprisingly low L/S ratio would suggest an earlier gestational age rather than fetal growth restriction. In cases of symmetric growth restriction, a late amniocentesis may also be employed to obtain amniotic fluid for a fetal karyotype.

To review, if growth restriction is suspected or anticipated, appropriate fetal testing and daily maternal assessment of fetal activity should be instituted. Ultrasound examinations to assess fetal growth should be scheduled every 3 weeks. As long as studies show continued fetal head growth and test results remain reassuring, no intervention is required. If the patient fails a primary surveillance tool such as the NST, follow-up testing must be done. If the CST result is positive or the fetal biophysical profile score is either 6 with oligohydramnios or 4 or less, delivery should be considered. An assessment of fetal lung maturity should be made if possible. In the face of a mature L/S ratio and ominous antepartum test results, delivery should be effected. If the patient has an immature L/S ratio and abnormal test findings, then consideration can be given to steroid administration with continuous heart rate monitoring and oxygen supplementation until delivery or until antepartum test results improve. If amniotic fluid cannot be obtained for an L/S ratio as a result of oligohydramnios and the clinical picture supports the diagnosis of severe IUGR, early delivery should be considered. In these difficult cases, the pediatricians who will care for the baby should be included in the decision-making process.

Because a large proportion of growth-restricted infants suffer intrapartum asphyxia, intrapartum management demands continuous fetal heart rate monitoring. During labor, a tracing without late decelerations is predictive of a good outcome in cases complicated by IUGR. However, with late decelerations, the incidence of asphyxia in growth-restricted infants is far greater than in normally grown infants. Therefore, earlier intervention may be indicated.[164] An unfavorable cervix may also preclude internal fetal heart rate monitoring. In the face of an inadequate external tracing, cesarean delivery may be necessary.

Neonatal Outcome

Neonatal morbidity must be anticipated when the growth-restricted fetus is delivered. Because immediate attention to the many neonatal problems experienced by these infants is essential, appropriate pediatric support should be present in the delivery room when an infant suspected of being growth restricted is to be delivered. These infants suffer more frequently from meconium aspiration than do appropriately grown infants. At delivery, careful suctioning of the nasopharynx and oropharynx with the DeLee catheter decreases the incidence of this complication.[166] Further clearing of the airway can be accomplished by direct laryngoscopy and aspiration by an experienced pediatrician.

Hypoglycemia is a frequent problem in growth-restricted infants and should be anticipated in all such infants. Polycythemia is observed three to four times more frequently in the growth-restricted infant than in weight-matched controls. Polycythemia leads to increased red blood cell breakdown, accounting in part for the high incidence of hyperbilirubinemia in these infants. Polycythemia may also contribute to hyperviscosity. Hypothermia is another common problem for the growth-restricted infant. It results from decreased body fat stores secondary to intrauterine malnourishment.[167]

Have recent improvements in obstetric and pediatric care favorably affected the outcome of the growth-restricted infant? The perinatal mortality rate for those infants who receive optimal intrapartum and neonatal management is decreased when compared with that for age-matched controls who did not have intensive care.[172] The ultimate growth potential for these infants also appears to be good. These infants can be expected to have normal growth curves and normal, albeit slightly reduced, size as adults. In general, those infants suffering growth restriction near the time of delivery do tend to catch up. However, those neonates with earlier onset and more longstanding growth restriction in utero continue to lag behind.

In summary, neurologic outcome depends on the degree of growth restriction, its time of onset, and the immaturity of the infant at birth. An early intrauterine insult, between 10 and 17 weeks' gestation, could limit neuronal cellular multiplication and would obviously have a profound effect on neurologic function.[184] Recovery after a period of impaired growth in the third trimester is more likely to occur. Thus the preterm appropriately grown infant has more normal neurologic development and fewer severe neurologic deficits than its preterm growth-restricted counterpart. Developmental milestones and neurologic development of mature infants with IUGR and mature infants of normal birth weight are similar. Presumably, this also reflects heightened physician awareness of the growth-restricted infant that allows detection, appropriate antepartum management, intrapartum therapy, and early pediatric intervention.[185–187] The premature growth-restricted infant suffers from increased susceptibility to intrauterine asphyxia and all of the neonatal complications of the premature, as well as those of the infant with IUGR. If growth restriction is associated with lagging head growth before 26 weeks, even mature infants have significant developmental delay at 4 years of age.

Key Points

- Fetal growth restriction is the second leading cause of perinatal morbidity and mortality. Intrauterine growth restriction is currently defined by fetal size alone.

- Characterization of fetal size should be performed using growth curves that are population specific and appropriate.
- The definition of fetal growth restriction has not been based on correlations with short- and long-term morbidity.
- Preterm delivery is associated with an increased incidence of fetal growth restriction.
- Fundal height measurements have low sensitivity in the identification of fetal growth restriction.
- Mortality resulting from fetal growth restriction can be reduced with appropriate antenatal surveillance strategies, which may include early delivery.
- The use of fetal umbilical Doppler flow studies in the management of the growth-restricted fetus reduces perinatal morbidity and mortality.
- Fetal growth restriction is associated with high rates of intrapartum asphyxia.
- Intrauterine growth restriction can result in both short-term and lifelong morbidities.

Postdate Pregnancy

Roger K. Freeman and
David C. Lagrew, Jr.

Postdate pregnancy is a common problem in obstetric practice. Through the use of first- and second-trimester ultrasound, this group now contains fewer patients with poor dating; therefore, these patients as a whole are at higher risk for complications. Comprehensive management of postdate pregnancy involves both fetal testing and consideration for delivery, with the choice for each individual pregnancy dependent on several clinical factors.

Background

In 1963, McClure-Brown's data[2] showed a twofold increase in fetal mortality when the patient reached 42 weeks' gestation. For this reason, British clinicians recommended routine induction of labor between the 42nd and 43rd weeks to prevent poor outcome. They demonstrated beneficial birth results from such aggressive management.[2]

Definition and Incidence

In this chapter, the terms *postdate* and *post-term* will be used interchangeably. Most authors define a postdate pregnancy as that which has reached 42 weeks of amenorrhea. The incidence of morbidity increases after 40 weeks (Fig. 18-1).[2] At 42 weeks, perinatal mortality doubles, making this an appropriate cutoff point.

Accurate diagnosis of post-term pregnancy depends on proper clinical dating of the pregnancy. Early prenatal examination and ultrasound clearly improve the accuracy of dating. Approximately 50 percent of patients deliver by their estimated date of confinement,

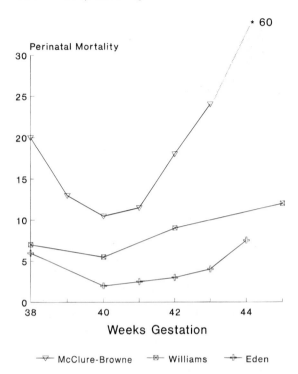

Fig. 18-1 Comparison of perinatal mortality rates versus gestational age through the past three decades. (From McClure-Browne JC: Postmaturity. Am J Obstet Gynecol 85:373, 1963 data collected in 1958, Williams RL, Creasy RK, Cunningham CG et al: Fetal growth and perinatal viability in California. Obstet Gynecol 59:624, 1982 in 1970–1976, and Eden RD, Seifert JS, Winegar A: Perinatal characteristics of uncomplicated postdate pregnancies. Obstet Gynecol 69: 296, 1987, with permission).

and about 35 to 40 percent deliver within the following 2 weeks. Three percent of all patients reach the 42nd week.

Morbidity and Mortality

The rate of maternal, fetal, and neonatal complications increases exponentially with gestational age.[2-4] The primary maternal risk is cesarean delivery, with an associated increased incidence of postpartum infections, hemorrhage from uterine atony, prolonged hospitalization, wound complications, and pulmonary emboli. The cesarean delivery rate more than doubles when passing the 42nd week compared with term (38 to 40 weeks). This increase can be attributed to cephalopelvic disproportion resulting from larger infants. Some cesarean deliveries are accounted for by attempted induction of patients with unripe cervices. The overall incidence of nonreassuring heart rate patterns during labor is minimally elevated compared with term populations.[10] Maternal complications also include trauma from the vaginal delivery of large babies.[11]

Neonatal complications from postmaturity include placental insufficiency, birth trauma from macrosomia, and meconium aspiration syndrome.

The incidence of growth restriction or dysmaturity reaches 10 percent by the 43rd week.[8] Clifford[3] described these infants as withered, meconium stained, long nailed, and fragile, with a small placenta and at risk for stillbirth. In the neonatal period there is an increased risk of hypoglycemia, heat instability, and meconium aspiration.[3] Growth restriction from postmaturity is the result of uteroplacental insufficiency.[12] Antenatal surveillance is necessary in *all* post-term pregnancies regardless of growth. Fortunately, long-term problems appear to arise less with postmaturity than with other forms of growth restriction.

Meconium is found in 25 to 30 percent of post-term pregnancies, double the incidence at term.[9,15] The diminished amniotic fluid causes the meconium to be thicker and more likely to obstruct airways. Aspiration into the alveoli can cause significant respiratory embarrassment and death.

Management

Diagnosis

The accurate diagnosis of postdate pregnancy can be made only by proper dating. A major problem of determining gestational age is that all methods of estimating gestational age lose accuracy in the third trimester, when fetal growth diminishes. Since we cannot predict who will be undelivered by 42 weeks, we must accurately date all prenatal patients (see Ch. 4).

It is important to review clinical parameters in all patients since they are helpful in establishing gestational age at minimal cost. The regularity, date, amount, and length of menses are important clinical factors in gestational age estimation. First-trimester pelvic examination can be helpful in confirming menstrual dates. Other clinical parameters include date of first pregnancy test, first fetal heart tones (12 weeks with Doppler, 18 weeks with fetoscope), timing of the fundal height reaching the umbilicus (20 weeks), and quickening.

Routine first- or second-trimester ultrasound of all pregnant patients decreases the incidence of post-term pregnancy.[20] In patients with regular menses, confirmation by a first-trimester pelvic examination, ovulation data, or timed insemination, ultrasound is of less importance. Ultrasound is clearly beneficial in patients without known or reliable clinical data. Ultrasound is most accurate in early gestation. Measurement of crown–rump length between 6 and 10 weeks can define gestational age within 3 to 5 days.[21] A screening ultrasound at 16 to 20 weeks also allows review of fetal anatomy and dating within ± 1.5 weeks. The most cost-effective period for ultrasound dating, therefore, is between 16 and 20 weeks.

The Choice: Expectant Management Versus Induction of Labor

The first major decision in management is dependent on the certainty of the dates. Patients with unsure dates should be managed in a less aggressive fashion when considering delivery if the cervix is not clearly inducible. However, these patients should receive the same program of antenatal surveillance as well-dated pregnancies. There are two basic schemes of management for well-dated postdate patients (Fig. 18-2).

Patients with favorable cervices benefit from induction of labor. Unfortunately, these are the minority of postdate pregnancies. There are two major reasons for inducing patients with favorable cervices. First, some fetuses will continue growing after term and may develop macrosomia and cephalopelvic disproportion. Second, although antenatal surveillance with appropriate methods is quite reliable, there are occasional mispredictions that result in 0.5 to 1/1,000 unexpected stillbirths in nonanomalous fetuses even with good patient compliance.[24] Therefore, if the cervix is favorable, delivery provides the safest alternative for mother and baby. Induction is a reasonable option in such patients after the 41st week has passed and spontaneous labor has not ensued.

With confirmed dates and an unfavorable cervix there are two major management methods. The most established method is to initiate antepartum surveillance while awaiting spontaneous labor[25] and/or spontaneous cervical ripening. The other method is to administer prostaglandin gel for cervical ripening and proceed with induction.[26]

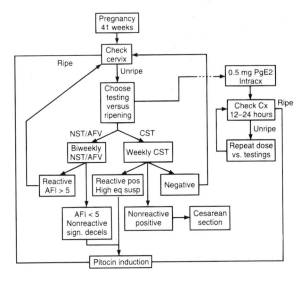

Fig. 18-2 Postdate pregnancy management flow chart. The scheme depicts the various decision-making processes involved in the management of the post-term pregnancy with respect to delivery. The decision whether to use intracervical prostaglandin should be based on clinical data regarding patient safety and ripeness of the cervix. It has been our practice to attempt a trial of induction in well-dated pregnancies at 43 weeks' gestation.

There are clinical problems with both management schemes that must be considered. The purpose of expectant management with testing is to await cervical ripening and spontaneous labor, which should decrease the need for cesarean delivery.

An American trial randomized 440 patients to induction versus expectant management.[27] The induction group was then subdivided into those receiving a single insertion of intracervical prostaglandin gel or placebo. There were no differences in incidences of adverse perinatal outcomes, macrosomia, or cesarean delivery between the groups. It was concluded that either management protocol was acceptable.[27] A Canadian trial randomized 3,407 women at 41 weeks.[28] The induction group received three doses of prostaglandin gel followed by oxytocin induction. These patients had a significantly lower cesarean delivery rate (21.2 vs. 24.5 percent) when compared with women managed expectantly due to a reduced incidence of fetal distress. There was no statistical difference in the rate of stillbirth. A meta-analysis of 11 trials has revealed that routine induction has a lower rate of perinatal mortality, cesarean delivery, and meconium staining.

Cervical Ripening with Prostaglandin

Prostaglandin gel can improve the likelihood of successful induction. Prostaglandin E_2 gel applied locally to the cervix softens, dilates, and effaces the cervix. The clinical effects are shortened labor, fewer failed inductions, and less need for artificial amniotomy.[26]

Prostaglandin ripening should be used in patients with an unripe cervix at or beyond 41 weeks' gestation when induction is elected. The gel is given on the afternoon or evening before scheduled induction. Before administration, a reassuring fetal heart rate and uterine activity pattern is documented. If the fetus has a nonreassuring fetal heart rate tracing or there is excessive uterine activity, the use of prostaglandin gel may not be advisable. After evaluating cervical status, 0.5 mg of prostaglandin E_2 gel is placed intracervically. The patient is observed on the monitor for approximately 2 hours or until uterine activity has subsided. When needed, oxytocin induction should be started the next morning after examination has documented ripening of the cervix. If the cervix remains unfavorable, a second dose of prostaglandin gel may be given or expectant management with fetal surveillance initiated while awaiting cervical ripening.

Expectant Management with Antenatal Surveillance

Most expectant management schemes require antenatal surveillance of fetal well-being. The general trend in the United States has been to begin testing during the 41st week of pregnancy. This practice appears to be reasonable in light of the increased incidence of perinatal mortality following 40 weeks. Since cost effectiveness becomes an issue, fetal movement charting may be reasonable prior to the 41st week (see Ch. 5).

Most antepartum testing in the United States is done with the nonstress test (NST). The NST yields few equivocal results, and interventions are rarely necessary for an abnormal test result.[33] The major concern using this modality has been falsely reassuring results. Weekly NSTs appear to have a false-negative rate of 6.1/1,000 (stillbirth within 1 week of a reassuring test).[34] Twice-weekly testing decreases the false-negative rate from

6.1 to 1.9/1,000. Therefore, to improve predictability, NSTs are performed twice weekly. Spontaneous decelerations are significant. Poor perinatal outcomes are increased in patients with decelerations on their NST.

Another surveillance choice is the contraction stress test (CST). The major benefit of the CST is that negative results appear to predict fetal well-being for 7 days. Weekly CSTs are effective in preventing stillbirth and have a false-negative rate of only 0.71/1,000.[24] The major problem of the CST is the high rate of equivocal results.[24,33] Patients with equivocal tests require repeat testing in 24 hours. For positive and highly suspicious tests, attempted delivery is indicated. If the CST result is reactive and positive, a trial of labor may be attempted, since many of these patients will deliver vaginally.[24] Should the test result be nonreactive and positive, the patient should have constant electronic fetal monitoring while preparations for cesarean delivery are made. If the fetus remains nonreactive, a cesarean delivery is preferred.[24] With clinically significant oligohydramnios, cord compression may occur as manifested by variable decelerations. Variable decelerations should be evaluated with an estimate of amniotic fluid volume.

Some investigators have advocated the modified biophysical profile (mBPP). This twice-weekly test uses the NST and amniotic fluid volume. Post-term patients are five times more likely to develop oligohydramnios in 3 to 4 days following a normal amniotic fluid index (AFI).[47] These data suggest the AFI should be repeated *twice weekly* in post-term patients.[47]

If the patient remains undelivered by the 43rd week of gestation, it has been our policy to attempt induction of labor.

Intrapartum Management

The major complications in the intrapartum period are meconium staining, macrosomia, and fetal intolerance to labor. The key to proper management is timely recognition, prompt reaction, and skilled actions.

Meconium staining is four times more common in the post-term pregnancy than in term gestations. Before the institution of suctioning techniques, meconium aspiration syndrome was the leading cause of mortality in infants over 2,500 g.

When minimal fluid is encountered at the time of membrane rupture, the risk for thick, tenacious meconium is increased. Amnioinfusion dilutes meconium, improves 1-minute Apgar scores, and decreases the number of infants with meconium below the cords.[52] Instillation of normal saline through an intrauterine pressure catheter is a relatively benign procedure and may reduce variable decelerations (see Ch. 7).[53]

Meconium aspiration syndrome may be reduced by aggressive suctioning at the time of delivery of the head. This technique should be combined with neonatal tracheal aspiration when meconium is present at or below the vocal cords.[55] While these techniques have been shown to make meconium aspiration syndrome less common, they will *not* prevent the disease completely. It has become evident that fetal asphyxia in utero before labor may lead to pulmonary injury such that the lungs cannot clear meconium. This problem combined with pulmonary vascular damage followed by persistent fetal circulation after birth can lead to significant neonatal morbidity and mortality (see Ch. 13).[56]

Another important aspect of management is preventing birth trauma associated with macrosomia. Macrosomia should be suspected in all post-term gestations. Fetal weight should be estimated immediately before or in the early stages of labor of all post-term pregnancies in which vaginal delivery is considered.

There are several steps to take with suspected macrosomia. Midpelvic operative vaginal delivery should be avoided, particularly with a prolonged second stage. The pediatrician and anesthesiologist should be notified so they can prepare for delivery. Someone skilled in the various maneuvers for dealing with shoulder dystocia should be present for the delivery. Finally, cesarean delivery should be considered for suspected macrosomia in patients with an estimated fetal weight greater than 4,500 g, a marginal pelvis, or previous difficult vaginal delivery with the same or smaller sized infant.

Intrapartum asphyxia is also more common in the post-term pregnancy; therefore, close observation of the fetal heart rate is necessary.

Conclusion

While postdate pregnancy increases the risks to the fetus and mother, satisfactory outcome can be expected with appropriate pregnancy dating, fetal surveillance, intervention when necessary, and careful intrapartum and neonatal management.

Key Points

- Postdatism has not always been of universal concern, but with improving gestational age assessment and closer follow-up, the problem has become more well defined.

- The primary risk to the mother from postdatism includes an increase in postpartum infections, hemorrhage from uterine atony, prolonged hospitalization, wound complications, and an increased incidence of cesarean delivery.

- Neonatal complications from postmaturity include placental insufficiency, birth trauma from macrosomia, and meconium aspiration syndrome.

- The accuracy of diagnosis of the post-term pregnancy can be made only by proper dating, since all methods of estimating gestational age lose accuracy in the third trimester. It is important to determine an accurate estimated delivery date in early pregnancy.

- Post-date management can be divided into two clear choices, (1) expectant management and (2) induction of labor.

- Patients with favorable cervices benefit from induction of labor.

- When the cervix is uninducible, consideration of cervical ripening is weighed against expectant management with antepartum testing.

- Recent prospective randomized trials have suggested that a slightly decreased cesarean delivery rate is associated with induction of labor. Expectant management should be accompanied by antepartum testing.

- Oligohydramnios is an important clinical development in the post-date pregnancy. All pregnancies should be followed closely for this development.

- Intrapartum management should include careful fetal surveillance, identification of and prevention of trauma from macrosomia, and suctioning of meconium-stained fluid at delivery.

Rhesus Isoimmunization in Pregnancy

Marc Jackson and
D. Ware Branch

This chapter reviews the causes and management of isoimmunization in pregnancy: Rhesus (Rh) isoimmunization, sensitization caused by other erythrocyte antigens, and platelet isoimmunization. Rh isoimmunization is emphasized because it remains a leading cause of fetal or neonatal death from hemolytic disease. The principles of pathophysiology and management discussed under Rh isoimmunization also generally apply to the other causes of isoimmunization. Throughout this chapter, the traditional term *sensitization* is used interchangeably with *isoimmunization*.

Genetics and Biochemistry of the Rh Antigen

Genetics

The Rh gene complex has eight allele complexes. Listed in decreasing order of frequency in the white population, they are CDe, cde, cDE, cDe, Cde, cdE, CDE, and CdE. Genotypes are indicated as pairs of gene complexes, such as CDe/cde. Certain haplotypes, and thus certain phenotypes, are more common in the population than others (Table 19-1).[8] Genotypes CDe/cde and CDe/CDe are the most common, with approximately 55 percent of all whites having the CcDe or CDe phenotype. Genotype CdE has actually never been demonstrated.[7] Although the alleles are always written in the order C(c), D(d), E(e), the actual order of the genes on chromosome 1 is D, C(c), E(e).

The genetic locus for the Rh antigen is on the short arm of chromosome 1.[11,12] The Rh locus has molecularly been shown to consist of two distinct structural

Table 19-1 Frequency of Rh Phenotypes and Genotypes Among Whites

Phenotype	Population Frequency (%)	Frequency Within:	
		Genotype	(%)
CcDe	35	CDe/cde (R^1/r)	94
		CDe/cDe (R^1/R^0)	6
		cDe/Cde (R^0/r')	<1
CDe	20	CDe/CDe (R^1/R^1)	95
		CDe/Cde (R^1/r')	5
ce	16	cde/cde (r/r)	100
CcDEe	13	CDe/cDE (R^1/R^2)	89
		CDe/cdE (R^1/r'')	7
		cDE/Cde (R^2/r')	2
		CDE/cde (R^z/r)	1
		CDE/cDe (R^z/R^0)	<1
cDEe	10	cDE/cde (R^2/r)	93
		cDE/cDe (R^2/R^0)	6
		cDe/cdE (R^0/r'')	1
cDE	3	cDE/cDE (R^2/R^2)	86
		cDE/cdE (R^2/r'')	14
cDe	2	cDe/cde (R^0/r)	97
		cDe/cDe (R^0/R^0)	3
Cce	1	Cde/cde (r'/r)	100

genes adjacent to one another, RhCcEe and RhD. These two genes likely share a single genetic ancestor, as they are identical in more than 95 percent of their coding sequences.[13] The first gene codes for the C/c and E/e antigens, and the second gene codes for the D antigen; patients who are D-negative lack the RhD gene on both their chromosomes. Thus, D-negative patients have a deletion of the D gene on both their chromosomes 1.

Gene dosage has an effect on the number of specific Rh antigen sites that express antigen; individuals homozygous for a particular genotype have up to twice as many antigen sites as individuals who are heterozygous.[16]

Allelic interaction on Rh antigen sites has been described: erythrocytes of genotype CDe/cde express less D antigen than do the erythrocytes of genotype cDE/cde.[18] Thus the presence of the C antigen seems to affect the expression of the D antigen. Similarly, individuals of genotype CDe/cDE express less C antigen than individuals of genotype CDe/cde.[8] In addition, genes other than those coding for the Rh antigen may affect the final antigenic expression; two independently segregating regulator genes have been described.[10]

Causes of Rh Isoimmunization

For Rh isoimmunization to occur in a pregnancy, at least three circumstances must exist:

1. The fetus must have Rh-positive erythrocytes and the mother must have Rh-negative erythrocytes.
2. A sufficient number of fetal erythrocytes must gain access to the maternal circulation.
3. The mother must have the immunogenic capacity to produce antibody directed against the D antigen.

Incidence of Rh-Incompatible Pregnancy

About 15 percent of whites of European extraction are Rh negative; only 5 to 8 percent of American blacks and 1 to 2 percent of Asians and Native Americans are Rh negative. In the white population, an Rh-negative woman has about an 85 percent chance of mating with an Rh-positive man. About 60 percent of Rh-positive men are heterozygous and 40 percent are homozygous at the D locus. Given that one-half of conceptions due to heterozygous men will be Rh positive, the overall chance of an Rh-positive man producing an Rh-positive fetus is about 70 percent. Thus, without knowing the father's blood type, an Rh-negative woman has about a 60 percent chance of bearing an Rh-positive fetus (0.85×0.70). Among whites, the net result is that about 10 percent of pregnancies are Rh incompatible (0.15×0.60). However, because sufficient fetomaternal hemorrhage and a subsequent maternal antibody response do not occur in every case, less than 20 percent of incompatible pregnancies eventuate in maternal sensitization. Thus, in the era before Rh immune globulin prophylaxis, about 1 percent of pregnant women had anti-D antibody.

Fetomaternal Hemorrhage

Fetal red cells can gain access to the maternal circulation during pregnancy and the immediate postpartum period. Fetomaternal hemorrhage in a volume sufficient to cause isoimmunization is most common at delivery, occurring in about 15 to 50 percent of births.[33–36] In more than half of these intrapartum fetomaternal bleeds, the amount of fetal blood entering the maternal circulation is 0.1 ml or less.[36,37] However, in

0.2 to 1 percent of cases, the estimated volume of feto-maternal hemorrhage is 30 ml or more.[34,38,39] Such factors as cesarean delivery, multiple gestation, bleeding placenta previa or abruption, manual removal of the placenta, and intrauterine manipulation may increase the chance of substantial hemorrhage. However, the majority of excessive fetomaternal hemorrhages occur in patients without risk factors who have an uncomplicated vaginal delivery.[39,40]

The amount of fetomaternal hemorrhage necessary to cause isoimmunization varies from patient to patient, probably due to the immunogenic capacity of the Rh-positive erythrocytes and the immune responsiveness of the mother. As little as 0.1 ml of Rh-positive red blood cells has been shown to sensitize some Rh-negative volunteers, and about 3 percent of women found to have 0.1 ml of fetal erythrocytes in their circulation after an Rh-incompatible delivery develop anti-D antibodies within 6 to 12 months.[36]

Overall, about 16 percent of Rh-negative women will become isoimmunized by their first Rh-incompatible (ABO-compatible) pregnancy if not treated with Rh immune globulin.[37] Half of these women respond with the production of sufficient anti-D antibody to be detectable within the first 6 months after delivery; in the remainder, anti-D is not detected until early in the next incompatible pregnancy. In this latter group, sensitization likely occurred during the first pregnancy, but the primary immune response was too slight for detectable antibody levels to develop. Although not all Rh-negative women bearing Rh-positive infants will become sensitized, the risk of sensitization approaches 50 percent after several incompatible pregnancies.

Even without labor or obvious disruption of the choriodecidual junction, antepartum fetomaternal hemorrhage occurs in sufficient volume to result in isoimmunization in a small percentage of cases. In one large series, fetomaternal hemorrhage was detected in 7 percent of patients in the first trimester, in 16 percent of patients during the second trimester, and in 29 percent of the third trimester determinations.[33] The result of this antepartum fetomaternal hemorrhage is an overall rate of Rh sensitization of about 1 to 2 percent before delivery.[41] However, antepartum sensitization rarely occurs before the third trimester.

Fetomaternal hemorrhage leading to isoimmunization has also been described with abortion and tubal pregnancy.[42-45] Fetal Rh antigens are present at least by the thirty-eighth day after conception. Assuming that as little as 0.1 ml of fetal blood can cause isoimmunization, a fetomaternal hemorrhage leading to sensitization could occur by the seventh week after the last menses.[46]

For the unsensitized Rh-negative woman, a spontaneous first-trimester abortion carries a 3 to 4 percent risk of isoimmunization.[48] Induced abortions are also likely to produce detectable fetomaternal hemorrhage. In the second trimester, pregnancy termination by saline injection and hysterotomy is associated with significant fetomaternal hemorrhage.[44,45] Threatened abortion in the first trimester also appears to increase the risk of sensitization. All Rh-negative unsensitized women should receive 50 μg of Rh immune globulin within 72 hours of induced or spontaneous first-trimester abortion. Patients in the midtrimester, 13 weeks or more, are routinely given a full dose, 300 μg.

Ectopic pregnancy can result in isoimmunization in a susceptible woman.[42] The risk of significant fetomaternal hemorrhage may be greater in cases of ruptured tubal pregnancy, presumably because of the absorption of fetal erythrocytes into the maternal circulation across the peritoneum.[52]

Amniocentesis in any trimester is associated with fetomaternal hemorrhage in 15 to 25 percent of cases, even when ultrasound is used to identify placental location.[53,54] Isoimmunization occurring after amniocentesis has been reported.[55] Similar statements apply to chorionic villus sampling.

Maternal Immunologic Response

Two major factors determine whether isoimmunization will occur in a susceptible Rh-negative woman. First, as many as 30 percent of Rh-negative individuals appear to be immunologic "nonresponders" who will not become sensitized, even when challenged with large volumes of Rh-positive blood.[56,57] Second, ABO incompatibility exerts a protective effect against the development of Rh sensitization.[58]

Two mechanisms explaining the protective effect of ABO incompatibility have been proposed. One suggests that the ABO-incompatible fetal cells are more rapidly cleared from the maternal circulation so that trapping of the antigen in the spleen, where sensitization can be initiated, does not occur. A second mechanism for the protective effect of ABO incompatibility proposes that maternal anti-A or anti-B antibodies damage or alter the fetal Rh antigen so that it is no longer immunogenic.[59]

Irrespective, ABO incompatibility diminishes the risk of isoimmunization to about 1.5 to 2 percent after the delivery of an Rh-positive fetus.[60] This effect is most pronounced in matings in which the mother is type O and the father is type A, type B, or type AB.[61]

The Use of Rh Immune Globulin

The principle that a passively administered antibody will prevent active immunization by its specific antigen is termed *antibody-mediated immune suppression* (AMIS) and was well known to immunologists for decades before being applied to the prevention of Rh disease. During the early 1960s, Freda et al.[62] in the United States and Clarke et al.[63] in Great Britain simultaneously undertook to evaluate AMIS in humans. Both groups achieved a high degree of protection from isoimmunization by administering anti-D immune globulin (Rh immune globulin) to Rh-negative male volunteers who had been infused with Rh-positive red cells.[62,63] In 1963, Pollack et al.[64] established that 300 µg of Rh immune globulin would reliably prevent isoimmunization in male volunteers who had received 10 ml of Rh-positive cells. By an extrapolation of the data, Pollack et al. showed that 20 µg of Rh immune globulin per milliliter of fetal erythrocytes or 10 µg/ml of whole fetal blood was required to prevent isoimmunization; thus the rule was established that 10 µg Rh immune globulin should be given for every 1 ml of fetal blood in the maternal circulation. Although in early trials 300 µg or more of Rh immune globulin was used, it has subsequently been shown that a dose of 100 to 150 µg is probably adequate for routine use.[67,68] Nonetheless, the standard approved dose for Rh prophylaxis in the United States remains 300 µg.

The 72-hour time limit set for the postpartum administration of Rh immune globulin is an artifact of the design of the early male prisoner volunteer studies. Prison officials would only allow the investigators to visit the volunteers at 3-day intervals[69]; thus the use of Rh immune globulin at intervals of more than 3 days after a challenge with Rh-positive cells was never extensively evaluated. However, to be effective, Rh immune globulin must be given before the primary immune response is established. The time required to mount a primary immune response doubtlessly varies from case to case, and it is prudent to administer Rh immune globulin to appropriate mothers as soon as possible after delivery. If for some reason the neonatal Rh status is unknown by the third day after delivery, it is preferable to administer Rh immune globulin to an Rh-negative mother rather than to continue to await the neonatal results. Finally, if an Rh-negative mother who is a candidate for Rh immune prophylaxis is mistakenly not treated within the recommended 72 hours following delivery, she may be given Rh immune globulin up to 14 to 28 days after delivery in an effort to avoid sensitization.

Antepartum Prophylaxis

Early trials showed that 1 to 2 percent of susceptible women became sensitized in spite of postpartum Rh immune prophylaxis. The majority of these "prophylaxis failures" resulted from antepartum fetomaternal hemorrhage. In an effort to address this problem, Bowman and colleagues[70] in Canada conducted an antepartum Rh prophylaxis trial in which 300 μg of Rh immune globulin was given at 28 and 34 weeks' gestation. Antenatal sensitization was reduced from 1.8 to 0.1 percent. Subsequently, it was shown that 300 μg of Rh immune globulin given only at 28 weeks' gestation is nearly as effective.[71] This policy is now recommended.

Management of the Unsensitized Rh-Negative Pregnant Woman

At the first prenatal visit of each pregnancy, every patient should have her ABO blood group, Rh type, and antibody screen checked (Fig. 19-1). It is essential that

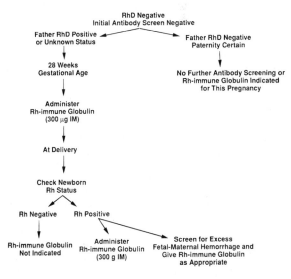

Fig. 19-1 Flow diagram outlining the management of Rh-negative, non-immunized pregnancies.

these determinations are made in each subsequent pregnancy, as previous maternal antibody screening is not an adequate assessment.

If the patient is Rh negative, D^u negative, and has no demonstrable antibody, she is a candidate for Rh immune globulin prophylaxis at 28 weeks' gestation and again immediately postpartum. Before administration of 300 μg of Rh immune globulin at the beginning of the third trimester, an antibody screen is usually recommended to ensure that the patient is not already sensitized and producing anti-D.[84] A repeat antepartum antibody screen at 35 to 36 weeks' gestation is unwarranted.

When the Rh-negative, unsensitized patient is admitted for delivery, an antibody screen is routinely done. If the antibody screen is negative and the newborn is Rh positive or D^u positive, the patient should again be given Rh immune globulin.

Because up to 1 percent of deliveries result in a fetomaternal hemorrhage of greater than 30 ml (the largest volume of fetal blood adequately covered by a standard 300-μg dose of Rh immune globulin), Rh-negative patients with an Rh-positive or D^u-positive newborn should be screened for "excessive" fetomaternal hemorrhage immediately postpartum.[85] An erythrocyte rosette test has been shown to be a simple and sensitive method for detecting excessive fetomaternal bleeding,[39] and most laboratories use one of the commercially available versions of the erythrocyte rosette test as a screening test. For patients with a positive screen, Kleihauer-Betke testing can be used to quantitate the volume of fetal red cells in the maternal circulation. In this way, the appropriate dose of Rh immune globulin can be calculated. If the volume of hemorrhage is estimated to be greater than 30 ml whole blood, a dose of Rh immune globulin calculated at 10 μg/ml of whole fetal blood should be administered.

Management of the D^u-positive patient is sometimes confusing. A D^u-positive mother who delivers an Rh-positive infant is not at significant risk of Rh sensitization, probably because the D^u antigen is actually a weakly expressed D antigen. Thus, D^u-positive mothers may be clinically treated as if they were Rh positive. However, occasionally a woman previously typed as Rh negative is unexpectedly found to be D^u positive during pregnancy or after delivery. In this situation, the clinician should be suspicious that the patient's "new" D^u-positive status is actually due to a large number of fetal cells in the maternal circulation. Appropriate diagnostic studies should be performed, and if fetomaternal

Table 19-2   Recommended Doses of Rh Immune
              Globulin

Indication	Dose (μg) of Rh Immune Globulin
First-trimester spontaneous or induced abortion	50
First-trimester chorionic villus sampling	50
Ectopic pregnancy	
Prior to 12 weeks' gestation	50
After 12 weeks' gestation	300
Amniocentesis or second-trimester chorionic villus sampling	300
Fetomaternal hemorrhage	10 per estimated ml of whole fetal blood

From American College of Obstetricians and Gynecologists:
Prevention of D Isoimmunization (ACOG Technical Bulletin
147). Washington, DC, American College of Obstetricians and
Gynecologists, 1990, with permission.

hemorrhage is found, the mother should be treated
with Rh immune globulin.

Because of the risk of significant fetomaternal hemorrhage with abortion or ectopic pregnancy, Rh immune globulin prophylaxis is indicated if the patient
is Rh negative and unsensitized. If the pregnancy loss
occurs at 12 weeks' gestation or less, a 50-μg dose of
Rh immune globulin is adequate to cover the entire
fetal blood volume[86] (Table 19-2). If the gestational age
is unknown or beyond 12 weeks, a full 300-μg dose of
Rh immune globulin is indicated.

An Rh-negative, unsensitized patient who has antepartum bleeding or suffers an unexplained second- or
third-trimester fetal death should be evaluated for the
possibility of massive fetomaternal hemorrhage. If fetal
cells are found in the maternal circulation, Rh immune
globulin is indicated at a dose of 10 μg per estimated
milliliter of whole fetal blood (Table 19-2).

Antenatal Rh immune globulin is indicated at the
time of chorionic villus sampling or amniocentesis in
an Rh-negative, unsensitized patient. For first-trimester procedures, 50 μg of Rh immune globulin is protective. However, for second- or third-trimester procedures, a full 300-μg dose is indicated even if the
procedure is not associated with detectable hemorrhage (Table 19-2). When amniocentesis is performed
within 72 hours of delivery, such as for the determination of fetal pulmonary maturity, Rh immune globulin

may be withheld and administered immediately post-partum if the infant is found to be Rh positive or D^u positive; if delivery is to be delayed for more than 72 hours, Rh immune globulin should be given.

The Rh-Isoimmunized Pregnancy: Assessment of the Fetus

Any patient with an anti-D antibody titer of greater than 1:4 should be considered Rh sensitized and her pregnancies managed accordingly. The eventual goal of management is to minimize fetal and neonatal morbidity and mortality. Patients (fetuses) can be roughly categorized as (1) those who are unlikely to require intrauterine intervention and who can be delivered when they achieve pulmonary maturity, and (2) those who will likely have moderate to severe hemolytic disease and require intrauterine transfusion and early delivery. An accurate assignment of gestational age using menstrual dates and early ultrasound is crucial in management of the Rh-isoimmunized pregnancy, as the timing of amniocentesis, umbilical cord blood sampling, in utero treatment, and delivery will depend on it.

Determination of the Fetal Antigen Status

When first confronted with an Rh-immunized pregnancy, the possibility that the fetus might be Rh negative and therefore not need expensive and potentially hazardous procedures should be considered. If the woman might have become sensitized during a pregnancy fathered by another partner or by a mismatched blood transfusion, determining the paternal Rh antigen status is reasonable since the father of the current pregnancy might be Rh negative. If he is Rh negative (and it is certain that he is the father of the fetus), further assessment and intervention are unnecessary. If the father is Rh positive, the blood bank laboratory can reliably estimate the probability that he is heterozygous for the D antigen by using Rh antisera to determine his most likely genotype (Table 19-1). Alternatively, DNA analysis can be used to determine his zygosity with a high degree of certainty.[89] Of course, if the man has fathered Rh-negative children, he is a known heterozygote.

If the father is homozygous for the D antigen, all his children will be Rh positive; if he is heterozygous, there is a 50 percent likelihood that each pregnancy will have an Rh-negative fetus who is at no risk of anemia and does not require further assessment or treatment.

In the past, cordocentesis with analysis of fetal red blood cells was required to determine fetal antigen status. Some have advocated routine fetal blood sampling for fetal Rh antigen status at 18 to 20 weeks' gestation in all Rh-immunized pregnancies with a heterozygous father.[90] However, this approach never gained widespread acceptance, probably because of the increased risks of fetal loss and fetomaternal hemorrhage associated with cordocentesis.[91]

Recently, advances in molecular genetics have made it possible to determine fetal Rh status without analysis of fetal red blood cells. The Rh locus on chromosome 1p34-p36 has been cloned,[92] and polymerase chain reaction (PCR) now allows determination of fetal Rh status from the uncultured amniocytes in 2 ml of amniotic fluid or as little as 5 mg of chorionic villi.[93,94]

One can routinely analyze DNA of fetal cells. If an Rh-sensitized patient (with a partner who is heterozygous or whose status is unknown) is having a chorionic villus sampling or second-trimester amniocentesis for another, unrelated indication, one can perform fetal Rh typing at that time. In other cases, fetal Rh typing is performed at the time of the first amniocentesis for amniotic fluid bilirubin analysis. In cases where the PCR results indicate an Rh-negative fetus, one approach is use of fetal kick counts and serial ultrasounds, after a full discussion and explanation that the sensitivity and specificity of the PCR technique are still uncertain.

Because of the added risk and expense, chorionic villus sampling or early amniocentesis should not be offered solely for Rh typing, except for patients with severe Rh sensitization who would consider termination of an Rh-positive pregnancy. Fetal Rh status has been determined from analysis of fetal cells in the maternal circulation, but this is not yet routine. Preimplantation genetic diagnosis of RhD type on single blastomeres is also possible, allowing transfer only of RhD-negative embryos and hence avoiding Rh isoimmunization.

Antibody Titer

In the first sensitized pregnancy, the level of the anti-D antibody titer determines the need for amniocentesis. Severe erythroblastosis or perinatal death does not occur when the antibody levels remain below a certain "critical titer."[59,100,101] This titer varies from laboratory to laboratory but is usually 1:16 or 1:32. An anti-D titer of 1:8 or greater is usually considered an indication for amniocentesis to manage the sensitized pregnancy

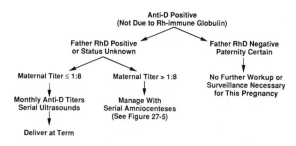

Fig. 19-2 Flow diagram outlining the management of a first Rh-sensitized pregnancy.

(Fig. 19-2). If the initial anti-D titer is less than 1/8, and if the patient does not have a history of a previously affected infant, the pregnancy may be followed with anti-D titers every 2 to 4 weeks and serial ultrasound assessment of the fetus.

Except for using the "critical titer" to establish the need for amniocentesis in the first sensitized pregnancy, maternal serum anti-D titers are not particularly useful in the management of most Rh-isoimmunized pregnancies; indeed, titers may remain stable throughout gestation in as many as 80 percent of the severely affected pregnancies.[101]

Obstetric History

A well-documented obstetric history can be an important management guide for the Rh-isoimmunized patient. Fetal hemolytic disease tends to be either as severe or more severe in subsequent pregnancies. A history of previous intrauterine or neonatal death from hemolytic disease carries a particularly grave prognosis.[100,102] As a general rule of thumb, if a mother has had a hydropic fetus, the chance that the next Rh-incompatible fetus will become hydropic (if left untreated) is more than 80 percent. Only occasionally will an Rh-incompatible fetus be less severely affected than its previous sibling.

In general, hemolysis and hydrops develop at about the same time or somewhat earlier in subsequent pregnancies; this can be used as a rough guide for timing initial fetal studies and transfusions. However, the history is not particularly helpful if the previous pregnancy was the first sensitized pregnancy, since relatively few fetuses develop hydrops in a first sensitized pregnancy.

Amniotic Fluid Analysis

Assessment of amniotic fluid in Rh immunization is based on the original observations of Bevis[103] that spectrophotometric determinations of amniotic fluid bilirubin correlated with the severity of fetal hemolysis. The bilirubin in amniotic fluid is a by-product of fetal hemolysis that reaches the amniotic fluid primarily by excretion into fetal pulmonary and tracheal secretions and diffusion across the fetal membranes and the umbilical cord. Using a semilogarithmic plot, the curve of optical density of normal amniotic fluid is approximately linear between wavelengths of 525 and 375 nm. Bilirubin causes a shift in the spectrophotometric density with a peak at a wavelength of 450 nm. The amount of shift in optical density from linearity at 450 nm (the ΔOD_{450}) is used to estimate the degree of fetal red cell hemolysis (Fig. 19-3).

Liley[104] provided a framework for the management of Rh-immunized pregnancies based on ΔOD_{450} values in the third trimester. Retrospectively, he correlated amniotic fluid ΔOD_{450} values with newborn outcome by dividing the graph of gestational age versus ΔOD_{450} into three zones. Unaffected fetuses and those with mild anemia had ΔOD_{450} values in zone I (the lowest zone), while severely affected fetuses had ΔOD_{450} values in zone III (the highest zone). Fetuses with zone II values (the middle zone) had disease ranging from mild to severe, indicated primarily by the trend of the amniotic fluid bilirubin determinations. There is a normal tendency for amniotic fluid bilirubin to decrease as pregnancy advances; thus the boundaries of the zones slope downward as gestational age increases (Fig. 19-4).

It became clear with further study that a single measurement of ΔOD_{450} was poorly predictive of fetal condition unless it was very high or very low.[105] Also, because of the wide range of severity of disease in the middle zone, Liley emphasized the need for repeating the amniotic fluid analyses to establish the ΔOD_{450} trend. Queenan[106] subsequently analyzed serial amniotic fluid ΔOD_{450} values in patients delivering unaffected (Rh negative), mildly affected (cord hemoglobin greater than 14 g/dl), severely affected (cord blood hemoglobin less than 10 g/dl), and stillborn infants. There was a clear downward trend in the ΔOD_{450} values in unaffected and mildly affected infants, and values from the severely affected fetuses showed a mixed pattern of higher values. The amniotic fluid ΔOD_{450} values from infants who died in utero from erythroblastosis showed upward trends except in a single case that was compli-

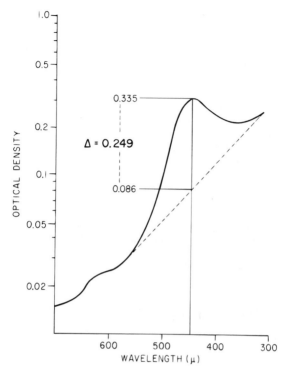

Fig. 19-3 Graph of spectrophotometric analysis of amniotic fluid taken from an Rh-sensitized pregnancy with fetal hydrops. The solid line is the plot of the optical density of the bilirubin-containing fluid across the wavelengths on the x-axis. The interrupted line represents the curve expected from amniotic fluid without increased bilirubin. The difference between the optical density of the solid line and the interrupted line at 450 nm is the ΔOD_{450} value.

cated by polyhydramnios. Thus a horizontal or rising trend is ominous and indicates the need for intervention either by intrauterine transfusion or delivery. Management now includes serial amniocenteses to determine the trend of ΔOD_{450} values over time.[106,107]

However, others have found amniotic fluid bilirubin analysis before 28 weeks to be useful. Ananth and Queenan[112] studied ΔOD_{450} values and trends in 32 Rh-immunized pregnancies between 16 and 20 weeks' gestation. They found that ΔOD_{450} values greater than or trending above 0.15 predicted severe isoimmunization, whereas ΔOD_{450} values below 0.09 indicated mild or absent disease. They concluded that umbilical blood sampling is necessary only in pregnancies with ΔOD_{450}

values greater than 0.15; fetuses with ΔOD_{450} values below 0.15 can be managed with serial amniocenteses to determine whether the trend indicates severe disease.

In a subsequent analysis of nearly 800 amniotic fluid bilirubin levels obtained between 14 and 40 weeks' gestation, Queenan et al.[113] defined the trends in ΔOD_{450} values in unffected and Rh-immunized pregnancies. In unaffected pregnancies, normal amniotic fluid ΔOD_{450} values trend upward between 14 and 22 weeks, level off until 26 weeks, then decline steadily until term. Using the mean and standard deviation of values across the gestational age range, these authors proposed a new graphic framework for assessment of ΔOD_{450} values in Rh-sensitized pregnancies, with four zones: Rh negative, indeterminate, Rh positive (affected), and intrauterine death risk. Although valuable in assessing Rh-sensitized pregnancies prior to 28 weeks, further work and independent confirmation of this new management scheme will be necessary before it supplants the Liley curve.

Fetal Blood Analysis

Fetal blood sampling allows determination of the presence or absence of the offending antigen on the fetal

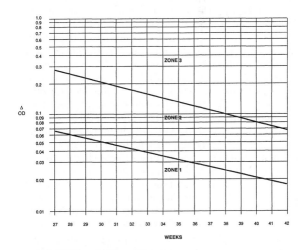

Fig. 19-4 Liley graph used to determine severity of immunization. (Modified from Liley AW. Liquor amnii analysis in the management of the pregnancy complicated by rhesus sensitization. Am J Obstet Gynecol 82:1359, 1961, with permission.)

erythrocytes when the antigen status or zygosity of the father is unknown or uncertain.[90,117] As a result, direct fetal blood sampling is now considered by many to be a first step in the analysis of the fetus at risk for severe hemolytic disease.

Adoption of routine umbilical cord blood sampling has not been universal because of concern for potential fetal and maternal morbidity. The procedure is successful in greater than 95 percent of cases, but attributable fetal loss rates between 0.5 and 2 percent per procedure have been reported even by experienced investigators.[117,119,120] In approximately 5 percent of patients, other morbidity occurs; complications such as acute refractory fetal distress, umbilical cord hematoma, amnionitis with maternal adult respiratory distress syndrome, and placental abruption have been described.[121–123]

Additionally, there appears to be a significant risk of fetomaternal bleeding with umbilical cord blood sampling, with the potential for worsened maternal sensitization and fetal involvement.[124–126]

Because of the technical difficulty and increased hazard (both immediate and remote) associated with the procedure, umbilical cord blood sampling should be used with caution and performed only by properly trained personnel.

Ultrasound and Doppler Studies

Ultrasonographic examination of the fetus has become an extremely important adjunct in the management of the Rh-sensitized pregnancy, primarily as a guide to amniocenteses and intrauterine transfusions. Ultrasound has also been studied in an effort to identify sonographic findings that might predict the severity of erythroblastosis fetalis so as to avoid the need for invasive assessments. Polyhydramnios, placental thickness greater than 4 cm, pericardial effusion, dilation of the cardiac chambers (especially the right atrium), chronic enlargement of the spleen and liver, visualization of both sides of the fetal bowel wall, and dilation of the umbilical vein have all been proposed as indicators of significant prehydropic fetal anemia.[127–134] However, sonographic findings other than hydrops are not reliable in distinguishing mild from severe hemolytic disease even in experienced hands, and the role of ultrasound in the monitoring of fetuses with severe Rh immunization is limited to the establishment of gestational age, monitoring for hydropic changes, and guidance for amniocentesis, umbilical blood sampling, and transfusion.

Doppler flow velocity waveforms have also been extensively investigated as noninvasive predictors of fetal anemia[135-143] and acidosis.[144,145] In general, fetal blood flow velocity waveforms have not been predictive of acid–base status in Rh-isoimmunized pregnancies. Similarly, although many studies have found significant differences in blood flow indices between anemic and nonanemic fetuses, the wide range and overlap of values in both groups of patients have limited the utility of Doppler technology.

At present, neither ultrasound nor Doppler blood flow analysis can be recommended in lieu of amniotic fluid ΔOD_{450} determinations or fetal blood sampling for determining the need for intrauterine transfusion or delivery in Rh-immunized pregnancies.

Determining the Need for Intrauterine Transfusion

About one-half of susceptible infants of Rh-immunized pregnancies do not require intrauterine transfusion or extensive extrauterine therapy. Such fetuses are considered to have mild to moderate hemolytic disease. In general, mild to moderate fetal hemolysis is expected when (1) the involved pregnancy is the first sensitized pregnancy or (2) previously delivered Rh-positive infants have been mildly to moderately affected (mild to moderate anemia without hydrops). In such cases, we perform ultrasound examinations of the fetus every 2 to 4 weeks from 18 weeks' gestation until delivery. If the fetus shows no evidence of hydrops, we use amniotic fluid ΔOD_{450} determinations for the initial management, performing the first amniocentesis at 24 to 28 weeks' gestation. The timing of repeat amniocenteses and determination of the need for intrauterine transfusion or delivery are based on the ΔOD_{450} values and trend (Fig. 19-5). If the values fall within the low zone or the lower half of the middle zone, amniocentesis is repeated every 2 to 4 weeks, depending on the ΔOD_{450} trend. Severe anemia requiring intrauterine transfusion is suspected when the ΔOD_{450} values rise into the upper quarter of the middle zone or into zone III, especially before 30 weeks' gestation. Depending on the clinical situation, a single ΔOD_{450} value in zone III also may be taken as an indication of severe anemia. If at any time the fetus has evidence of hydrops by ultrasound, one can assume a fetal hematocrit less than 15 percent,[16,131] and fetal blood sampling and transfusion should be arranged immediately.

The need for cordocentesis in the management of nonhydropic fetuses with ΔOD_{450} values indicative of

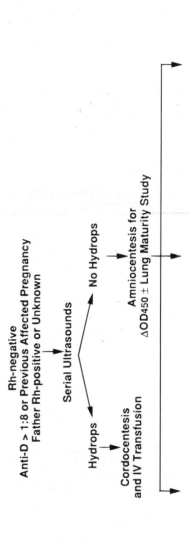

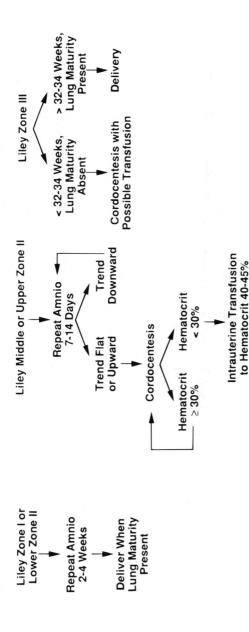

Fig. 19-5 Flow diagram outlining the management of an Rh-sensitized pregnancy. The timing of the first amniocentesis is based on the history, maternal titer, and gestational age. In addition to assessment of amniotic fluid bilirubin or umbilical cord hematocrit, all patients monitor fetal movements on a daily basis after 26 to 28 weeks and have nonstress tests one to two times weekly and ultrasound exams every 1 to 2 weeks.

severe anemia (and requiring intrauterine transfusion) is controversial. As discussed below, there is no proven advantage to cordocentesis and intravascular transfusion in nonhydropic fetuses, and experienced practitioners have described excellent perinatal outcomes using amniotic fluid ΔOD_{450} values with intraperitoneal transfusions.[146–148] However, because of the morbidity associated with fetal transfusion regardless of route, it seems appropriate to obtain umbilical cord blood when practical to determine fetal Rh status and to confirm anemia prior to transfusion.

When the obstetric history suggests that the fetus is at risk for moderate to severe hemolysis and hydrops, we search for fetal anemia earlier in the pregnancy. In this situation, we usually follow the trend of ΔOD_{450} values, using a modification of the Liley curve, with the understanding that interpretation of ΔOD_{450} values before 24 weeks is difficult. Between 18 and 24 weeks, we stress ΔOD_{450} trends over single values and typically use Queenan's data from second-trimester pregnancies as a guide to interpretation.[112,113] In some cases, especially those with a history of severe second-trimester disease or previous severe disease with misleading ΔOD_{450} values, cordocentesis to determine the fetal hematocrit and antigen status is a reasonable first step. Again, the optimum management in an individual case will be determined by history, clinical findings, and the experience and expertise of the management team.

At any gestational age, the presence of fetal hydrops should be taken as evidence of severe fetal anemia, and cordocentesis with immediate intravascular transfusion is indicated.

ABO Incompatibility

Twenty to 25 percent of pregnancies are ABO incompatible, meaning that the mother's serum contains anti-A or anti-B, while the erythrocytes of the fetus contain the respective antigen. This results in ABO incompatibility being a common cause of hemolytic disease of the newborn, accounting for over 60 percent of all cases.[204] Fortunately, the disease is nearly always manifested as no worse than moderate neonatal anemia and mild to moderate neonatal hyperbilirubinemia, and less than 1 percent of cases require exchange transfusion. ABO incompatibility has never clearly been shown to be a cause of fetal hemolysis and can generally be regarded as a pediatric rather than an obstetric problem.[205]

There are several reasons why ABO incompatibility rarely results in severe hemolytic disease. Individuals with group A or B blood type produce predominantly IgM anti-B or anti-A, both of which cross the placenta poorly. Also, there are fewer A and B antigen sites on the fetal erythrocyte than on the adult erythrocyte; thus less antibody can bind to fetal red cell membranes. Finally, maternal and fetal tissues other than erythrocytes contain the A and B antigens, and some investigators believe that anti-A or anti-B antibodies are absorbed by these sites so that less of the antibodies are available for erythrocyte binding.[204]

The A and B antigens are "naturally occurring" antigens; that is, they occur widely in nature unassociated with erythrocyte membranes. Therefore, A or B sensitization does not require prior exposure to red cells through pregnancy or by transfusion, and it is not unusual for ABO hemolytic disease to affect the firstborn child. Clinically apparent hemolytic disease of the newborn resulting from ABO incompatibility is mostly confined to the situation wherein the mother is type O and the infant is type A or B, because group O individuals produce anti-A and anti-B that is predominantly of the IgG class and can therefore cross the placenta to bind to the fetal erythrocytes.[204]

ABO hemolytic disease usually manifests itself as mild to moderate hyperbilirubinemia during the first 24 to 48 hours of life. It is rarely associated with significant anemia. High levels of bilirubin can cause kernicterus, with preterm neonates being most susceptible. Phototherapy is the first line of treatment, although exchange transfusion may be indicated according to the degree of hyperbilirubinemia.

Because ABO incompatibility is likely to occur in subsequent pregnancies, the delivery of an affected newborn should be documented in the patient's record. However, since significant fetal hemolysis does not occur, screening for anti-A or anti-B antibodies in the mother's serum and analysis of the amniotic fluid for bilirubin are not required.

Key Points

- To reduce the incidence of Rh sensitization, Rh immune globulin should be given to Rh-negative unsensitized women at 28 weeks' gestational age and again after delivery if the newborn is Rh positive. Rh immune globulin is also indicated for these patients in cases of miscarriage, ectopic pregnancy, chorionic villus sampling, amniocentesis, or fetomaternal hemorrhage.

- The gene coding for the D antigen has been cloned, and prenatal determination of fetal Rh status is available from uncultured amniocytes obtained at amniocentesis.
- Measurement of amniotic fluid bilirubin remains the standard for assessment of pregnancies at risk for significant fetal anemia. Neither ultrasound alone nor Doppler is adequately sensitive to identify anemic fetuses.
- The timing of the first amniocentesis is based on history, maternal anti-D titers, gestational age, and ultrasound findings. The timing of subsequent amniocenteses is based on the ΔOD_{450} values and trends.
- Analysis of amniotic fluid bilirubin before 26 weeks is controversial. Although most data suggest that ΔOD_{450} values and trends are accurate before the third trimester, more liberal use of cordocentesis may be appropriate.
- Fetal transfusion can be performed using either the intraperitoneal or intravascular route. For hydropic fetuses, intravascular transfusion is clearly superior. For nonhydropic fetuses, perinatal survival rates are similar with either method.
- With the reduction in Rh disease through widespread use of Rh immune globulin prophylaxis, sensitization to the minor or atypical antigens has become relatively more common. A number of these minor antigens can cause severe fetal anemia.
- The optimal management scheme for pregnancies affected with platelet sensitization is unclear. One protocol involves (1) cordocentesis at 24–28 weeks for documentation of thrombocytopenia (2) weekly maternal administration of intravenous immunoglobulin, and (3) cordocentesis at about 37 weeks to determine platelet count before delivery.

Pregnancy and Coexisting Disease

Chapter 20

Hypertension in Pregnancy

Baha M. Sibai

Hypertensive disorders are the most common medical complications of pregnancy, with a reported incidence ranging between 5 and 10 percent.[1] The term *hypertension in pregnancy* is usually used to describe a wide spectrum of patients who may have only mild elevations in blood pressure or severe hypertension with various organ dysfunctions.

Definitions

Preeclampsia and Eclampsia

The diagnosis of preeclampsia is based on blood pressure criteria, as well as proteinuria or edema or both. Blood pressure must increase by at least 30 mm Hg systolic or 15 mm Hg diastolic. Readings of 140/90 mm Hg after 20 weeks' gestation, if prior blood pressure is unknown, are considered sufficiently elevated for the diagnosis of preeclampsia. The elevation must be present on two measurements taken 6 hours apart. Either an increase in mean arterial pressure of 20 mm Hg or, if the prior blood pressure is unknown, a mean arterial pressure of 105 mm Hg are indications of hypertension. Mean arterial pressure is one-third the pulse pressure plus the diastolic pressure. Edema is diagnosed as clinically evident generalized swelling or rapid increase in weight. Proteinuria is defined as a concentration of 0.1 g/L or more in at least two random urine specimens collected 6 hours or more apart or 0.3 g in a 24-hour collection. In mild preeclampsia, the diastolic blood pressure remains below 110 mm Hg. The criteria for severe preeclampsia are given in the box on p 438.[4]

Clinical Manifestations of Severe Disease in Patients with Pregnancy-Induced Hypertension

1. Blood pressure >160–180 mm Hg systolic or >110 mm Hg diastolic
2. Proteinuria of >5 g/24 hours (normal <300 mg/24 hours)
3. Elevated serum creatinine
4. Grand mal seizures (eclampsia)
5. Pulmonary edema
6. Oliguria <500 ml/24 hours
7. Microangiopathic hemolysis
8. Thrombocytopenia
9. Hepatocellular dysfunction (elevated alanine aminotransferase, aspartase aminotransferase)
10. Intrauterine growth retardation or oligohydramnios
11. Symptoms suggesting significant end-organ involvement: headache, visual disturbances, or epigastric or right-upper quadrant pain

From American College of Obstetricians and Gynecologists, Hypertension in Pregnancy (Technical Bulletin No. 219). Washington, DC, American College of Obstetricians and Gynecologists, 1996, with permission.

Eclampsia is the occurrence of seizures not attributable to other causes.

Chronic Hypertension

Chronic hypertension is defined as hypertension present before the pregnancy or that diagnosed before the 20th week of gestation. Hypertension is a blood pressure greater than 140/90 mm Hg. Hypertension that persists beyond 42 days postpartum is also classified as chronic hypertension.

Chronic Hypertension with Superimposed Preeclampsia

Women with chronic hypertension may also show the development of superimposed preeclampsia. The diagnosis is made on the basis of an elevation of blood pressure (30 mm Hg systolic or 15 mm Hg diastolic or 20 mm Hg mean arterial pressure) together with the appearance of proteinuria or generalized edema.

Transient Hypertension

Transient hypertension is the development of an elevated blood pressure during pregnancy or in the first 24 hours postpartum without other signs of preeclampsia or preexisting hypertension. The blood pressure must return to normal within 10 days after delivery.

Edema as a Criterion

Generalized edema is common in normal pregnancy, although it does not occur as frequently and is not as marked as when associated with preeclampsia. In addition, one-third of eclamptic women never demonstrate the presence of edema.[7]

Preeclampsia

The incidence ranges between 10 and 14 percent in primigravidas and between 5.7 and 7.3 percent in multiparas.[13,14] The incidence is significantly increased in patients with twin pregnancies[15] and in those with previous preeclampsia.[16]

The etiology of preeclampsia is unknown. Many theories have been suggested, but most of them did not withstand the test of time.

Laboratory Abnormalities in Preeclampsia

Women with preeclampsia may exhibit a symptom complex ranging from minimal blood pressure elevation to derangements of multiple organ systems. The renal, hematologic, and hepatic systems are most likely to be involved.

Renal Function

In preeclampsia, vasospasm and glomerular capillary endothelial swelling lead to an average reduction in GFR of 25 percent below the rate for normal pregnancy.[111] Serum creatinine is rarely elevated in preeclampsia, but uric acid is commonly increased.[112]

Hepatic Function

Hepatic involvement is seen in only 10 percent of women with severe preeclampsia.[116] When liver dysfunction occurs in preeclampsia, mild elevation of serum transaminase is most common[118] and bilirubin is rarely increased. Elevated liver enzymes are part of the syndrome of hemolysis, elevated liver enzymes, and low platelets (HELLP), a variant of severe preeclampsia.

Hematologic Changes

Thrombocytopenia is the most common hematologic abnormality in women with preeclampsia. A platelet count less than 150,000/mm^3 is found in 50 percent and a count of less than 100,000/mm^3 is found in 36 percent of the women with severe preeclampsia. The admission platelet count is an excellent predictor of subsequent coagulation studies, and fibrinogen levels, prothrombin time, and partial thromboplastin time need be obtained only in women with a platelet count of less than 100,000/mm^3.

The HELLP Syndrome

The syndrome of hemolysis, elevated liver enzymes, and low platelets (HELLP) is a variant of severe preeclampsia. Thrombocytopenia (platelet count <100,000/mm^3) has been the most consistent finding in this syndrome.

There is a strong association between the presence of HELLP syndrome and eclampsia, with HELLP syndrome present in 30 percent of patients.

Hemolysis, defined as the presence of microangiopathic hemolytic anemia, is the hallmark of the HELLP syndrome. HELLP syndrome is not a variant of disseminated intravascular coagulation (DIC), since coagulation parameters such as prothrombin time, partial thromboplastin time, and serum fibrinogen are normal. DIC is defined as the presence of thrombocytopenia, low fibrinogen levels (plasma fibrinogen <300 mg/dl), and fibrin split products above 40 μg/ml. DIC is seen in 20 to 40 patients with HELLP syndrome. The majority of cases occur in women who have antecedent abruptio placentae, peripartum hemorrhage, or subcapsular liver hematomas. In the absence of these complications, the frequency of DIC is only 5 percent.[134] The laboratory criteria to establish the diagnosis are presented in the box on p 441.

The patient is usually seen remote from term complaining of epigastric or right upper-quadrant pain (65 percent), nausea or vomiting (50 percent), or nonspecific viral syndrome–like symptoms. The majority of patients will give a history of malaise for the past few days before presentation; some may present with hematuria or gastrointestinal bleeding. Hypertension and proteinuria may be absent or minimal.[135,136] Physical examination will demonstrate right upper-quadrant tenderness and significant weight gain with edema.

Severe hypertension is not a constant or even a frequent finding in HELLP syndrome. Patients are often

Criteria to Establish the Diagnosis of HELLP Syndrome

Hemolysis
   Abnormal peripheral blood smear
   Increased bilirubin (≥1.2 mg/dl)
   Increased lactate dehydrogenase (>600 IU/L)

Elevated liver enzymes
   Increased SGOT (≥72 IU/L)
   Increased lactate dehydrogenase (>600 IU/L)

Low platelets
   Platelet count <100,000/mm³

misdiagnosed as having various medical and surgical disorders. It is therefore recommended that all pregnant women having any of these symptoms should have a complete blood count and platelet and liver enzyme determinations irrespective of maternal blood pressure.

The management of preeclamptic patients presenting with the HELLP syndrome is similar to that used in the management of severe preeclampsia remote from term.[127] The majority of these patients will demonstrate deterioration in either maternal or fetal condition within 1 to 10 days after conservative management. It is doubtful that such a limited pregnancy prolongation will result in improved perinatal outcome, especially when maternal and fetal risks are substantial.

The reported perinatal mortality has ranged from 7.7 to 60 percent and maternal mortality from 0 to 24 percent. Maternal morbidity is common. Most of these patients have required transfusions of blood and blood products and are at increased risk for the development of acute renal failure, pulmonary edema, ascites, pleural effusions, hepatic rupture,[132,134,144–146] abruptio placentae, and DIC.

Seventy percent of the patients have evidence of the syndrome antepartum, and 30 percent develop the manifestations postpartum, with the majority developing within 48 hours postpartum. Eighty percent of the postpartum patients have evidence of preeclampsia prior to delivery, whereas 20 percent have no such evidence. Patients in this group are at increased risk for the development of pulmonary edema and acute renal failure. The differential diagnosis in these patients

Medical and Surgical Disorders Confused with the HELLP Syndrome

Acute fatty liver of pregnancy

Appendicitis

Diabetes

Gallbladder disease

Gastroenteritis

Glomerulonephritis

Hemolytic–uremic syndrome

Hepatic encephalopathy

Hyperemesis gravidarum

Idiopathic thrombocytopenia

Kidney stones

Peptic ulcer

Pyelonephritis

Systemic lupus erythematosus

Thrombotic thrombocytopenic purpura

Viral hepatitis

should include exacerbation of systemic lupus erythematosus, thrombotic thrombocytopenic purpura (TTP), and hemolytic–uremic syndrome.

Patients with the HELLP syndrome who are remote from term should be referred to a tertiary care center and initial management should be as for any patient with severe preeclampsia. The first priority is to assess and stabilize maternal condition, particularly coagulation abnormalities. The next step is to evaluate fetal well-being using the nonstress test and biophysical profile. The patient may be given steroids to accelerate fetal lung maturity and then delivered 24 hours later. Patients presenting with well-established labor should be allowed to deliver vaginally as indicated, and labor may be initiated with oxytocin in those with a favorable cervix.

The majority of these patients will have spontaneous resolution of their disease. Some have recommended that a trial of plasma exchange with fresh frozen plasma be considered in HELLP syndrome that persists past 72 hours from delivery and in which there is evidence of a life-threatening microangiopathy.

Subcapsular Hematoma of the Liver in HELLP Syndrome

The diagnosis of a subcapsular hematoma of the liver in pregnancy is often overlooked because of its rarity. The differential diagnosis should include acute cholecystitis with sepsis, acute fatty liver of pregnancy, ruptured uterus, placental abruption with DIC, and TTP. In addition to the signs and symptoms of preeclampsia, physical examination findings consistent with peritoneal irritation and hepatomegaly may be present. Profound hypovolemic shock with hypotension in a previously hypertensive patient is a hallmark of rupture of the hematoma.

An ultrasound or computed tomography scan of the liver should be performed to rule out the presence of subcapsular hematoma and assess for the presence of intraperitoneal bleeding. Paracentesis confirms the presence of intraperitoneal hemorrhage suspected by examination or radiographic imaging.

Surgical repair has been recommended for hepatic hemorrhage without liver rupture. More recent experience suggests, however, that this complication can be managed conservatively in patients who remain hemodynamically stable.[148,149] Serial assessment of the subcapsular hematoma with ultrasound or computed tomography is necessary, with immediate intervention for rupture or worsening of maternal status. It is important with conservative management to avoid exogenous sources of trauma to the liver, such as abdominal palpation, convulsions, or emesis, and to use care in transportation of the patient.

In the literature, there is an 82 percent overall survival for the 27 cases managed by packing and drainage, whereas only 25 percent of eight patients undergoing hepatic lobectomy survived.

The Management of Preeclampsia

Definitive therapy in the form of delivery is the only cure for preeclampsia. The decision between immediate delivery and expectant management will depend on the severity of the disease process, maternal and fetal status at the time of initial evaluation, and fetal gestational age.

Mild Preeclampsia

Patients with diagnosed preeclampsia should ideally be hospitalized at the time of diagnosis for evaluation of maternal and fetal conditions. The mother is at increased risk for the development of abruptio placentae or convulsions, particularly in cases remote from term. Thus women with mild disease who have a favorable cervix at or near term should undergo induction of labor. The pregnancy should not continue past term, even if conditions for induction of labor are unfavorable, because the uteroplacental blood flow becomes suboptimal.

The optimal management of mild preeclampsia before term (<37 weeks' gestation) is controversial. Management of these patients with bedrest in the hospital for the duration of pregnancy enhances fetal survival and diminishes the frequency of progression to severe disease. In many such instances, this treatment arrests the clinical course of the disease or at least improves it long enough to achieve fetal maturity and reduces maternal morbidity.[172,173] However, the benefits of prolonged antepartum hospitalization for women with mild gestational hypertension (without proteinuria) were challenged by European investigators who reported that most of these women can be safely managed on an ambulatory basis or in a day care facility.

Outpatient management includes automated blood pressure measurement four times daily and daily assessment of weight, proteinuria, and fetal movement.

No studies of drug therapy have reported a better perinatal outcome than the respective outcomes in studies using hospitalization alone.

At our institution, all patients with mild preeclampsia are initially hospitalized at the time of their diagnosis. During hospitalization, patients receive a regular diet with no salt restriction and no activity limits. Diuretics and antihypertensive drugs are not prescribed, and sedatives are not used. Patients initially undergo evaluation of maternal and fetal well-being. The frequency of subsequent testing usually depends on the fetal gestational age and maternal response following hospitalization. Subsequent fetal evaluation includes serial ultrasonography for fetal growth every 3 weeks, daily fetal movement count, nonstress testing every week, and biophysical profile if needed. Maternal evaluation includes blood pressure monitoring (every 4 hours during the day), maternal weight assessment, and checking for the presence of edema daily. In addition, women are questioned regarding symptoms of impending eclampsia (persistent headache, visual disturbances, or epigastric pain). Laboratory evaluation includes measurements of urine protein, hematocrit, and platelet count, and liver function tests, as patients may develop thrombocytopenia and elevated liver enzymes with minimal blood pressure elevation.[136]

Severe Preeclampsia

The clinical course of severe preeclampsia may be characterized by progressive deterioration in both maternal and fetal conditions. As a result, there is universal agreement that all such patients should be delivered if the disease develops after 34 weeks' gestation or prior to that time if there is evidence of maternal or fetal distress.[184] There is also agreement on delivery of such patients prior to 35 weeks' gestation in the presence of any of the following: premature rupture of membranes, labor, or severe fetal IUGR.

There is considerable disagreement about management of patients with severe disease prior to 34 weeks' gestation. Some authors consider delivery as the definitive therapy for all cases, regardless of gestational age, whereas others recommend prolonging pregnancy in all severe preeclamptic gestations remote from term until development of fetal lung maturity, fetal or maternal distress, or a gestational age of 34 weeks is achieved.[185–187]

Severe Preeclampsia at 28 to 32 Weeks' Gestation

Studies describing expectant management of women with severe preeclampsia at 28 to 32 weeks' gestation suggest that expectant management improves outcome in a selected patient population.[184]

In one study of preeclampsia at 28 to 34 weeks, the patients were treated initially with magnesium sulfate, hydralazine, and corticosteroids for fetal lung immaturity. All received intensive maternal and fetal care in a high-risk obstetrics ward. Nonstress tests were done at least three times daily, and laboratory tests were evaluated at least twice weekly. Twenty of the 58 women were delivered because of maternal or fetal reasons within 48 hours after hospitalization. The remaining 38 were then randomized to either aggressive or expectant management ($n = 20$). Patients assigned to the aggressive-management group received steroids and were delivered within 72 hours. Patients assigned to the expect-ant-management group were treated with hydralazine to maintain blood pressure between 140/90 and 150/100 mm Hg. In addition, they received frequent evaluations for maternal and fetal well-being. The authors found lower neonatal complications and lower number of days spent in the neonatal intensive care unit in the expectant-management group.[189]

Mid-Trimester Severe Preeclampsia

Aggressive management of patients with mid-trimester severe preeclampsia with immediate delivery will result in high neonatal mortality and morbidity. However, attempts to prolong pregnancy may result in fetal demise or damage in utero, and severe maternal morbidity and even mortality. All patients are first admitted to labor and delivery and are evaluated carefully for the presence of either maternal or fetal distress. Pregnancy termination is recommended for patients with gestation ages of 24 weeks or less, whereas aggressive expectant management is recommended for patients with gestational age over 24 weeks. Expectant management for women with severe preeclampsia should be selective and done only in a tertiary care center with adequate intensive care facilities.[193]

Patients with resistant severe hypertension or other signs of maternal or fetal deterioration are delivered within 24 hours, irrespective of gestational age or fetal lung maturity.[184] In addition, patients in labor, or those with fetuses with a gestational age older than 35 weeks, and those with evidence of fetal lung maturity (by amniocentesis) at 33 to 35 weeks also are delivered within 24 hours.[184] Patients at 33 to 35 weeks' gestation with immature amniotic fluid receive steroids to accelerate fetal lung maturity and are delivered 24 hours after the steroids in the absence of any change in maternal or fetal condition.

Corticosteroids are safe and effective drugs for preventing respiratory distress syndrome, treating thrombocytopenia, and improving perinatal outcome in severe preeclampsia. We administer betamethasone 12 mg as soon as possible, and the dose is repeated 24 hours later.

Patients at 28 to 32 weeks' gestation receive individualized management based on their clinical response during the observation period. All of these patients receive steroids to accelerate fetal lung maturity, as there is still benefit even if the delivery occurs less than 24 hours or more than 1 week later. If the blood pressure remains below 100 mm Hg diastolic (without antihypertensive therapy) after the observation period, magnesium sulfate is discontinued and the patients are followed closely on the high-risk ward until fetal maturity is achieved. During hospitalization, they receive antihypertensive drugs (usually oral nifedipine 40 to 120 mg/day) to keep their diastolic blood pressure between 90 and 100 mm Hg, with daily evaluation of maternal and fetal well-being.

We believe that all women who meet the blood pressure criteria for preeclampsia should receive intravenous magnesium sulfate to prevent eclamptic convulsions.[196] Our rationale for this approach is the observation that, in most series of eclampsia, 20 percent of the women had only minimal blood pressure elevation, frequently without edema or proteinuria.

Magnesium sulfate is administered by a controlled continuous intravenous infusion with a loading dose of 6 g in 100 ml over 15 to 20 minutes. The intravenous route for magnesium therapy permits more precise control of the patient's blood level and avoids the pain of intramuscular injections. Maintenance therapy is given at a rate of 2 g in 100 ml of fluid per hour. Serum magnesium levels are obtained 4 to 6 hours later, with the rate of infusion adjusted to keep serum magnesium levels between 4.8 and 9.6 mg/dl (4 to 6 mEq/L). Treatment is continued for 24 hours postdelivery.

Magnesium is excreted in the urine, so an accurate record of maternal urine output must be maintained. In patients with normal renal function, the half-life for magnesium excretion is about 4 hours.

In the therapeutic range (4.8 to 9.6 mg/dl), magnesium sulfate slows neuromuscular conduction and depresses central nervous system irritability. For this reason, maternal respiratory rate, deep tendon reflexes, and state of consciousness must be frequently monitored to detect magnesium toxicity. An ampule of calcium gluconate, 1 g (10 ml of 10 percent solution) should be drawn up in a syringe and clearly labeled and be kept at the bedside in case of magnesium toxicity. If respiratory depression occurs, the magnesium sulfate should be stopped and the calcium gluconate should be given intravenously over 3 minutes.

We carefully monitor the amount of intravenous fluids used in women with preeclampsia or eclampsia. Intake and output should be assessed hourly. Our goal is to maintain the urine output at 30 ml/hr. If urine output drops below 100 ml in 4 hours, the dose of magnesium sulfate and intravenous fluids should be reduced accordingly. Another cause of decreased urine output is a drop in maternal blood pressure due to the repeated injections of hydralazine. Hydralazine has a

Magnesium Toxicity

Loss of patellar reflex	8–12 mg/dl
Feeling of warmth, flushing	9–12 mg/dl
Somnolence	10–12 mg/dl
Slurred speech	10–12 mg/dl
Muscular paralysis	15–17 mg/dl
Respiratory difficulty	15–17 mg/dl
Cardiac arrest	30–35 mg/dl

relatively long duration of action and, when multiple bolus injections of hydralazine are used to control blood pressure, the diastolic blood pressure may be reduced more than intended, that is, below 90 mm Hg. This will frequently reduce urine output for 2 to 3 hours. One of the potential problems when attempting to limit intravenous fluids to 125 ml/hr is that high concentrations of drugs must be used if the woman is receiving intravenous magnesium sulfate, oxytocin, and hydralazine.

To control severe maternal hypertension intrapartum, we use bolus injections of hydralazine 5 to 10 mg every 20 to 30 minutes to lower the diastolic blood pressure to 90 to 100 mm Hg range. This requires monitoring of blood pressure every 5 minutes for at least 30 minutes after the drug is given. An alternative regimen is to use bolus injections of labetalol hydrochloride 20 to 50 mg. Unlike hydralazine, labetalol does not cause maternal tachycardia, flushing, or headaches.

Counseling Women Who Have Had Preeclampsia in Prior Pregnancies

There is a strong familial predisposition for preeclampsia. In 273 primigravidas whose sisters did not have preeclampsia, the incidence of severe preeclampsia was 4.5 percent. The incidence of severe preeclampsia was 13.8 percent for women whose sisters had severe preeclampsia during their first pregnancies. The incidence of severe preeclampsia was 15.9 percent in the 126 mothers of primigravidas who had severe preeclampsia, compared with a 4.4 percent incidence of severe preeclampsia in the 136 mothers-in-law.

We have examined the pregnancy outcomes and incidences of preeclampsia in subsequent pregnancies, as well as the incidences of chronic hypertension and diabetes in women who had severe preeclampsia or eclampsia in their first pregnancies, compared with 409 women who remained normotensive during their first pregnancies. The incidence of chronic hypertension was significantly higher in the preeclampsia group (14.8 vs. 5.6 percent; $p < 0.001$). This difference became even greater for those women followed for more than 10 years (51 vs. 14 percent; $p < 0.001$). The incidence of severe preeclampsia was also significantly higher in the second pregnancies (25.9 vs. 4.6 percent) as well as in the subsequent pregnancies (12.2 vs. 5.0 percent) of women with preeclampsia.[207] In women who have had severe preeclampsia in the second trimester,[208] 65 percent of subsequent pregnancies are complicated by preeclampsia. In addition, these women have a high incidence of chronic hypertension on follow-up, with the highest incidence being in those who had recurrent severe preeclampsia in the second trimester (55 percent).

The risk of abruptio placentae increases significantly in those with severe preeclampsia before 34 weeks' gestation, and particularly in those who have severe preeclampsia in the second trimester.[209] The risk of subsequent abruptio ranges from 5 to 20 percent. Women with severe preeclampsia remote from term may have underlying renal disease for which they should be evaluated after delivery.

Eclampsia

Eclampsia is the occurrence of convulsions or coma unrelated to other cerebral conditions with signs and symptoms of preeclampsia. Magnesium sulfate is the drug of choice for this disease.

Pathophysiology

The pathophysiologic events leading to convulsions remain unknown. There is a functional derangement of multiple organ systems, such as the central nervous system and hematologic, hepatic, renal, and cardiovascular systems.[217] Women in whom eclampsia develops exhibit a wide spectrum of signs and symptoms.

Eclampsia usually begins with rapid weight gain and ends with the onset of generalized convulsions. Excess weight gain (with or without clinical edema) of more than 2 pounds per week during the last trimester may be the first warning sign. Hypertension is the hallmark of eclampsia, and excess weight gain or edema are not necessary for the diagnosis.[7] In about 20 percent of cases, hypertension may be "relative," signified by any rise in blood pressure that is 30 mm Hg systolic or 15 mm Hg diastolic above the nonpregnant blood pressure reading. Eclampsia is usually associated with significant proteinuria. In eclamptic women, headache, visual disturbances, and right upper quadrant/epigastric pain are the most common premonitory symptoms before convulsions. Of interest is the absence of edema (32 percent) and proteinuria (19 percent) in 254 eclamptic women.

Convulsions may occur antepartum, intrapartum, or postpartum. One-half of cases of eclampsia occur before the onset of labor, with the other 50 percent equally divided between the intrapartum and postpartum periods. Although rare, atypical eclampsia may occur before the 20th week of gestation and more than 48 hours after delivery.[218,219] Maternal death occurs in approximately 1/250 eclamptic women. This can be from magnesium toxicity or cardiorespiratory arrest after multiple seizures. The main risks to the fetus of the eclamptic woman are abruptio placentae, prematurity, IUGR, and hypoxic episodes during the convulsions.[7,238,261]

Management of Labor and Delivery in Eclampsia

The woman with eclampsia should undergo continuous intensive monitoring. The guard rails should be up on the bed and a padded tongue blade kept at the bedside. A large-bore peripheral intravenous line should be in place. No other anticonvulsants should be left at the bedside except for a syringe containing 2 to 4 g magnesium sulfate. No more than 8 g magnesium sulfate should be given over a short period of time to control convulsions.

Once convulsions have been controlled and the woman has regained consciousness, her general medical condition is assessed. When she is stable, induction of labor is initiated. Delivery is the treatment for eclampsia. Fetal heart rate and intensity of uterine contractions should be closely monitored.

Fetal bradycardia can occur during an eclamptic seizure with fetal tachycardia occurring frequently after the prolonged bradycardia.

Uterine hyperactivity demonstrated by both increased uterine tone and increased frequency of uterine contractions occurs during an eclamptic seizure. The duration of the increased uterine activity varies from 2 to 14 minutes.

Fetal outcome is generally good after an eclamptic convulsion. The mechanism for the transitory fetal distress may be a decrease in uterine blood flow caused by intense vasospasm and uterine hyperactivity, or the absence of maternal respiration during the convulsion. Since the fetal heart rate pattern usually returns to normal after a convulsion, other conditions should be considered if an abnormal pattern persists, such as IUGR or placental abruption.

Treatment of Eclamptic Convulsions

Eclamptic convulsions are a life-threatening emergency and are tonic–clonic in type. The woman usually bites her tongue unless it is protected. Respirations are absent throughout the seizure. Coma follows the convulsion, and the woman usually remembers nothing of the recent events. If she has repeated convulsions, some degree of consciousness returns after each convulsion. She may enter a combative state and be very agitated and difficult to control. Rapid and deep respirations usually begin as soon as the convulsions end. Maintenance of oxygenation is usually not a problem after a single convulsion; the risk of aspiration is low in the well-managed patient.

Several steps should be taken in managing an eclamptic convulsion:

1. *Do not attempt to shorten or abolish the initial convulsion.* Drugs such as diazepam should not be given, especially if the patient does not have an intravenous line in place and someone skilled in intubation is not immediately available. Rapid administration of diazepam may lead to apnea or cardiac arrest, or both.[242]

2. *Prevent maternal injury during the convulsion.* A padded tongue blade should be inserted between the patient's teeth to prevent biting of the tongue. Place the woman on her left side and then suction the foam and secretions from her mouth.

3. *Maintain adequate oxygenation.* After the convulsion has ceased, the patient begins to breathe again and oxygenation is rarely a problem. Difficulty with oxygenation may occur in women who have had repetitive convulsions or who have received drugs in an attempt to abolish the convulsions. Such women should have a chest radiograph to rule out aspiration pneumonia.

4. *Minimize the risk of aspiration.* Aspiration may be

caused by forcing the padded tongue blade to the back of the throat, stimulating the gag reflex with resultant vomiting and aspiration. The use of sedative drugs to try to control the convulsions increases the risk of aspiration.

5. *Give adequate magnesium sulfate to control the convulsions.* As soon as the convulsion has ended, a large-bore secure IV line should be inserted and a loading dose of magnesium sulfate given intravenously. In our institution, we use a 6-g intravenous loading dose given over *15 to 20 minutes.* If the patient has a convulsion after the loading dose, another bolus of 2 g magnesium sulfate can be given intravenously over 3 to 5 minutes. Approximately 10 to 15 percent of women will have a second convulsion after receiving the intravenous loading dose of magnesium sulfate.

We use serum magnesium levels in the clinical management of the eclamptic woman. If the initial level, obtained 4 hours after the loading dose, is over 10 mg/dl, we reduce the 2-g/hr maintenance dose of magnesium sulfate. This will occasionally occur in women with renal compromise. Similarly, in the rare patient with a brisk urine output, we give a maintenance dose of 3 g/hr to keep levels in the therapeutic range.

An occasional patient will have recurrent convulsions while receiving therapeutic doses of magnesium sulfate. In these cases, a short-acting barbiturate such as sodium amobarbital can be given in a dose of up to 250 mg IV over 3 to 5 minutes, or a pentothal drip can be used.

Magnesium toxicity should be considered in those women who do not regain consciousness, as accidental overdoses have been reported.

6. *Correct maternal acidemia.* Blood oxygenation and pH should be in the normal range. Patients who have had repeated convulsions may be acidotic, and a low Po_2 may indicate aspiration pneumonitis. Sodium bicarbonate is not given unless the pH is below 7.10. Abnormal blood gases may be the result of respiratory depression.

7. *Avoid polypharmacy.* Polypharmacy is extremely hazardous in the woman with eclampsia, as addition of diazepam or phenytoin may lead to respiratory depression or arrest. No alternate drugs have been shown to be as effective as magnesium sulfate in treating eclamptic convulsions.

Atypical Eclampsia

Eclampsia occurring before the 20th week of gestation or after 48 hours postpartum is called *atypical eclampsia.*

Eclampsia occurring before the 20th week of gestation has usually been reported with molar or hydropic degeneration of the placenta. These women may be misdiagnosed as having hypertensive encephalopathy or a seizure disorder. Women in whom convulsions develop in association with hypertension and proteinuria during the first half of pregnancy should be considered to have eclampsia. They should be treated with parenteral magnesium sulfate to control convulsions, with termination of pregnancy as the definitive therapy. Late postpartum eclampsia accounts for 16 percent of eclampsia cases.

Can Eclampsia Be Prevented?

Eclampsia may often be a preventable complication of pregnancy. Severe forms of preeclampsia should be preventable by appropriate prenatal care. However, 38 to 42 percent of cases are not preventable.

Counseling Women with Eclampsia and Their Relatives

Long-term follow-up of women who had eclampsia found no increase in hypertension in these patients above that expected in the general female population. Eclampsia does not cause hypertension. However, women who had eclampsia as multiparas died at a rate which was significantly higher than the expected mortality rate. Eighty-two percent of the remote deaths were due to cardiovascular-renal disease.

The prognosis for future pregnancies after eclampsia is good. Preeclampsia/eclampsia recurred in 34.5 percent of the women and in 20.6 percent of their subsequent pregnancies. When hypertension occurred in a future pregnancy, it was usually mild. Eclampsia developed in 1 percent of pregnancies beyond 20 weeks' gestation.

The sisters and daughters of eclamptic women are at increased risk for the development of preeclampsia and eclampsia.[266] Preeclampsia developed in 25 percent and eclampsia occurred in 3 percent of the daughters. Preeclampsia occurred in 37 percent and eclampsia developed in 4 percent of the sisters. The incidence of preeclampsia is much higher in future pregnancies in women who have had eclampsia remote from term. The overall incidence of chronic hypertension on follow-up is only 9.5 percent in women who were normotensive before the eclamptic pregnancy.

Chronic Hypertension

Diagnosis of Chronic Hypertension

The diagnosis of chronic hypertension in pregnancy is usually made on the basis of either of the following:

1. Documented history of high blood pressure antedating pregnancy
2. Persistent elevation of blood pressure (at least 140/90 mm Hg) on two occasions more than 24 hours apart before the 20th week of gestation

Other findings might be suggestive of the presence of chronic hypertension:

Retinal changes on funduscopic examination
Cardiac enlargement on chest x-ray and electrocardiogram (ECG)
Compromised renal function or associated renal disease
Presence of medical disorders known to lead to hypertension
Multiparity with previous history of hypertensive pregnancies
Evidence of persistent hypertension beyond the 42nd day postpartum.

Sometimes the diagnosis is difficult to make because of the marked and variable changes seen with blood pressure during midpregnancy. During midpregnancy the blood pressure can be in the normal range in women who were severely hypertensive prior to pregnancy.

Etiology and Classification of Chronic Hypertension

Essential hypertension is by far the most common cause of chronic hypertension during pregnancy. Chronic hypertension in pregnancy is classified as mild or severe depending on the systolic or diastolic blood pressure reading. Hypertension is severe if either systolic pressure is more than 160 mm Hg or diastolic pressure is above 110 mm Hg.

Superimposed preeclampsia is defined as exacerbation of hypertension of at least 30 mm Hg in systolic or at least 15 mm Hg in diastolic blood pressure, together with the development of generalized edema, or proteinuria during the course of the pregnancy (at least 300 mg/24 hr), or exacerbation of preexisting proteinuria (at least 2 g/24 hr), and elevation of serum uric acid levels (at least 6 mg/dl) during the second half of the pregnancy.

Maternal and Fetal Risks of Chronic Hypertension

Pregnancies complicated by chronic hypertension are at increased risk for the development of superimposed preeclampsia, abruptio placentae, and poor perinatal outcome. Some pregnant chronic hypertensives may have silent undiagnosed chronic renal disease and may experience urinary protein excretion that increases with advancing gestation, particularly in the third trimester; many such women will demonstrate an increase in either their systolic or diastolic blood pressure with advancing gestation. It is recommended that superimposed preeclampsia be diagnosed on the basis of exacerbated hypertension plus the development of either substantial proteinuria (>1 g/24 hr) or elevated serum uric acid levels. In women on antihypertensive medications where exacerbation of blood pressure is less common, the diagnosis should be based on the development of substantial proteinuria.

The incidence of abruptio placentae is reportedly increased and ranges between 0.45 and 10 percent depending on the duration and the severity of hypertension. This incidence is not influenced by the use of antihypertensive medications.[275] Of note also is the compounding effect of superimposed preeclampsia in cases complicated by abruptio placentae, where its presence was associated with higher perinatal mortality than when preeclampsia was absent. Also, this incidence is substantially increased in those with a history of abruption in previous pregnancies.[282]

The above-mentioned complications are responsible for most of the perinatal deaths as well as the increased incidence of fetal growth retardation and premature delivery in such pregnancies. In addition, these pregnancies are reportedly associated with increased frequency of midtrimester losses, particularly in those not receiving antihypertensive therapy.[278,283,284] In general, perinatal mortality and morbidity are not increased in patients with uncomplicated mild chronic hypertension, whereas they are markedly increased in patients with severe disease, in those with renal disease, and in those complicated by superimposed preeclampsia.[275]

Pregnancy Outcome in Relation to Treatment of Chronic Hypertension

There is general agreement that chronic antihypertensive therapy will decrease the incidence of cardiovascular complications and cerebrovascular accidents in nonpregnant patients with diastolic blood pressures exceeding 105 mm Hg. However, it is not clear if antihypertensives are equally beneficial in pregnancies with mild uncomplicated hypertension. In addition, no studies have shown any reduction in the incidence of superimposed preeclampsia or abruptio placentae when antihypertensives were used.[275]

Superimposed preeclampsia and abruptio placentae are responsible for most of the poor perinatal outcome in women with mild chronic hypertension. Antihypertensive drugs do not reduce the frequency of either of these complications. Most patients with mild chronic hypertension will have a good outcome with proper obstetric follow-up without the use of antihypertensive agents.

Antihypertensive Drugs in Pregnancy

Methyldopa

Methyldopa is the only antihypertensive drug whose long-term safety for the mother and the fetus has been adequately assessed. No adverse fetal effects have been noted. It reduces systemic vascular resistance without causing physiologically significant changes in heart rate or cardiac output, while renal blood flow is maintained. If used in mild hypertension, the usual dose is 250 mg three times daily. The fall in blood pressure is maximal about 4 hours after an oral dose. It is considered a weak antihypertensive best suited for cases with mild hypertension, and if adequate blood pressure control is not achieved with the maximum dosage of 4 g/day additional antihypertensive agents may be added.

Clonidine

Clonidine is used primarily for treatment of mild to moderate hypertension. The usual oral dose in pregnancy is 0.1 to 0.3 mg/day given in two divided doses, which can be increased up to 1.2 mg/day as needed. A randomized study in 100 pregnant hypertensive women comparing clonidine to methyldopa found no significant difference in blood pressure control or maternal and fetal outcome.

Prazosin

Prazosin reduces both systolic and diastolic blood pressures, while producing significantly less tachycardia and sodium retention than methyldopa. It causes vasodilation of both the resistance and capacitance vessels, thereby reducing cardiac preload and afterload without reducing renal blood flow or glomerular filtration rate. In addition, it produces a decrease in plasma renin activity and it is probably the drug of choice for treatment of hypertension characterized by high plasma renin levels. The usual dose of prazosin is 1 mg twice daily; however, the drug has been used in doses as high as 20 mg/day. The first dose in some individuals can produce syncope due to exaggerated hypotension "first pass," and this can be avoided by decreasing the first dose. In 80 women with chronic hypertension who were treated with either prazosin or methyldopa, both drugs were effective in controlling hypertension, and the incidence of superimposed preeclampsia was similar in both groups. There were no differences in perinatal outcome between the two groups.

Calcium Channel Blockers

Calcium channel blockers cause vasodilation and reduction in the peripheral resistance. They have rapid onset of action following oral administration. Nifedipine has potent vasodilating properties without reduction in cardiac output. The drug is effective in controlling maternal blood pressure, and no adverse fetal or neonatal effects have been noted. However, there is limited experience with nifedipine treatment of chronic hypertension. Care should be exercised when using nifedipine with magnesium sulfate (which is a calcium channel blocker itself), since the use of both agents together could potentiate the antihypertensive action.

Angiotensin-Converting Enzyme Inhibitors

Angiotensin-converting enzyme (ACE) inhibitors (captopril, enalapril) induce vasodilation without reflex increase in the cardiac output. Because of their efficacy and low side effects, these agents are becoming widely used as first-line therapy for chronic hypertension in the nonpregnant state. In human pregnancy, the chronic use of ACE inhibitors has been associated with oligohydramnios, neonatal anuria and renal failure, and neonatal death.[298–301] Thus it is recommended that the use of these agents in pregnancy be avoided.[299]

Hydralazine

Hydralazine is a potent vasodilator that acts directly on the vascular smooth muscle. Hydralazine is the agent most commonly used to control severe hypertension in preeclampsia, where it is given intravenously in bolus injections. After its intravenous use, the hypotensive effect of this drug develops gradually over 15 to 30 minutes, peaking at 20 minutes. The usual bolus dose is 5 to 10 mg to be repeated every 20 to 30 minutes as needed. Because oral hydralazine when used as a monotherapy is a weak antihypertensive, it is usually combined with diuretics, methyldopa, or β-blockers. The usual oral dose is 10 mg given four times daily, but this can be increased up to 300 mg/day.

β-Blockers

β-Blockers have been extensively used and are felt to be safe in pregnancy. They have been reportedly associated with neonatal bradycardia and hypoglycemia when given to the mother within 2 hr of delivery. There is increased risk of intrauterine growth restriction and so ultrasound monitoring is prudent.

Thiazide Diuretics

In the first 3 to 5 days of treatment, these drugs result in reduction in both plasma and extracellular fluid volumes with a concomitant decrease in the cardiac output and lowering of the blood pressure. However, these changes return to pretreatment levels within 4 to 6 weeks. These effects are followed by a long-term reduction in peripheral resistance. The usual dose of hydrochlorothiazide is a single 25-mg dose in the morning. Neonatal adverse effects are electrolyte imbalance and thrombocytopenia.

Pregnant patients with chronic hypertension treated with diuretics have a marked reduction in plasma volume. However, plasma volume expansion is normal after the discontinuation of diuretics.

Prophylactic thiazide therapy does not reduce the incidence of preeclampsia. Because the initiation of diuretic therapy causes a decrease in blood volume and cardiac output, adding a diuretic late in pregnancy is contraindicated unless it is needed for treatment of pulmonary edema. Since plasma volume depletion is associated with poor perinatal outcome, we have cautioned against the use of diuretics in pregnancies complicated by chronic hypertension. Furthermore, when diuretics are discontinued, few patients require additional medications during the remainder of the pregnancy.[309]

Preconceptional Evaluation of Chronic Hypertension

Management of patients with chronic hypertension should ideally begin before pregnancy, when evaluation is undertaken to assess the etiology and the severity of the hypertension, the presence of other medical illnesses, and to rule out the presence of target organ damage. Diuretics or ACE inhibitors should be changed to those with well-documented safety.

Pregnancies in women with chronic hypertension and renal insufficiency are associated with increased perinatal loss and higher incidence of superimposed preeclampsia, preterm delivery, and fetal growth retardation.[313-315] These risks rise in proportion to the severity of the renal insufficiency. Thus, women with renal disease desiring pregnancy should be counseled to conceive before renal insufficiency becomes severe. For women with hypertension and severe renal insufficiency in the first trimester, the decision to continue pregnancy should not be made without extensive counseling regarding the potential maternal and fetal risks.

Initial and Subsequent Prenatal Visits for Patients with Chronic Hypertension

Early prenatal care will ensure accurate determination of gestational age as well as the severity of hypertension in the first trimester. Initial counselling should include:

1. Instruction by a nutritionist regarding nutritional requirements, weight gain, and sodium intake
2. Instruction regarding the negative impact of maternal anxiety, smoking, and caffeine, as well as drugs, on maternal blood pressure and perinatal outcome
3. Instruction regarding the positive impact of adequate rest during the day and at night on maternal blood pressure and pregnancy outcome
4. Counselling regarding the possible adverse effects and complications of hypertension during pregnancy
5. Counselling regarding the importance of frequent prenatal visits and their impact on preventing or minimizing the above adverse effects

If the patient is well motivated, she can be instructed in self-determination of blood pressure, which avoids the phenomenon of "white coat hypertension." It is recommended that patient-recorded measurements of blood pressure be used to supplement those recorded in the doctor's office.

Maternal evaluation should include serial measurements of hematocrit, serum creatinine, and 24-hour urinary excretion of protein at least once every trimester. The occurrence of one or more of the following is an indication for prompt maternal hospitalization:

1. Pyelonephritis
2. Significant elevations in blood pressure with levels in the range of severe hypertension
3. Significant elevation in serum uric acid level and new onset of substantial proteinuria (>1 g/24 hr). This finding is usually an early sign of developing superimposed preeclampsia
4. Severe fetal IUGR

Managing Low-Risk Chronic Hypertension

Most patients with uncomplicated mild chronic hypertension will have a good perinatal outcome irrespective of the use of antihypertensive drugs. Only 13 percent of patients will require antihypertensive medications for exacerbation of hypertension during the third trimester. Most of the poor outcome is related to the development of superimposed preeclampsia. Thus it is our policy to discontinue all antihypertensive medications in all such patients at the time of the first prenatal visit. Antihypertensive therapy is subsequently started only if the blood pressure exceeds 160 mm Hg systolic or 110 mm Hg diastolic. These patients are usually treated with methyldopa (750 to 4,000 mg/day) given as needed to keep diastolic blood pressure consistently at or below 105 mm Hg. The development of exacerbated hypertension alone is not an indication for delivery. The pregnancy in these patients may be continued until term or until the onset of superimposed preeclampsia. Superimposed preeclampsia or suspected fetal growth retardation is an indication for hospitalization and close evaluation of maternal and fetal well-being. Mild superimposed preeclampsia is an indication for delivery if the gestational age is at least 37 weeks.

There are short-term maternal benefits from treating women with mild hypertension and target organ damage such as diabetes mellitus, renal disease, and cardiac dysfunction. As a result, we recommend treating mild chronic hypertension in pregnant women with these complications.

Managing High-Risk Chronic Hypertension

Patients with chronic renal disease (serum creatinine >2.5 mg/dl) should be managed in consultation with a nephrologist and maternal fetal medicine specialist. Antihypertensive medications should be used to keep systolic blood pressure between 140 and 160 mm Hg and diastolic blood pressure between 90 and 105 mm

Hg. Maternal blood pressure can be controlled with methyldopa, labetalol, or nifedipine.

These women need close monitoring throughout pregnancy and may require multiple hospital admissions for control of blood pressure or associated medical complications. Fetal evaluation should be started as early as 26 weeks and repeated as needed. Superimposed preeclampsia is an indication for immediate hospitalization. Severe superimposed preeclampsia is an indication for delivery in all patients with gestational age beyond 34 weeks. If preeclampsia develops before this time, the pregnancy may be followed conservatively with daily evaluation of maternal and fetal well-being.

Hypertensive Emergencies in Chronic Hypertension

Life-threatening clinical conditions require immediate control of blood pressure, such as hypertensive encephalopathy, acute left ventricular failure, acute aortic dissection, or increased circulating catecholamines (pheochromocytoma, clonidine withdrawal, cocaine ingestion). Although a diastolic blood pressure of 115 mm Hg or greater is usually considered as a hypertensive emergency, this level is actually arbitrary and the rate of change of blood pressure may be more important than absolute level.[317]

Hypertensive encephalopathy is usually seen in patients with systolic blood pressure above 250 mm Hg or diastolic blood pressure above 150 mm Hg.[318] Patients with acute onset of hypertension may develop encephalopathy at pressure levels that are generally tolerated by those with chronic hypertension. Severe hypertension may result in abruptio placentae with resultant DIC.

Lowering Blood Pressure. There are risks associated with a too rapid or excessive reduction of elevated blood pressure, which can produce cerebral ischemia, stroke, or coma. The aim of therapy is to lower mean blood pressure by no more than 15 to 25 percent. Small reductions in blood pressure in the first 60 minutes, working toward a diastolic level of 100 to 110 mm Hg, have been recommended.[317,321] If the hypertension proves increasingly difficult to control, this is an indication to end the pregnancy.

The drug of choice in hypertensive crisis is sodium nitroprusside. Other drugs such as diazoxide, labetalol, and hydralazine can also be used.

Sodium nitroprusside causes arterial and venous relaxation and is given as an intravenous infusion of 0.25 to 8.0 µg/kg/min. The onset of action is immediate, and its effect may last 3 to 5 minutes after discontinuing the infusion. Hypotension caused by nitroprusside should resolve within a few minutes of stopping the infusion.

Nitroglycerin is an arterial and venous dilator (mostly venous). It is given as an intravenous infusion of 5 μg/min that is gradually increased every 3 to 5 minutes up to a maximum dose of 100 μg/min. It is the drug of choice in preeclampsia associated with pulmonary edema and for control of hypertension associated with tracheal manipulation. It is contraindicated in hypertensive encephalopathy because it increases cerebral blood flow and intracranial pressure.[318]

Key Points

- Hypertension is the most common medical complication during pregnancy.
- Preeclampsia is a leading cause of maternal mortality and morbidity worldwide.
- The pathophysiologic abnormalities of preeclampsia are numerous, but the etiology is unknown.
- At present, there is no proven method to prevent preeclampsia.
- The HELLP syndrome may develop in the absence of maternal hypertension.
- Expectant management improves perinatal outcome in a select group of women with severe preeclampsia before 32 weeks' gestation.
- Magnesium sulfate is the ideal agent to prevent or treat eclamptic convulsions.
- Rare cases of eclampsia can develop before 20 weeks' gestation and beyond 48 hours postpartum.
- Antihypertensive agents do not improve pregnancy outcome in women with mild uncomplicated chronic hypertension.
- Methyldopa is the drug of choice for the treatment of chronic hypertension; ACE Inhibitors should be avoided.

Chapter 21

Medical Complications

Philip Samuels and
Mark B. Landon

The management of medical complications in pregnancy represents one of the most demanding and rewarding areas of obstetrics. The clinician must first be familiar with the normal physiologic changes brought about by pregnancy. This information must then be integrated with the pathophysiology of the disease itself. In short, one must ask how pregnancy affects this medical disorder and how this medical disorder affects pregnancy. In addition, the obstetrician must be aware of the consequences of the medical complication for both the mother and her fetus. These considerations encompass not only the consequences of the disease itself, but the risks associated with the treatment of the disorder as well.

Cardiac and Pulmonary Disease

Mark B. Landon and Philip Samuels

Heart Disease

Mark B. Landon

Cardiac disease complicates approximately 1 percent of all pregnancies. It remains a major nonobstetric cause of maternal death in the United States.[1]

Labor and Delivery

Maternal pain and anxiety result in increased adrenergic stimulation that is accompanied by a rise in blood pressure and heart rate, particularly during the second stage of labor. Thus anesthesia can greatly influence the hemodynamic changes observed during labor. Epidural anesthesia may attenuate the normal increase in cardiac output and heart rate because it acts as an analgesic as well as a peripheral vasodilator, which reduces venous return to the heart. These changes result in a diminished preload or ventricular end-diastolic volume. Similar effects may be observed with spinal anesthesia, if a patient is not adequately hydrated prior to its administration. Regional anesthesia may be used effectively in most patients with cardiac disease. For patients undergoing cesarean delivery, consideration of potentiating right-to-left shunting with diminished preload must be weighed against the risk of myocardial depression of general anesthetic agents, as well as acute hypertension associated with intubation and extubation.

Both epidural and spinal anesthesia may produce a fall in cardiac output and blood pressure prior to elective cesarean delivery. Hypotension is generally corrected by employing left-lateral uterine displacement and infusing appropriate intravenous fluids. Correction of hypotension with ephedrine is inadvisable in patients who cannot tolerate tachycardia.

Diagnosis and Detection of Cardiac Disease

Interpreting the results of standard techniques used to investigate cardiac disease may be difficult in preg-

Signs and Symptoms of Cardiac Disease

History
Progressive or severe dyspnea
Dyspnea at rest
Paroxysmal nocturnal dyspnea
Angina or syncope with exertion
Hemoptysis
Physical examination
Loud systolic murmur or click
Diastolic murmur
Cardiomegaly, including parasternal heave
Cyanosis or clubbing
Persistent jugular venous distention
Features of Marfan syndrome
Electrocardiogram
Dysrhythmia

nancy. Chest radiographs will often demonstrate cardiomegaly and increased pulmonary vascular markings. Therefore, more significant changes must be present to suggest hemodynamically significant cardiac disease. Electrocardiographic findings may aid in the preliminary diagnosis of valvular disease or anatomic defects if chamber hypertrophy is suggested. However, myocardial ischemia must not be confused with the ST-T segment depression and flattening of T waves in the precordial leads, which may be present in normal pregnant women. Premature atrial and ventricular beats are also common in pregnancy.

Because it does not expose the mother and the fetus to radiation, echocardiography has become the preferred technique for detection and management of cardiac abnormalities during pregnancy. The internal dimensions of the left ventricle, ejection fraction, and stroke volume are all increased in pregnant women after the first trimester.[13,14]

General Considerations in Management

The successful management of heart disease in pregnancy requires close cooperation between the cardiologist and the obstetrician. In the best circumstances, cardiac disease is identified *prior* to pregnancy so that appropriate counseling regarding risks and outcome can be undertaken. Certain conditions including Eisenmenger syndrome and primary pulmonary hypertension have been associated with such high maternal mortality rates that pregnancy is not advised. Patients with mitral stenosis may elect to undergo cardiac catheterization and possible valve replacement earlier in their illness if contemplating pregnancy. In such patients, a porcine valve may be preferred since it reduces the need for anticoagulation.

The specific cardiac lesion present will also determine the need for antibiotic prophylaxis during labor and delivery. Although the efficacy of antibiotic prophylaxis against infective endocarditis has not been proven, the low risk of drug toxicity when weighed against the dangers of endocarditis makes such prophy-

---

Maternal Mortality Risk Associated With Specific Cardiac Diseases

Group I: mortality <1%
  Atrial septal defect (uncomplicated)
  Ventricular septal defect (uncomplicated)
  Patient ductus arteriosus (uncomplicated)
  Pulmonic/tricuspid disease
  Corrected tetralogy of Fallot
  Porcine valve
  Mitral stenosis (mild)
Group II: mortality 5–15%
  Mitral stenosis with atrial fibrillation
  Artificial valve
  Mitral stenosis (moderate to severe)
  Aortic stenosis
  Coarctation of aorta, uncomplicated
  Uncorrected tetralogy of Fallot
  Previous myocardial infarction
Group III: mortality 25–50%
  Pulmonary hypertension
  Coarctation of aorta (complicated)
  Marfan syndrome with aortic involvement

Adapted from Clark SL: Structural cardiac disease in pregnancy. In Clark SL, Phelan JP, Cotton DB (eds): Critical Care Obstetrics. Montvale, NJ, Medical Economics Books, 1987, p 92, with permission.

laxis the recommended practice. Manual removal of the placenta is an absolute indication for antibiotic prophylaxis in patients with structural heart disease. For some patients, including those with prosthetic valves, mortality rates are particularly high should they become infected. Prophylaxis usually includes the intravenous administration of aqueous penicillin G and an aminoglycoside at the start of true labor, with continuation every 8 hours until one dose postdelivery has been given. Vancomycin may be substituted in patients who are allergic to penicillin (Table 21-1).

Antibiotic prophylaxis for rheumatic fever should be used in patients with a positive past history, especially if they demonstrate valvular disease. The American Heart Association recommends a monthly injection of 1.2 million units of benzathine penicillin G. Alternative regimens include daily oral administration of penicillin or erythromycin.

Anticoagulation may be required in individuals with prosthetic valves as well as those with arrhythmias who may be at risk for an arterial embolus. Patients with mitral stenosis and associated atrial fibrillation should also be anticoagulated. Oral anticoagulants are contraindicated, as fetal exposure to Coumadin during the first 2 months of gestation may result in a significant malformation rate. Heparin does not cross the placenta, and it is the preferred anticoagulant.

Table 21-1   Recommended Regimen for Antibiotic Prophylaxis

For labor and delivery	Ampicillin 2.0 g IM or IV plus gentamicin 1.5 mg/kg IM or IV given in active labor; one follow-up dose given 8 hours later and postpartum
Oral regimen for minor or repetitive procedures in low-risk patients	Amoxicillin 3.0 g orally 1 hr before procedure and 1.5 g 6 hr later
Penicillin-allergic patients	Vancomycin 1.0 g IV slowly over 1 hour, plus gentamicin 1.5 mg/kg IM or IV given 1 hr before procedure; repeat once 8 hr later

Adapted from Shulman ST, Amren DP, Bisno AL et al: Prevention of bacterial endocarditis. Circulation 70:1125A, 1984; and Dajani AS, Bisno A, Chung KJ: Prevention of bacterial endocarditis. JAMA 264:2919, 1990, with permission.

Careful assessment by both the cardiologist and obstetrician should ensure that the patient's hemodynamic status remains optimal during pregnancy. Monitoring of weight, blood pressure, and pulse as well as a detailed cardiovascular examination should be performed at each visit. It is important to consider conditions such as anemia and infection that may stress patients with significant cardiac disease. In a patient who demonstrates worsening symptoms, it is often necessary to institute changes in diet, activity, or medication.

Specific Cardiac Diseases

Despite the declining incidence of rheumatic fever in the United States, rheumatic heart disease remains the most common cardiac problem encountered in pregnancy. The prognosis for patients with rheumatic disease who receive optimal care is generally good. In patients who survive pregnancy, life expectancy is not shortened.[19]

Acquired Valvular Disease

Mitral Stenosis

This lesion is the most common form of rheumatic heart disease found in pregnancy. It can be isolated or accompany aortic or right-sided valvular lesions. Mitral stenosis is usually a sequel of rheumatic fever. In patients who develop carditis, mitral insufficiency often precedes the development of stenosis. Symptoms may not appear for over a decade, at which time a reduction in cardiac output causes patients to become easily fatigued. Obstruction to left atrial outflow produces a rise in atrial pressure and eventually pulmonary capillary wedge pressure. Pulmonary congestive and right ventricular failure are seen 5 to 10 years after the onset of symptoms.[21] The normal cross-sectional area of the mitral valve is greater than 4 cm^2. Patients generally remain asymptomatic until the area decreases to less than 2.5 cm^2. In patients with a valve area of less than 1 cm^2, mild exercise will produce symptoms. In symptomatic patients, the maternal mortality rate during pregnancy is sufficiently high to recommend surgical correction prior to pregnancy.

The augmented cardiac output of pregnancy, including tachycardia and increased circulatory volume, imposes a tremendous stress on patients with significant mitral disease. Any condition, such as pregnancy, that increases cardiac output and shortens diastolic filling time may raise the diastolic gradient across the mitral valve, thereby elevating left atrial pressure and pulmonary capillary pressure.

Symptoms of reduced cardiac output should be treated with limitation of activity and, if the patient is volume overloaded, cautious diuresis. Control of arrhythmias, particularly atrial fibrillation, is essential. In hemodynamically stable patients, digitalis is initially used to slow the ventricular rate prior to cardioversion.

If medical measures are unsuccessful in the treatment of symptoms, valve commissurotomy or replacement must be considered. Commissurotomy should ideally be performed in patients who do not have significant regurgitation and who have limited calcification of the mitral valve. No other valvular disease should be present.

Labor and delivery is a hazardous process for the patient with mitral stenosis. Patients with significant disease require invasive monitoring of pulmonary capillary wedge pressure and cardiac output using a Swan-Ganz catheter. The volume of fluids administered should be monitored carefully during both labor and the immediate postpartum period. Patients should be given oxygen and should labor in the semi-Fowler position. Although epidural anesthesia is the preferred anesthetic technique, a decline in cardiac output has been associated with its use.[27] Ventricular rate must be monitored closely to avoid tachycardia, which can result in decreased cardiac output. It should be remembered that stenosis of the mitral valve is accompanied by a relatively fixed stroke volume, which may not rise with an increase in heart rate. Rapid heart rates further decrease diastolic filling time and elevate left atrial pressure. Verapamil or digitalis may be required to slow the ventricular rate in cases of atrial arrhythmias. If sinus tachycardia becomes excessive (> 140 bpm), the use of anesthetics to alleviate pain or cautious use of propranolol may be employed. Patients who receive epidural anesthesia should be carefully observed for hypotension, which may precipitate tachycardia. Systemic vascular resistance is best maintained with the α-agonist metaraminol. The β-agonist component of ephedrine will result in tachycardia, and its use should therefore be avoided. In patients delivering vaginally, the second stage of labor, including intense Valsalva efforts, may be shortened by the use of outlet forceps or vacuum extraction. A large bolus of intravenous oxytocin should be avoided, as it may precipitate hypotension.

The most hazardous time for women with mitral stenosis is the postpartum period.[18] A rise in wedge pressure is common, and careful attention must be given to changes in cardiac output that accompany fluid shifts following delivery. In general, a requirement for frequent administration of furosemide is to be anticipated.[27] Antibiotic prophylaxis is required in patients with mitral stenosis.

Mitral Regurgitation

The hemodynamic changes of pregnancy are usually well tolerated in patients with minimal mitral insufficiency. Patients with longstanding disease may develop atrial enlargement and fibrillation. The risk for arrhythmias may be increased during pregnancy.[32] Reduction of left ventricular afterload may therefore become an important therapeutic maneuver in patients with impaired cardiac output. Patients with chronic disease, including those with a large left ventricle, may require inotropic support if the afterload is substantially reduced.

During labor and delivery, patients with significant mitral insufficiency may benefit from central monitoring to direct fluid and drug therapy. Pain may be associated with an increase in blood pressure that is due to enhanced sympathetic activity. If systemic vascular resistance also rises, pulmonary congestion may follow. Epidural analgesia is recommended to prevent this occurrence. Regional anesthesia may impair venous return to the heart and often requires careful administration of intravenous fluids to maintain filling of the enlarged left ventricle. Patients with this lesion should also receive antibiotic prophylaxis during labor and delivery.

Congenital Lesions

Left-to-Right Shunts

Left-to-right shunting may occur through an atrial septal defect, ventricular septal defect, or patent ductus arteriosus. During pregnancy, right-sided and left-sided resistances decrease in a similar manner; therefore, the degree of shunting is not significantly altered. Small defects are usually associated with a good pregnancy outcome. In patients who have developed pulmonary hypertension that has led to shunt reversal, as in Eisenmenger syndrome, maternal mortality rates of up to 50 percent have been reported.

Ventricular Septal Defect

Patients with small ventricular septal defects (VSDs) generally tolerate pregnancy well. The degree of left-to-right shunting is not significantly altered if baseline pulmonary vascular resistance is normal.[36] Hemodynamic changes of pregnancy may increase left-to-right shunting to a critical level. Once pulmonary vascular resistance rises, right ventricular failure develops and reverse shunting with cyanosis may occur.

Increases in systemic vascular resistance that accompany the stress of labor may increase the degree of left-to-right shunting. Continuous epidural anesthesia is an effective method to relieve pain and lower systemic resistance. Patients with VSDs do require antibiotic prophylaxis during labor and delivery.

Atrial Septal Defect

Atrial septal defect (ASD) is the most common congenital heart lesion found in the adult population, accounting for 30 percent of such lesions. Young women with an ASD are often asymptomatic or may experience mild fatigue.

Prophylactic antibiotics are often administered, although the risk of bacterial endocarditis is low and routine anticoagulation is not recommended. Uncomplicated patients may be managed during labor and delivery without invasive monitoring. Epidural anesthesia is a well-accepted analgesic technique.

Right-to-Left Shunts

Eisenmenger Syndrome

Eisenmenger syndrome is defined as right-to-left or bidirectional shunting at either the atrial or ventricular level, combined with elevated pulmonary vascular resistance. Maternal mortality ranges from 12 to 70 percent, and fetal mortality approaches 50 percent.[22] At least 30 percent of fetuses will be growth restricted. Because of these risks, termination of pregnancy is strongly recommended in patients with Eisenmenger syndrome complicated by significant pulmonary hypertension. Women who continue pregnancy require strict limitation of activity with strong consideration for anticoagulation.

It is imperative that Swan-Ganz monitoring be employed for management during labor and delivery. There appears to be no advantage to cesarean delivery compared with vaginal delivery in women with Eisenmenger syndrome.[39]

Developmental Cardiac Lesions

Marfan Syndrome

Marfan syndrome is an autosomal dominant disorder of connective tissue marked by joint deformities, arachnodactyly, dislocations of the ocular lens, and cardiac manifestations, including weakness of the aortic root and wall. Mitral valve prolapse is found in 90 percent of cases.

Patients with Marfan syndrome must receive genetic counseling and be made aware of the risks of pregnancy with their particular condition. The variability in the clinical expression of this disorder makes it imperative to study the cardiovascular system of these patients before counseling them about the dangers of pregnancy. Transesophageal echocardiographic measurement of the width of the aorta has been helpful in selecting patients at greatest risk for aortic dissection, although serial measurements of aortic root diameter may occasionally fail to detect a patient at risk for dissection.[47] Dilatation of the aorta greater than 40 mm is a contraindication to pregnancy. Mortality rates of up to 50 percent have been associated with Marfan disease in pregnancy in cases with significant maternal cardiovascular disease prior to conception.

The management of patients with Marfan disease includes efforts to minimize hypertension as well as the contractile force transmitted to the aortic wall. β-Blockade using propranolol may be efficacious. Regional anesthesia for labor and delivery is generally well tolerated.[49]

Mitral Valve Prolapse

Mitral valve prolapse (MVP) is the most common congenital heart lesion found in young women of childbearing age. The incidence in this population is approximately 12 percent.[51] The dysfunctional characteristic of MVP is abnormal prolapse of one or both mitral leaflets into the left atrium during ventricular systole; while most women with MVP are asymptomatic, others experience palpitations, atypical chest pain, and syncope.

Most women with MVP have uneventful pregnancies. It is possible that the increased intravascular volume of pregnancy that increases left ventricular end-diastolic volume results in less prolapse of the mitral valve leaflets. Debate still exists as to whether routine antibiotic prophylaxis is warranted during pregnancy in patients with MVP. Because of the relative safety of therapy, it is recommended that prophylactic antibiotics be administered until this issue is further resolved.

Other Cardiac Diseases
Peripartum Cardiomyopathy

Peripartum cardiomyopathy has classically been defined as congestive failure with cardiomyopathy found in the last month of pregnancy or in the first 5 months postpartum.[59,60] Symptoms of left-sided failure occur in association with a dilated hypocontractile heart in patients who have no previous history of cardiac disease. The overwhelming majority (82 percent) of patients present with cardiac failure in the first 3 months postpartum.[59] Most reports have documented the higher frequency of this lesion among older black multiparas, particularly in association with twins or preeclampsia.

Primary therapy of peripartum cardiomyopathy should include bedrest, sodium restriction, digitalis, and diuretics.[65] Thromboembolic complications stemming from mural thrombi are not uncommon. Anticoagulation may be necessary, particularly in patients with massively enlarged cardiac chambers.

It is generally accepted that the clinical course of this disease can be predicted by the size of the heart several months after the diagnosis has been made. Approximately 50 percent of affected women will continue to have symptoms of failure and cardiomegaly beyond 6 months. These women should be advised against pregnancy as the incidence of recurrent disease is high, with mortality rates approaching 100 percent.[66] Persistent cardiomegaly has been associated with a 5-year mortality rate exceeding 50 percent.[59,60]

Key Points

- The presence of underlying cardiac disease should be suspected in any pregnant woman with (1) a progressive limitation of physical activity due to worsening dyspnea, (2) chest pain that accompanies exercise or increased activity, and (3) syncope that is preceded by palpitations or physical exertion.
- Women who develop right-to-left shunting with increased pulmonary vascular pressure (Eisenmenger syndrome) may exhibit maternal mortality rates approaching 50 percent.
- Treatment of mitral stenosis involves limitation of activity, cautious diuresis, and control of arrhythmias. Tachycardia is poorly tolerated as stroke volume is relatively fixed. If medical treatment fails to control symptoms, valvuloplasty or replacement must be considered.
- Marfan syndrome, when accompanied by a significantly dilated aortic root (>40 mm), is associated with mortality rates up to 50 percent. Pregnancy is contraindicated with significant aortic root dilatation.
- Peripartum cardiomyopathy is a congestive cardiomyopathy found in the last month of pregnancy or

in the first 5 months postpartum. It is more common in blacks and twin gestations. Half of affected women will continue to have failure or cardiomegaly beyond 6 months.

- Myocardial infarction, when it occurs during pregnancy, is often observed in older gravidas with a history of chronic hypertension. Mortality rates are highest during the third trimester and when delivery occurs within 2 weeks of the event. Cesarean delivery is reserved for obstetric indications.

Pulmonary Disease

Philip Samuels

Tuberculosis

Pregnancy should not be a deterrent to the accurate diagnosis and treatment of tuberculosis. Tuberculin skin testing with subcutaneous administration of intermediate-strength purified protein derivative (PPD) is the mainstay of testing for tuberculosis in the United States. In high-risk areas and populations, it should be administered at the first prenatal visit. A positive PPD only means that the patient has been previously exposed to tuberculosis and that there are dormant organisms present. Less than 10 percent of patients with a positive PPD and an intact immune system will progress to active disease. This method, however, has several drawbacks. Only 80 percent of patients with a reactivation of tuberculosis will have positive skin tests. In addition, any patient who has previously received the bacillus Calmette-Guérin (BCG) vaccine will retain a positive tuberculin skin test for life. Although this vaccine is rarely used in the United States, it is administered routinely in countries where tuberculosis is endemic.

If a differential diagnosis of tuberculosis is entertained in a patient presenting with respiratory symptoms and lethargy, a chest x-ray with abdominal shielding should be obtained without hesitation. A chest x-ray should also be taken without delay if the patient's previously negative tuberculin skin test becomes positive, if it cannot be determined when a patient's skin test became positive, or if a patient has persistent respiratory or constitutional symptoms.[2] If possible, chest x-rays should be delayed until after the first trimester. The definitive diagnosis of tuberculosis is based on identifying *Mycobacterium tuberculosis* by culture or by acid–fast or fluorescent stain of the sputum.

When adequate treatment is implemented, tuberculosis appears to have no adverse effect on pregnancy, and, conversely, pregnancy does not alter the natural history of the disease.[5–7]

Highly effective chemotherapeutic agents have been developed for the treatment of tuberculosis (Table 21-2). Although the prognosis for tuberculosis during pregnancy is excellent, severe complications such as miliary, renal, and meningeal tuberculosis have developed.[10] Treatment has become more complex as resistant strains of *M. tuberculosis* have developed. It is paramount that cultures and sensitivities be obtained on all patients.

Current standard therapy for pregnancy is isoniazid in a single daily dose of 300 mg and rifampin 600 mg/day.[11] If a resistant strain is suspected, ethambutol should be added.[11] This therapy should be continued for 9 months. The major adverse effects of isoniazid include toxic hepatitis, peripheral neuropathy, and hypersensitivity reactions. Transient elevations of the serum transaminases are seen in approximately 20 percent of patients. Transaminase levels should therefore be monitored monthly. Peripheral neuropathy appears to be related to a deficiency of pyridoxine (vitamin B_6). Patients taking isoniazid should receive a 25- to 50-mg

Table 21-2   Antituberculosis Agents

Drug	Dosage	Maternal Side Effects
Isoniazid	300 mg/day (single dose) PO	Toxic hepatitis, peripheral neuropathy (prevented with pyridoxine)
Ethambutol	15 mg/kg/day (single dose) PO	Optic neuritis
Rifampin	600 mg/day (single dose) PO	Orange discoloration of body secretions, gastrointestinal disturbance, liver toxicity
Pyrazinamide	15 mg/kg PO	Hepatitis, hyperuricemia
Streptomycin	15 mg/kg/day (single dose) IM	Cranial nerve VIII toxicity, nephrotoxicity

supplement of pyridoxine daily to prevent this complication. Ethambutol also appears safe for use during gestation and has not been associated with an increase in congenital anomalies.[13] If possible, streptomycin should be avoided during pregnancy. Studies have shown damage to cranial nerve VIII in offspring of mothers treated with streptomycin. Rifampin readily crosses the placenta and should be used with caution during gestation.

Transplacental passage of tuberculosis is extremely rare. Most perinatal infections occur when a mother with active tuberculosis handles her neonate.[18] The risk to the child of contracting tuberculosis from a mother with active disease during the first year of life may be as high as 50 percent.[19] Daily administration of isoniazid chemoprophylaxis can be given to the newborn for the length of the mother's treatment,[20] or the neonate may be vaccinated with BCG.

Pneumonia

Most bacterial pneumonia in pregnant women is due to *Streptococcus pneumoniae*. Most of these patients are smokers.[28] The clinical hallmarks of pneumococcal pneumonia include sudden onset, productive cough, purulent sputum, tachypnea, and fever with shaking chills. The diagnosis should be made on the basis of chest x-ray, Gram stain of the sputum, and cultures of blood and sputum. The chest x-ray usually reveals lobar consolidation and air bronchograms. Gram stain shows numerous leukocytes and gram-positive diplococci.

Patients with pneumococcal pneumonia complicating pregnancy should be initially hospitalized and receive 600,000 units of aqueous penicillin G intravenously four times daily. Parenteral treatment should continue for several days after defervescence. The therapy can then be changed to an oral penicillin or ampicillin (500 mg four times daily). The treatment should be continued for a total of 10 to 14 days. For patients who are allergic to penicillin, either a cephalosporin or erythromycin can be used.

Mycoplasma pneumonia caused by *Mycoplasma pneumoniae* is common in young adults. In contrast to the sudden onset of pneumococcal pneumonia, patients with mycoplasma pneumonia usually have a slow, gradual onset of symptoms with a nonproductive cough. The diagnosis is usually made clinically. On chest x-ray, infiltrates are diffuse and patchy and can be either unilateral or bilateral. One must consider the diagnosis of mycoplasma pneumonia in any patient whose clinical symptoms are not responding to penicillin or to cephalosporins. During pregnancy, the treatment of mycoplasma pneumonia consists of the administration of erythromycin for 10 to 14 days. Azithromycin and clarithromycin can also be used. These medications may cause less gastrointestinal distress than erythromycin but are considerably more expensive. Tetracycline and its derivatives should be avoided.

Asthma

Asthma is the most common obstructive pulmonary disease that coexists with pregnancy. It is observed in 0.4 to 1.3 percent of pregnant women.[37,38] Pregnancy can have a varying effect on the course of asthma: 49 percent of pregnant patients have no change in the course of their asthma, 29 percent show improvement, and 22 percent experience an exacerbation of their disease.[40–43]

The goals in treating asthma during pregnancy are (1) reduction in the number of asthmatic attacks, (2) prevention of severe asthmatic attacks (status asthmaticus), and (3) assurance of adequate maternal and fetal oxygenation. Patients receiving allergen desensitization may continue this treatment throughout pregnancy.[53] The Centers for Disease Control and Prevention (CDC) recommends that patients with chronic bronchial asthma receive yearly influenza immunization.[54] This is a killed vaccine and can be administered safely during pregnancy.

Inhaled β-agonists have become the mainstay of acute and chronic therapy for asthma in pregnancy. The most widely used of these agents are albuterol and metaproterenol. This therapy can be used on an as-needed basis for mild cases or on a scheduled basis for severe patients. No adverse pregnancy outcome is seen in women who use β-agonist inhalers in the first trimester.[55] The most common side effects seen with these agents include cardiac arrhythmias and tachyphylaxis.

In addition to inhaled β-agonists, many patients require inhaled glucocorticoids. This therapy has helped control asthma on an outpatient basis over the past few years.[56,57] Beclomethasone is the most commonly used inhaled corticosteroid, but triamcinolone and flunisolide are also available. The main side effect is oropharyngeal candidiasis, but this is minimized if a spacer device is used in the inhaler. Cromolyn is usually used as adjunctive therapy with both β-agonists and glucocorticoids.

The use of aminophylline has declined during pregnancy, but many obstetricians still prescribe it because of their familiarity with this agent. If this therapy is used, the goal is to keep the theophylline level between 10 and 20 µg/ml. Theophylline toxicity is commonly manifested by nausea and vomiting, but increased levels of theophylline may also cause tachycardia and cardiac arrhythmias.

Oral or parenteral corticosteroids should be employed when the aerosolized forms are inadequate.

Status asthmaticus requires immediate therapeutic intervention. During this period of acute treatment, the patient should receive a 30 to 40 percent concentration of humidified oxygen and should be well hydrated. Subcutaneous catecholamines should be administered. In humans, there is no evidence that using epinephrine for the treatment of acute asthma has deleterious effects on the fetus. Terbutaline, a β_2-agonist that is more selective than epinephrine, is a better first-line drug in pregnancy. In the emergent situation, however, epinephrine can be used if terbutaline is not immediately available. If the patient does not improve rapidly after the subcutaneous administration of catecholamines, intravenous corticosteroids should be administered. Methylprednisolone in a dose of 100 mg every 6 to 8 hours or hydrocortisone in a dose of 100 mg every 4 hours is usually administered until the asthma attack clears. Nebulized β-agonists should also be used. Rarely, intravenous aminophylline in a loading dose of 5 mg/kg followed by 0.6 mg/kg/hr can be used in the poorly responsive patient. In the unusual patient who is resistant to these measures and has a falling Po_2, endotracheal intubation should be considered.

Acute asthma attacks are unusual during labor. Should they occur, however, they are treated in the usual fashion. Epidural anesthesia is preferred for labor, vaginal delivery, and cesarean delivery. General anesthesia carries the risks of atelectasis and subsequent chest infection.[74] If the patient has been receiving oral corticosteroids during pregnancy, intravenous dosages should be used for labor and delivery. Generally, 100 mg of hydrocortisone every 4 to 6 hours or 100 mg of methylprednisolone administered intravenously at 6- to 8-hour intervals during labor and for 24 hours after delivery should suffice. Thereafter the patient should resume her maintenance dose of oral glucocorticoids.

Pulmonary Embolus

Pulmonary embolus complicates between 0.09 and 0.7/1,000 pregnancies.[75,76] Prompt diagnosis and treatment are imperative, as untreated pulmonary emboli during pregnancy carry a 12.8 percent mortality rate, while treatment lowers this to 0.7 percent.[77] If untreated, more than one-third of these patients will have recurrent emboli.[78] The vast majority of pulmonary emboli arise from thrombophlebitis of the deep femoral and pelvic veins. It is now common for patients in preterm labor to be aggressively treated with prolonged bedrest. This approach places these patients at an increased risk for thrombophlebitis and pulmonary embolism.

The patient with an acute pulmonary embolus usually presents with chest pain and dyspnea. Occasionally, a pleural friction rub may be auscultated. The chest x-ray is often normal, but arterial blood gas values usually show a decreased Po_2 and a slightly more decreased Pco_2. Massive pulmonary emboli are easily diagnosed. Hypotension and cardiovascular collapse often complicate such cases. In contrast, patients with small emboli may only have subtle signs and symptoms. It is imperative to establish the proper diagnosis in affected patients, as these small clots may be the harbinger of a massive embolus.

Certain acquired disorders of coagulation place the patient at increased risk of developing thrombophlebitis and pulmonary embolism, including congenital deficiency of protein C, protein S, and antithrombin III.

Although impedance plethysmography is still occasionally used to detect lower extremity thrombosis, Doppler studies with compression sonography have made testing much more accurate. The positive predictive value is 94 percent compared with 83 percent for impedance plethysmography.

The diagnosis of pulmonary embolus must be established radiographically. Adequate technique is essential so that fetal exposure to ionizing radiation is minimized. Pulmonary ventilation and perfusion (V/Q) scans are useful in diagnosing pulmonary embolism only if the chest x-ray is normal. Calculations have shown that maximum fetal radiation exposure from this type of study is 50 mrem.[87] These isotopes are excreted through the maternal urinary tract. The fetus receives 85 percent of its radiation exposure from the maternal bladder. Brisk diuresis and frequent micturition should therefore theoretically lower fetal exposure.[87] If necessary, a Foley catheter can be used to empty the bladder. "High probability" V/Q scans with clinical symptoms carry a high likelihood that the patient actually had a pulmonary embolism.[88]

If the V/Q scan is equivocal or if the patient's chest x-ray is abnormal, selective pulmonary angiography should be immediately undertaken. In experienced hands, the procedure carries a morbidity of less than

1 percent. Abdominal shielding should be used during the procedure. The increased plasma volume and vasodilatation that occur during pregnancy should make the procedure faster and technically easier than in the nonpregnant patient. Because the risk to the fetus from such exposure is small in both relative and absolute terms, the diagnostic procedure should be undertaken without hesitation when necessary.

Once the diagnosis is established, therapy should be initiated without delay. Anticoagulation with heparin is the treatment of choice. Heparin, a large negatively charged protein with a molecular weight of 20,000, does not cross the placenta.[90] The main complication of heparin therapy is maternal bleeding. This can be reduced, however, with meticulous attention to dosage and frequent monitoring of the activated partial thromboplastin time (APTT). The anticoagulant activity of heparin can be quickly reversed with protamine sulfate. Other potential complications of heparin therapy include osteoporosis, alopecia, urticaria, bronchoconstriction secondary to histamine release, and profound thrombocytopenia.[94] Platelet counts should be checked twice weekly during the first 2 weeks of therapy. Bone demineralization can occur if more than 22,000 units of heparin is administered daily for more than 20 weeks.

An initial heparin loading dose of 70 units/kg is administered intravenously, followed by a continuous infusion of 1,000 units/hr. This dose must be adjusted to keep the APTT approximately twice normal or the heparin titer at 0.2 to 0.4 units/ml. The required maintenance dose of heparin can show large interpatient variation. This regimen is continued for approximately 10 days in clinically stable patients.

Low-molecular-weight heparin is gaining in popularity because there are fewer bleeding complications and no reason to follow the APTT. It can be administered in a fixed or weight-adjusted dose once or twice daily. Even though it is of low molecular weight, it does not cross the placenta because it is still strongly negatively charged.

For the remainder of pregnancy, patients should receive a moderate dose of subcutaneous heparin. A dose of 7,500 to 10,000 units of heparin administered every 8 to 12 hours is usually sufficient to keep the APTT about 1.5 times normal and the heparin titer approximately 0.1 to 0.2 units/ml.[96] The dosage must be individualized until the desired APTT is reached. With the increases in Factor VIII and most other coagulation factors that are normally seen in pregnancy, the subcutaneous dose may need to be increased rather frequently during gestation.[97] In the stable patient, therapy should be discontinued during labor and delivery but can be restarted several hours postpartum. If delivery is imminent and the patient is fully anticoagulated, protamine can be carefully administered to reverse the heparin. This is especially necessary if a cesarean delivery is anticipated. During the postpartum period, the patient can be given warfarin, even if breast-feeding. However, oral anticoagulants should not be used during gestation. These drugs are vitamin K antagonists that readily cross the placenta and are teratogenic when used in early pregnancy. Anticoagulant therapy should be continued for 6 to 10 weeks postpartum, at which time coagulation factors should have returned to pre-pregnant levels. After that time, the duration of therapy should be individualized.

There is no consensus on treatment of the patient with thrombophlebitis in a prior pregnancy. If the patient has never experienced an embolus, many obstetricians would give the patient prophylactic heparin beginning with a dose of 5,000 units twice daily and increasing the dose each trimester until the patient is receiving 10,000 units twice daily. In women with a past history of pulmonary embolus we recommend anticoagulation under careful supervision.

Key Points

- Tuberculosis is making a reappearance in the pregnant population in this country, and any patient with systemic or pulmonary symptoms of tuberculosis should be tested.
- Any pregnant individual with a newly converted PPD test should also be tested for HIV.
- Smokers are at the highest risk of developing pneumococcal pneumonia during pregnancy.
- Nebulized β-mimetics have become the keystone for treating asthma in pregnancy. Nebulized steroids should be used as second-line therapy.
- If a pregnant patient is suspected of having a pulmonary embolus, heparin therapy should be immediately instituted while awaiting definitive testing.

Renal Disease

Philip Samuels

Urolithiasis

The prevalence of urolithiasis during pregnancy is 0.03 percent, with an incidence no higher than that of the general population.[20] Colicky abdominal pain, recurrent urinary tract infection (UTI), and hematuria suggest urolithiasis. If the diagnosis is suspected, intravenous pyelography should be undertaken, limiting this study to the minimum number of exposures necessary to make the diagnosis. Ultrasound can often be used to establish the diagnosis without radiation exposure. Urine microscopy can often detect crystals and help distinguish the type of stone before it is passed. For any patient suspected or proved to have renal stones, serum calcium and phosphorus levels should be measured to rule out hyperparathyroidism. Serum urate should also be determined.

Because of the physiologic hydroureter characteristic of pregnancy, most patients with symptomatic urolithiasis will spontaneously pass their stones. Treatment should be conservative, consisting of hydration and narcotic analgesia for pain relief.[21]

CHRONIC RENAL DISEASE

Diagnosis

Chronic renal disease can be silent until its advanced stages. Because obstetricians routinely examine the patient's urine for the presence of protein, glucose, and ketones, they may be the first to detect chronic renal disease.

Any gravida with more than trace proteinuria should collect a 24-hour urine specimen for creatinine clearance and total protein excretion. Creatinine clearance is elevated in pregnancy and, during the first trimester, may exceed 140 ml/min. Before pregnancy, 24-hour urinary protein excretion should not exceed 0.2 g. During gestation, quantities up to 0.3 g/day may be normal. Moderate proteinuria (less than 2 g/day) is seen in glomerular disease, most commonly lipoid nephrosis, systemic lupus erythematosus, and glomerulonephritis. Microscopic examination of the urine can reveal much about the patient's renal status. If renal disease is suspected, a catheterized specimen should be obtained. More RBCs than one to two per high-power field or RBC casts are indicative of renal disease. RBCs usually indicate glomerular disease or collagen vascular disease. Less frequently, they suggest trauma or malignant hypertension. Increased numbers of white blood cells (WBCs) (more than one to two per high-power field) or the appearance of WBC casts is usually indicative of acute or chronic infection. Cellular casts are found in the presence of renal tubular dysfunction, and hyaline casts suggest significant proteinuria. A single bacterium seen in an unspun catheterized urine specimen is suggestive of significant bacteriuria, and a follow-up culture should be performed.

The obstetrician can easily be misled when relying solely on the blood urea nitrogen (BUN) and serum creatinine to assess renal function. A 70 percent decline in creatinine clearance, an indirect measure of glomerular filtration rate (GFR), can be seen before a significant rise in the BUN or serum creatinine occurs. In fact, little change in the serum creatinine or the BUN is seen until the creatinine clearance falls to 50 ml/min. Below that level, small decrements in creatinine clearance can lead to large increases in the BUN and creatinine. A single creatinine clearance value less than 100 ml/min is not diagnostic of renal diseases. An incomplete 24-hour urine collection is the most frequent cause of this finding. An abnormal clearance rate should therefore be restudied.

Effect of Pregnancy on Renal Function

Although baseline creatinine clearance is decreased in patients with chronic renal insufficiency, it should still increase during gestation.

The long-term effect of pregnancy on renal disease remains controversial. If the patient's serum creatinine is less than 1.5 mg/dl, pregnancy should have little effect on the long-term prognosis of the patient's kidney disease. Ideally, patients with chronic renal disease should be thoroughly counseled before conception about the possible consequences of pregnancy.

Severe hypertension is the greatest threat to the pregnant patient with chronic renal disease. Approximately 50 percent of these patients will have worsening hypertension as pregnancy progresses, and diastolic blood pressures of 110 mm Hg or greater will develop in about 20 percent of cases.[33] Blood pressure control is the cornerstone of successful treatment of chronic renal disease in pregnancy.

Worsening proteinuria is common during pregnancy complicated by chronic renal disease and often reaches the nephrotic range.[33] In general, massive proteinuria does not indicate an increased risk for mother or fetus.[34] Low serum albumin, however, has been correlated with low birth weight.[35] In late pregnancy it is often difficult to differentiate impending preeclampsia from worsening chronic renal disease.

Effect of Chronic Renal Disease on Pregnancy

More than 85 percent of women with chronic renal disease will have a surviving infant if renal function is well preserved. Antepartum fetal surveillance and advances in neonatal care have played important roles in improving perinatal outcome in these patients. Preterm birth and intrauterine growth restriction (IUGR) are frequently observed in women with severe renal insufficiency whose baseline serum creatinine level is more than 1.5 mg/dl.

Surveillance and Treatment

A 24-hour urine collection for creatinine clearance and total protein excretion should be obtained as soon as the pregnancy is confirmed. These parameters should be monitored monthly. The patient should be seen once every 2 weeks until 32 weeks' gestation and weekly thereafter. These are general guidelines, and more frequent visits may be necessary in individual cases.

Control of hypertension is critical in managing patients with chronic renal disease. β-Blockers, calcium channel blockers, and hydralazine can be used to treat blood pressure effectively as long as the dosages are monitored carefully. Clonidine is occasionally useful in refractory patients. Doxazosin and prazosin may be used if necessary. Angiotensin-converting enzyme inhibitors should be avoided during pregnancy. These drugs have been associated with fetal and neonatal oliguria/anuria.[39,40]

The use of diuretics in pregnancy is controversial.[41–43] For massive debilitating edema, a short course of diuretics can be helpful. Electrolytes must be monitored carefully. Salt restriction does not appear to be beneficial once edema has developed. Salt restriction, however, should be instituted without hesitation in pregnant women with true renal insufficiency.

Fetal growth should be assessed with serial ultrasonography, because IUGR is common. Antepartum fetal heart rate testing should be started at 28 weeks' gestation.[44]

Obstetricians should have a low threshold for hospitalizing patients with chronic renal disease. Increasing hypertension and decreasing renal function warrant immediate hospitalization. A sudden deterioration of renal function may be due to infection, dehydration, electrolyte imbalance, or obstruction.

The timing of delivery must be individualized. Maternal indications for delivery include uncontrollable hypertension, the development of superimposed preeclampsia, and decreasing renal function after fetal viability has been reached. Fetal indications are dictated by the assessment of fetal growth and fetal well-being.

Renal biopsy is rarely indicated during pregnancy.

Pregnancy in the Renal Transplant Recipient

Preeclampsia, preterm birth, and IUGR frequently complicate pregnancies of women who have had a renal transplant. The allograft rejection rate is not increased.

Infection can be disastrous for the renal allograft. Therefore, urine cultures should be obtained at least monthly during pregnancy, and any bacteriuria should be aggressively treated. Renal function, as determined

Table 21-3   Guidelines for Renal Allograft Recipients Who Wish To Conceive

---

Absolute criteria

Wait 2 years after cadaver transplant or 1 year after graft from living donor

Immunosuppression should be at maintenance levels

Relative criteria

Plasma creatinine <1.5 mg/dl

Absent or easily controlled hypertension

No or minimal proteinuria

No evidence of active graft rejection

No pelvicalyceal distention on a recent ultrasound or intravenous pyelogram

Prednisone dose ≤15 mg/day

Azathioprine dose ≤2 mg/kg/day

Cyclosporin A dose 2–4 mg/kg (available data on the use of this drug in pregnancy includes <150 patients)

Adapted from Lindheimer MD, Katz AI: Pregnancy in the renal transplant patients. Am J Kidney Dis 19:173, 1992, with permission.

by 24-hour creatinine clearance and protein excretion, should be assessed monthly. Approximately 15 percent of transplant recipients will exhibit a significant decrease in renal function in late pregnancy.[73]

As for patients with chronic renal disease, serial ultrasonography should be used to assess fetal growth, and antepartum fetal heart rate testing should be started at 28 weeks' gestation. Approximately 50 percent of renal allograft recipients will deliver preterm. Preterm labor, preterm rupture of membranes, and IUGR are common. Vaginal delivery should be accomplished when possible, with cesarean delivery reserved for obstetric indications. Allograft recipients may have an increased frequency of cephalopelvic disproportion from pelvic osteodystrophy,[74] resulting from prolonged renal disease with hypercalcemia or extended steroid use. The transplanted kidney, however, rarely obstructs vaginal delivery despite its pelvic location.

Suggested guidelines, for renal allograft recipients who wish to conceive are summarized in Table 21-3.

Acute Renal Failure in Pregnancy

Acute renal failure (ARF) is defined as a urine output of less than 400 ml in 24 hours. It is seen most frequently in septic first-trimester abortions and in cases of sudden severe volume depletion resulting from hemorrhage caused by placenta previa, placental abruption, or postpartum uterine atony.[76] It is also observed in the marked volume contraction associated with severe preeclampsia[77] and with acute fatty liver of pregnancy.[77,78]

Renal ischemia is the common denominator in all cases of ARF. With mild ischemia, quickly reversible prerenal failure results. With more prolonged ischemia, acute tubular necrosis occurs. This process is also reversible, as glomeruli are not affected. Severe ischemia, however, may produce acute cortical necrosis. This pathology is irreversible, although on occasion a small amount of renal function is preserved.[80]

Clinically, patients with reversible ARF first experience a period of oliguria of variable duration. Polyuria then occurs. It is important to recognize that BUN and serum creatinine levels continue to rise early in the polyuric phase. During the recovery phase, urine output approaches normal. In these patients, it is important to monitor electrolytes frequently and to treat any imbalance carefully.

The main goal of treatment is the elimination of the underlying cause. Volume and electrolyte balance must receive constant scrutiny. To assess volume requirements, invasive hemodynamic monitoring is useful. This is especially true during the polyuric phase. Central hyperalimentation may also be required if renal failure is prolonged.

Acidosis frequently occurs in cases of ARF. Arterial blood gases therefore should be followed regularly. Acidosis must be treated promptly to prevent hyperkalemia. Absolute restriction of potassium intake should be instituted immediately. Sodium bicarbonate, used to treat acidosis, may overload the patient with sodium and water. In this case, peritoneal or hemodialysis may be instituted. The main indications for dialysis in ARF of pregnancy are hypernatremia, hyperkalemia, severe acidosis, volume overload, and worsening uremia.

Key Points

- Patients with glomerulonephritis can have successful pregnancies, but pregnancy loss rates increase greatly if the patient has preexisting hypertension.
- Creatinine clearance can decline 70 percent before significant increases are seen in the BUN or serum creatinine level. Therefore, a 24-hour urine specimen for creatinine clearance should be collected from any patient in whom renal disease is suspected.
- The chance of successful pregnancy is reduced if the creatinine clearance is less than 50 ml/min or if the serum creatinine level is more than 1.5 mg/dl.
- Severe hypertension is the greatest threat to the pregnant woman with chronic renal disease.
- Growth restriction and preeclampsia are common in women with chronic renal disease. These patients should have frequent sonograms and should start antepartum fetal surveillance at 28 weeks' gestation.
- Patients with chronic renal disease are often anovulatory. After transplantation, as renal function returns, they ovulate and may become pregnant unexpectedly.
- Patients should wait 2 years after receiving a cadaver renal allograft and 1 year after receiving a living allograft before contemplating pregnancy. Furthermore, there should be no signs of allograft rejection.
- Renal transplant patients should remain on their immunosuppressive medications throughout gestation.

Diabetes Mellitus and Other Endocrine Diseases

Mark B. Landon

Diabetes Mellitus

If optimal care is delivered to the diabetic woman, the perinatal mortality rate excluding major congenital malformations is equivalent to that observed in normal pregnancies. While the benefit of careful regulation of maternal glucose levels is generally well accepted, failure to establish optimal glycemic control as well as other factors continue to result in significant perinatal morbidity.

Pathophysiology

During normal pregnancy, maternal metabolism adjusts to provide adequate nutrition for both the mother and the growing fetoplacental unit. Early in pregnancy, glucose homeostasis is affected by increases in estrogen and progesterone that lead to β-cell hyperplasia and increased insulin secretion.[1] Insulin-dependent diabetic women commonly experience periods of hypoglycemia in the first trimester. Fasting hypoglycemia may appear more rapidly in late pregnancy as the conceptus increases its glucose utilization coupled with a reduction in maternal gluconeogenic substrates and hepatic glucose production.

Rising levels of human placental lactogen (hPL) and other "contra-insulin" hormones modify maternal utilization of glucose and amino acids. The actions of hPL are responsible, in part, for the "diabetogenic state" of pregnancy. The blood glucose response to an oral or intravenous carbohydrate load is greater than in the nonpregnant state. In the normal pregnant woman, glucose hemostasis is maintained by an exaggerated rate and amount of insulin release, which accompanies decreased sensitivity to insulin.[4]

With placental growth, larger amounts of these contra-insulin factors are synthesized. A woman with overt diabetes cannot respond to this stress and requires additional insulin therapy as pregnancy progresses. Her increased insulin requirement, approximately 30 percent over the pre-pregnancy dose, is roughly equivalent to the endogenous increase seen in a normal gestation. If the pregnant woman has borderline pancreatic reserve, it is possible that her endogenous insulin production will be inadequate, particularly late in gestation. Diabetes will then be revealed for the first time.

Glucose transport across the placenta occurs by carrier-mediated facilitated diffusion. Therefore, glucose levels in the fetus are directly proportional to maternal plasma glucose concentrations. Glucose is the primary fuel utilized by the fetus for protein and fat synthesis. The placenta is essentially impermeable to protein hormones such as insulin, glucagon, growth hormone, and hPL. In addition to glucose transfer, many amino acids are actively transported across the placenta to the fetal compartment. Ketoacids appear to diffuse freely across the placenta and may serve as a fetal substrate during periods of maternal starvation.

Fetal glucose levels are normally maintained within narrow limits because maternal carbohydrate homeostasis is so well regulated. During pregnancy in the insulin-dependent diabetic woman, periods of hyperglycemia lead to fetal hyperglycemia. Persistent elevations of glucose and perhaps amino acids may then stimulate the fetal pancreas, resulting in β-cell hyperplasia and fetal hyperinsulinemia.[10]

Perinatal Morbidity and Mortality

Fetal Death

In the past, sudden and unexplained stillbirths occurred in 10 to 30 percent of pregnancies complicated by insulin-dependent diabetes mellitus (IDDM, or type 1 diabetes mellitus).[11] Although relatively uncommon today, such losses still plague the pregnancies of patients who do not receive optimal care. Stillbirths have been observed most often after the thirty-sixth week of pregnancy in patients with vascular disease, poor glycemic control, hydramnios, fetal macrosomia, or preeclampsia. Fetuses of women with vascular complications may develop intrauterine growth restriction (IUGR) and suffer intrauterine demise as early as the second trimester. In the past, prevention of intrauterine death led to a strategy of scheduled preterm deliveries for IDDM women. This empirical approach reduced the number of stillbirths, but errors in estimation of fetal size and gestational age as well as the functional immaturity characteristic of the infant of the diabetic mother (IDM) contributed to many neonatal deaths from hyaline membrane disease.

Congenital Malformations

With the reduction in intrauterine deaths and a marked decrease in neonatal mortality related to hyaline membrane disease and traumatic delivery, congenital malformations have emerged as the most important cause of perinatal loss in pregnancies complicated by IDDM.

Most studies have documented a two- to sixfold increase in major malformations in infants of insulin-dependent diabetic mothers. In general, the incidence of major malformations in worldwide studies of offspring of IDDM or type 1 mothers has ranged from 5 to 10 percent.

The insult that causes malformations in IDM impacts on most organ systems and must act before the seventh week of gestation.[22] Central nervous system malformations, particularly anencephaly, and open spina bifida, are increased 10-fold.[23] Cardiac anomalies, especially ventricular septal defects and complex lesions such as transposition of the great vessels, are increased fivefold. The congenital defect thought to be most characteristic of diabetic embryopathy is sacral agenesis, an anomaly found 200 to 400 times more often in offspring of diabetic women (Fig. 21-1).

Impaired glycemic control and associated derangements in maternal metabolism appear to contribute to abnormal embryogenesis. The profile of a woman most likely to produce an anomalous infant would include a patient with poor periconceptional control, long-standing diabetes, and vascular disease.[23]

Macrosomia

Excessive growth may predispose the IDM to shoulder dystocia, traumatic birth injury, and asphyxia. Newborn adiposity also may be associated with a significant risk for obesity in later life (Fig. 21-2).[32] Macrosomia has been observed in as many as 50 percent of pregnancies complicated by gestational diabetes mellitus (GDM) and 40 percent of IDDM pregnancies. Delivery of an infant weighing greater than 4,500 g occurs *10 times* more often in diabetic women than in a nondiabetic control population.[33]

Fetal macrosomia in the IDM is reflected by increased adiposity, muscle mass, and organomegaly. The disproportionate increase in the size of the trunk and shoulder compared with the head may contribute to the likelihood of a difficult vaginal delivery.[34] Good maternal glycemic control has been associated with a decline in the incidence of macrosomia.

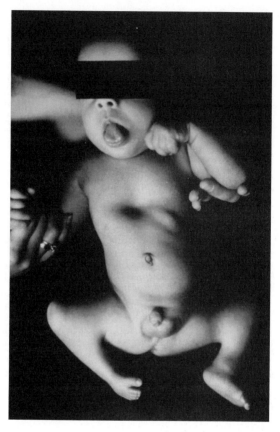

Fig. 21-1 Infant of a diabetic mother with sacral agenesis. The mother of this infant presented with class F diabetes at 26 weeks, in poor glycemic control. Ultrasound examination revealed absent lower lumbar spine and sacrum and hypoplastic lower extremities.

Hypoglycemia

Neonatal hypoglycemia, a blood glucose below 35 to 40 mg/dl during the first 12 hours of life, results from a rapid drop in plasma glucose concentrations following clamping of the umbilical cord. Presumably, prior poor maternal glucose control can result in fetal β-cell hyperplasia, leading to exaggerated insulin release following delivery. With near-physiologic control of maternal glucose levels during pregnancy, overall fetal hypoglycemia rates of 5 to 15 percent have been reported.[43,44] The degree of hypoglycemia may be influenced by at least two factors: (1) maternal glucose control during

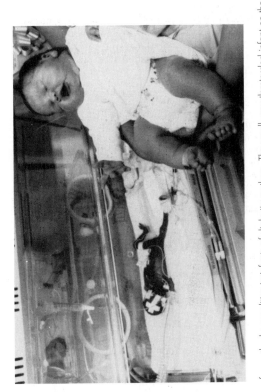

Fig. 21-2 Two extremes of growth abnormalities in infants of diabetic mothers. The small growth-retarded infant on the left weighed 470 g and is the offspring of a woman with nephropathy and hypertension, delivered at 28 weeks' gestation. The neonate on the right is the 5,100-g baby of a woman with suboptimally controlled class C diabetes.

the latter half of pregnancy and (2) maternal glycemia control during labor and delivery. Maternal capillary glucose levels greater than 100 mg/dl during delivery have been found to increase significantly the frequency of neonatal hypoglycemia.[48]

Respiratory Distress Syndrome

Hyperglycemia and hyperinsulinemia have been associated with delayed fetal pulmonary maturation. However, in well-controlled diabetic women delivered at term, the risk of neonatal respiratory distress syndrome (RDS) is no higher than that observed in the general population.[55,56]

Hyperbilirubinemia

Hyperbilirubinemia is frequently observed in the IDM. Neonatal jaundice has been reported in as many as 53 percent of pregnancies complicated by IDDM and 38 percent of pregnancies with GDM.[60,61]

Maternal Classification and Risk Assessment

Priscilla White[64] first noted that the patient's age at onset of diabetes, the duration of the disease, and the presence of vasculopathy significantly influenced perinatal outcome. Her pioneering work led to a classification system that has been widely applied to pregnant women with diabetes.[64] A modification of this scheme is presented in Table 21-4. Counseling a patient and formulating a plan of management requires assessment of both maternal and fetal risks. The White classification facilitates this evaluation.

Class A_1 diabetes mellitus includes those patients who have demonstrated carbohydrate intolerance during a 100-g 3-hour oral glucose tolerance test (GTT); however, their fasting and 2-hour postprandial plasma glucose levels are less than 105 mg/dl and 120 mg/dl, respectively. These patients are generally managed by dietary regulation alone. If the fasting value of the GTT is elevated ($\geq$ 105 mg/dl) or 2-hour postprandial plasma glucose levels exceed 120 mg/dl, patients are designated class A_2. It has recently been proposed that the cutoff values be lowered to a fasting capillary glucose of 95 mg/dl and a 2-hour capillary glucose of 120 mg/dl. Insulin is required for these women.

International Workshop Conferences on Gestational Diabetes sponsored by the American Diabetes Association (ADA) in cooperation with the American College

Table 21-4   Modified White Classification of Pregnant Diabetic Women

Class	Diabetes Onset Age (Year)		Duration (Year)	Vascular Disease	Insulin Need
Gestational diabetes					
A₁	Any		Any	0	0
A₂	Any		Any	0	+
Pregestational diabetes					
B	> 20		< 10	0	+
C	10–19	or	10–19	0	+
D	< 10	or	> 20	+	+
F	Any		Any	+	+
R	Any		Any	+	+
T	Any		Any	+	+
H	Any		Any	+	+

Modified from White P: Pregnancy complicating diabetes. Am J Med 7:609, 1949. Copyright 1949 Excerpta Medica Inc, with permission.

of Obstetricians and Gynecologists (ACOG) have recommended that the term *gestational diabetes* rather than *class A diabetes* be used to describe women with carbohydrate intolerance of variable severity with onset or recognition during the present pregnancy.[65,66] The term *gestational diabetes* fails to specify whether the patient requires dietary adjustment alone or treatment with diet and insulin. This distinction is important because those patients who are normoglycemic while fasting have a significantly lower perinatal mortality rate.[67] They do not appear to experience an increased incidence of intrauterine deaths in late pregnancy. Gestational diabetics who require insulin are at greater risk for a poor perinatal outcome than are those controlled by diet alone. This observation probably reflects more marked maternal hyperglycemia and, in some cases, a delay in the institution of insulin therapy.

Patients requiring insulin are designated by the letters B, C, D, R, F, and T (Table 21-4). Class D represents women whose disease is of 20 years duration or more, or whose onset occurred before age 10, or who have benign retinopathy. The latter includes microaneurysms, exudates, and venous dilatation.

Nephropathy

Class F describes the 5 to 10 percent of pregnant patients with underlying renal disease. This includes those with reduced creatinine clearance or proteinuria of at least 400 mg in 24 hours measured during the first 20 weeks of gestation. Two factors present prior to 20 weeks' gestation appear to be predictive of perinatal outcome in these women (e.g., preterm delivery, low birth weight, or preclampsia). These are (1) proteinuria above 3.0 g/24 hr and (2) serum creatinine above 1.5 mg/dl.

Several studies have failed to demonstrate a permanent worsening of diabetic renal disease as a result of pregnancy.[69-71] With improved survival of diabetic patients following renal transplantation, a small group of kidney recipients have now achieved pregnancy (class T).

Coronary Artery Disease

Class H diabetes refers to diabetic woman with coronary artery disease. Its incidence is increased in patients with longstanding nephropathy.

Retinopathy

Class R diabetes designates patients with proliferative retinopathy. Retinopathy may worsen significantly during pregnancy in spite of the major advances that have been made in diagnosis and treatment. Laser photocoagulation therapy during pregnancy with careful follow-up has helped to maintain many pregnancies to a gestational age at which neonatal survival is likely.

Progression to proliferative retinopathy during pregnancy rarely occurs in women with background retinopathy or in those without any eye ground changes. In contrast, most patients with untreated proliferative disease experienced worsening retinopathy during pregnancy.

Detection of Diabetes in Pregnancy

It has been estimated that 3 to 4 percent of pregnancies are complicated by diabetes mellitus and that 90 percent of the cases represent women with GDM.[85] Patients with GDM represent a group with significant risk for developing glucose intolerance, or type 2 diabetes mellitus, later in life. Approximately 50 percent of these patients will become diabetic in the 15 years following a pregnancy complicated by GDM.

GDM is a state restricted to pregnant women whose impaired glucose tolerance is discovered during pregnancy. Because in most cases patients with GDM have normal fasting glucose levels, some challenge of glucose tolerance must be undertaken.

The ADA[88] has recommended that most pregnant women should be screened for gestational diabetes with a 50-g oral glucose load followed by a glucose determination 1 hour later (Table 21-5). Women who have *all* of the following low-risk characteristics—less than 25 years of age, normal body weight, no family history of diabetes mellitus, not a member of a high-risk ethnic group (African American, Hispanic, Asian, Native

Table 21-5   Detection of Gestational Diabetes —
Upper Limits of Normal

	Plasma (mg/dl)	
Screening Test (50-g Load)	Threshold	140 mg/dl
Oral GTT[a]	NDDG[276]	Carpenter and Coustan[280]
Fasting	105	95
1-hour	190	180
2-hour	165	155
3-hour	145	140

[a] Diagnosis of gestational diabetes is made when any two values are met or exceeded.

American)—need *not* be screened. The ACOG[89] has suggested that, whereas selective screening for GDM may be appropriate in some clinical settings such as teen clinics (low-risk populations), universal screening may be more appropriate in other settings (high-risk populations).

The screening test for GDM, a 50-g glucose challenge, may be performed in the fasting or fed state; sensitivity is improved if the test is performed in the fasting state.[94,95] A plasma value of 140 mg/dl is used as a threshold for performing a 3-hour oral GTT.

Few false-negative results are obtained when the 50-g screening test is performed at 24 to 28 weeks' gestation.[96] Utilizing the plasma cutoff of 140 mg/dl, one can expect approximately 15 percent of patients with an abnormal screening value to have an abnormal 3-hour oral GTT. Patients whose 1-hour screening value exceeds 185 mg/dl rarely exhibit a normal oral GTT.[97] In these women, it is preferable to check a fasting blood glucose level before administering a 100-g carbohydrate load. If the fasting glucose is 95 mg/dl or greater, the patient is treated for GDM.

The criteria for establishing the diagnosis of gestational diabetes are listed in Table 21-5. These criteria have been recommended by the ACOG and recently by the ADA's Expert Committee on the Diagnosis and Classification of Diabetes Mellitus. Carpenter and Coustan[97] prefer to use another modification of these data (Table 21-5). Recent studies have confirmed that patients diagnosed according to the less stringent Carpenter criteria experience as much perinatal morbidity and fetal macrosomia as subjects diagnosed by the ACOG and ADA criteria.[99] For this reason, many experts advocate the use of the Carpenter values. In a patient who demonstrates a normal oral GTT despite significant risk factors, including obesity, advanced maternal age, or a previous history of GDM, a repeat test may be performed at 32 to 34 weeks' gestation.

Treatment of the Patient with Type 1 Diabetes Mellitus (Insulin-Dependent Diabetes Mellitus)

As fetal glucose levels reflect those of the mother, it is not surprising that clinical efforts aimed at optimizing maternal control are considered paramount in the decline in perinatal death seen in pregnancies complicated by type 1 diabetes. Self-monitoring of blood glucose levels combined with aggressive insulin therapy has made the maintenance of maternal normoglycemia (levels of 60 to 120 mg/dl) a therapeutic reality (Table

Table 21-6   Target Plasma Glucose Levels in
             Pregnancy

Time	Glucose (mg/dl)
Before breakfast	60–90
Before lunch, supper, bedtime snack	60–105
Two hours after meals	≤ 120
2 A.M. to 6 A.M.	> 60

21-6). Patients are taught to monitor their glucose control using glucose oxidase–impregnated reagent strips and a glucose reflectance meter.[105]

During pregnancy, conventional insulin therapy often needs to be abandoned in favor of intensive therapy. Insulin therapy must be individualized with dosage determinations tailored to diet and exercise. Insulin regimens have classically included one to two injections of insulin usually prior to breakfast and the evening meal, complemented by self-monitoring of blood glucose level and adjustment of insulin dose according to glucose profiles. Patients are instructed on dietary composition, insulin action, recognition and treatment of hypoglycemia, adjusting insulin dosage for exercise and sick days, as well as monitoring for hyperglycemia and potential ketosis. These principles form the foundation for intensive insulin therapy in which an attempt is made to simulate physiologic insulin requirements. Insulin administration is provided for both basal needs and meals, and rapid adjustments are made in response to glucose measurements. The treatment regimen often involves three to four daily injections or the use of continuous subcutaneous infusion devices (insulin pumps). With either approach, frequent self-monitoring of blood glucose is fundamental to achieve the therapeutic objective of physiologic glucose control. Glucose determinations are made in the fasting state and before lunch, dinner, and bedtime. Postprandial and nocturnal values are also helpful. Patients are instructed on an insulin dose for each meal and at bedtime if necessary. Mealtime insulin needs are determined by the composition of the meal, the premeal glucose measurement, and the level of activity anticipated following the meal. Basal or intermediate-acting insulin requirements are determined by periodic 2 A.M. to 4 A.M. glucose measurements as well as late afternoon values that reflect morning Neutral Protamine Hagedorn (NPH) or lente action. For patients who are not well controlled, a brief period of hospitalization is often necessary for the initiation of therapy.

Insulin is generally administered in two to three injections. We prefer a three-injection regimen, although most patients present taking a combination of intermediate-acting and regular insulin before dinner and breakfast. As a general rule, the amount of intermediate-acting insulin will exceed the regular component by a 2/1 ratio. Patients usually receive two-thirds of their total dose with breakfast and the remaining third in the evening as a combined dose with dinner or split into components with regular insulin at dinnertime and then intermediate acting insulin at bedtime in an effort to minimize periods of nocturnal hypoglycemia. Finally, some women may require a small dose of regular insulin before lunch, thus constituting a four-injection daily regimen.

Diet therapy is critical to successful regulation of maternal diabetes. A program consisting of three meals and several snacks is employed for most patients. Dietary composition should be 50 to 60 percent carbohydrate, 20 percent protein, and 25 to 30 percent fat with less than 10 percent saturated fats, up to 10 percent polyunsaturated fatty acids, and the remainder derived from monosaturated sources.[107] Caloric intake is established based on pre-pregnancy weight and weight gain during gestation. Weight reduction is not advised. Patients should consume approximately 35 kcal/kg ideal body weight. Obese women may be managed with an intake as low at 1,600 cal/day, although if ketonuria develops this allowance may be increased.

The presence of maternal vasculopathy should be thoroughly assessed early in pregnancy. The patient should be evaluated by an ophthalmologist familiar with diabetic retinopathy. Ophthalmologic examinations are performed during each trimester and repeated more often if retinopathy is detected. Baseline renal function is established by assaying a 24-hour urine collection for creatinine clearance and protein. An electrocardiogram and urine culture are also obtained.

Most patients with IDDM are followed with outpatient visits at 1- to 2-week intervals. At each visit, control is assessed and adjustments in insulin dosage are made. However, patients should be instructed to call at any time if periods of hypoglycemia (< 50 mg/dl) or hyperglycemia (> 200 mg/dl) occur. Family members should be instructed on the technique of glucagon injection for the treatment of severe hypoglycemic reactions.

Ketoacidosis

Diabetic ketoacidosis may develop in a pregnant woman with glucose levels barely exceeding 200 mg/dl (11.1 mmol/L). Thus diabetic ketoacidosis may be diagnosed during pregnancy with minimal hyperglycemia accompanied by a fall in plasma bicarbonate, a pH value less than 7.30, and serum acetone positive at a 1/2 dilution.

Diabetic ketoacidosis may occur in an undiagnosed diabetic woman receiving β-mimetic agents to arrest preterm labor and corticosteroids to accelerate fetal lung maturity. Because of the risk of hyperglycemia and diabetic ketoacidosis, magnesium sulfate has become the preferred tocolytic for preterm labor in patients with diabetes.

The general management of diabetic ketoacidosis in pregnancy is outlined in the box below. An attempt to treat any underlying cause for ketoacidosis, such as infection, should be instituted. Diabetic ketoacidosis does represent a substantial risk for fetal compromise. Successful fetal resuscitation will often accompany correction of maternal acidosis. Every effort should therefore be made to correct maternal condition before intervening and delivering a preterm infant.

Antepartum Fetal Evaluation

During the third trimester, when the risk of sudden intrauterine death increases, a program of fetal surveillance is initiated. Antepartum fetal monitoring tests have been used primarily to reassure the obstetrician and avoid unnecessary premature intervention. These techniques have few false-negative results, and allow the fetus to benefit from further maturation in utero.

Maternal assessment of fetal activity serves as a screening technique in a program of fetal surveillance. While the false-negative rate with maternal monitoring of fetal activity is low (about 1 percent), the false-positive rate may be as high as 60 percent.

The nonstress test (NST) has become the preferred method to assess antepartum fetal well-being in the patient with diabetes mellitus.[113] If the NST is nonreactive, a contraction stress test (CST) or biophysical profile (BPP) is then performed (Fig. 21-3). Heart rate monitoring is begun early in the third trimester, usually by 32 weeks' gestation. The NST should be done at least twice weekly once the patient reaches 32 weeks' gestation. In patients with vascular disease or poor control, in whom the incidence of abnormal tests and intrauterine deaths is greater, testing is often performed earlier and more frequently. The fetal BPP rather than

Management of Diabetic Ketoacidosis During Pregnancy

1. Laboratory assessment
   Obtain arterial blood gases to document degree of acidosis present; measure glucose, ketones, electrolytes, at 1- to 2-hr intervals.
2. Insulin
   Low dose, intravenous (IV)
   Loading dose: 0.2–0.4 units/kg
   Maintenance: 2.0–10.0 units/hr
3. Fluids
   Isotonic NaCl
   Total replacement in first 12 hours = 4–6 liters
   1 liter in first hour
   500–1,000 ml/hr for 2–4 hours
   250 ml/hr until 80% replaced
4. Glucose
   Begin 5% D/NS[a] when plasma level reaches 250 mg/dl (14 mmol/L).
5. Potassium
   If initially normal or reduced, an infusion rate up to 15–20 mEq/hr may be required; if elevated, wait until levels decline into the normal range, then add to IV solution in a concentration of 20–30 mEq/L.
6. Bicarbonate
   Add one ampule (44 mEq) to 1 liter of 0.45 NS if pH is <7.10.

[a] D/NS, dextrose in normal saline.

the CST is often employed to evaluate the significance of a nonreactive NST result.

It is important not only to include the results of antepartum fetal testing but also to weigh all the clinical features involving mother and fetus before a decision is made to intervene for suspected fetal distress, especially if this decision may result in a preterm delivery (Tables 21-7 and 21-8).

Ultrasound is a valuable tool in evaluating fetal growth, estimating fetal weight, and detecting hydramnios and malformations. A determination of maternal serum α-fetoprotein level at 16 weeks' gestation as part of triple analyte screening should be employed in association with a detailed ultrasound study at 18 weeks in an attempt to detect neural tube defects and other anomalies. Normal values of maternal α-fetoprotein for diabetic women are lower than for the non-diabetic population.[123] Fetal echocardiography is performed at 20 to 22 weeks' gestation for the investigation of possible cardiac anomalies.

Ultrasound examinations may be repeated at 32 weeks' gestation to assess fetal growth. The detection of fetal macrosomia, the leading risk factor for shoulder dystocia, is important in the selection of patients who are best managed by cesarean delivery. An increased rate of cephalopelvic disproportion and shoulder dystocia accompanied by significant risk of traumatic birth injury and asphyxia have been consistently associated with the vaginal delivery of large infants. The risk of such complications is greater for the fetus of a diabetic

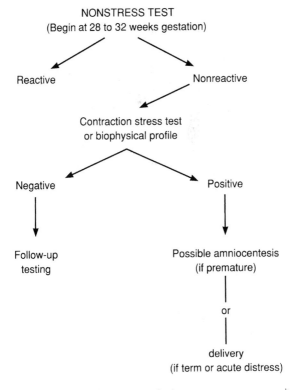

Fig. 21-3 Scheme for antepartum fetal testing in pregnancy complicated by diabetes mellitus.

Table 21-7 Antepartum Fetal Surveillance in Low-Risk Insulin-Dependent Diabetes Mellitus[a]

Study	
Ultrasonography at 4- to 6-week intervals	Yes
Maternal assessment of fetal activity, daily at 28 weeks	Yes
Nonstress test (NST) weekly at 28 weeks	Yes
	Twice weekly at 34 weeks
Contraction stress test or biophysical profile if NST nonreactive, lecithin/sphingomyelin ratio, lung profile	Yes, if elective delivery planned prior to 39 weeks

[a] Low-risk IDDM: excellent glucose control (60–120 mg/dl), no vasculopathy (classes B, C), no prior stillbirth.

Table 21-8   Antepartum Fetal Surveillance In High-Risk Insulin-Dependent Diabetes Mellitus[a]

Study	
Ultrasonography at 4- to 6-week intervals	Yes
Maternal assessment of fetal activity, daily at 28 weeks	Yes
Nonstress test (NST)	Minimum twice weekly
Contraction stress test or biophysical profile if NST nonreactive, lecithin/sphingomyelin ratio, lung profile at 37–38 weeks	Yes

[a] High-risk IDDM: poor glucose control (macrosomia, hydramnios), vasculopathy (classes D, F, R), prior stillbirth.

mother than for the fetus with similar weight whose mother does not have diabetes because of excessive fat deposition in the shoulders and chest.

Timing and Mode of Delivery

Delivery should be delayed until fetal maturation has taken place, provided that the patient's diabetes is well controlled and antepartum surveillance remains normal. In our practice, elective induction of labor is often planned at 38 to 40 weeks' gestation in well-controlled patients without vascular disease. Patients with vascular disease are delivered prior to term only if hypertension worsens or fetal growth restriction mandates early delivery. Before elective delivery prior to 39 weeks' gestation, an amniocentesis may be performed to document fetal pulmonary maturity. A low incidence of RDS is observed with a mature lecithin/sphingomyelin (L/S) ratio of 2.0 or greater. The presence of the acidic phospholipid phosphatidylglycerol (PG) is the final marker of fetal pulmonary maturation. The clinician must be familiar with the laboratory methodology in his or her institution and the neonatal outcome for the IDM at various L/S ratios in the presence or absence of PG.

When antepartum testing suggests fetal compromise, delivery must be considered. If the L/S ratio is mature, delivery should be accomplished promptly. In the presence of an immature L/S ratio, the decision to proceed with delivery should be based on confirmation of deteriorating fetal condition by several abnormal tests. For example, if the NST and the CST indicate fetal compromise, delivery is indicated. Finally, there remain several maternal indications for delivery, including preeclampsia, worsening renal function, or deteriorating vision secondary to proliferative retinopathy.

The route of delivery for the diabetic patient remains controversial. Cesarean delivery usually is favored when fetal compromise has been suggested by antepartum heart rate monitoring. If a patient reaches 38 weeks' gestation with a mature fetal lung profile and is at significant risk for intrauterine demise because of poor control or a history of a prior stillbirth, an elective delivery is planned. Elective cesarean delivery for a fetus estimated to weigh ≥4,250 g may be indicated to reduce the risk of shoulder dystocia.

During labor, continuous fetal heart rate monitoring is mandatory.

Glucoregulation During Labor and Delivery

As neonatal hypoglycemia is in part related to maternal glucose levels during labor, it is important to maintain

Insulin Management During Labor and Delivery

Usual dose of intermediate-acting insulin is given at bedtime.

Morning dose of insulin is withheld.

Intravenous infusion of normal saline is begun.

Once active labor begins or glucose levels fall below 70 mg/dl, the infusion is changed from saline to 5 percent dextrose and delivered at a rate of 2.5 mg/kg/min.

Glucose levels are checked hourly using a portable reflectance meter allowing for adjustment in the infusion rate.

Regular (short-acting) insulin is administered by intravenous infusion if glucose levels exceed 100 mg/dl.

(Adapted from Jovanovic L and Peterson CM: Insulin and glucose requirements during the first stage of labor in insulin-dependent diabetic women. Am J Med 75: 607, 1983, with permission.)

maternal plasma glucose levels at approximately 100 mg/dl. The patient is given nothing by mouth after midnight of the evening before induction or elective cesarean delivery. The usual bedtime dose of insulin is administered. Upon arrival to labor and delivery, early in the morning the patient's capillary glucose level is assessed with a bedside reflectance meter. Continuous infusion of both insulin and glucose are then administered based on maternal glucose levels. Ten units of regular insulin may be added to 1,000 ml of solution containing 5 percent dextrose. An infusion rate of 100 to 125 ml/hr (1 unit/hr) will, in most cases, result in good glucose control. Insulin may also be infused from a syringe pump at a dose of 0.25 to 2.0 units/hr and adjusted to maintain normal glucose values. Glucose levels are recorded hourly, and the infusion rate is adjusted accordingly.

When cesarean delivery is to be performed, it should be scheduled for early morning. This simplifies intrapartum glucose control and allows the neonatal team to prepare for the care of the newborn. The patient is given nothing by mouth, and her usual morning insulin dose is withheld. If her surgery is not performed early in the day, one-third to one-half of the patient's intermediate-acting dose of insulin may be administered. Epidural anesthesia is preferred because an awake patient permits earlier detection of hypoglycemia. Following surgery, glucose levels are monitored every 2 hours and an intravenous solution of 5 percent dextrose is administered.

Following delivery, insulin requirements are usually significantly lower than were pregnancy or pre-pregnancy needs. The objective of "tight control" used in the antepartum period is relaxed, and glucose values of 150 to 200 mg/dl are acceptable. Patients delivered vaginally who are able to eat a regular diet are given one-third to one-half of their end-of-pregnancy dose of NPH insulin the morning of the first postpartum day. Frequent glucose determinations are used to guide insulin dosage. If the patient has been given supplemental regular insulin in addition to the morning NPH dose, the amount of NPH insulin on the following morning is increased in an amount equal to two-thirds of the additional regular insulin. Most patients are stabilized on this regimen within a few days after delivery.

Women with diabetes are encouraged to breast-feed. The additional 500 kcal required daily are given as approximately 100 g of carbohydrate and 20 g of protein.[132] The insulin dose may be lower in lactating diabetic women.

Management of the Patient with GDM

The mainstay of treatment of GDM is nutritional counseling and dietary intervention. Women with GDM generally do not need hospitalization for dietary instruction and management. Once the diagnosis is established, patients are begun on a dietary program of 2,000 to 2,500 kcal daily.[132] This represents approximately 35 kcal/kg present pregnancy weight.

Once the patient with GDM is placed on an appropriate diet, surveillance of blood glucose levels is necessary to be certain that good glycemic control has been established. The patient should perform daily self-monitoring of blood glucose levels, including fasting and postprandial levels after breakfast, lunch, and dinner.

Fasting capillary glucose levels should be maintained below 95 mg/dl and 2-hour postprandial values should be less than 120 mg/dl in women with GDM. If a patient repetitively exceeds these thresholds, then insulin therapy is suggested.

Exercise has been recommended as an adjunctive treatment for GDM, as physical training increases insulin sensitivity. Patients may walk briskly for 20 minutes three times weekly.

Patients with GDM who are well controlled are at low risk for an intrauterine death. For this reason, we do not routinely institute antepartum fetal heart rate testing in uncomplicated diet-controlled GDM patients unless the patient has a hypertensive disorder or a history of a prior stillbirth.[148] Instituting a program of fetal surveillance once these pregnancies reach 40 weeks' gestation does, however, seem prudent. Women who require insulin treatment undergo twice-weekly heart rate testing at 32 weeks' gestation for GDM.

Counseling the Diabetic Patient

Anomalies of the cardiac, renal, and central nervous systems arise during the first 7 weeks of gestation, a time when it is most unusual for patients to seek prenatal care. Therefore, the management and counseling of women with diabetes in the reproductive age group should begin prior to conception. A reduced rate of major congenital malformations in patients optimally managed before conception has been observed in many centers.

Glycosylated hemoglobin levels obtained during the first trimester may be used to counsel diabetic women regarding the risk for an anomalous infant. Overall, the risk of a major fetal anomaly may be as high as 25 to 30 percent when the glycosylated hemoglobin level is several percent above normal values. Regardless of the glycosylated hemoglobin value obtained, all patients require a careful program of surveillance, as outlined earlier, to detect fetal malformations. The risk for spontaneous abortion also appears to be increased with marked elevations in glycosylated hemoglobin. However, for diabetic women in good control, there appears to be no greater likelihood of miscarriage.[157]

Physicians who care for young women with diabetes must be aware of the importance of preconception counseling. As a conservative recommendation, the patient should attempt to achieve a glycosylated hemoglobin level within two standard deviations of the mean for the reference laboratory,[162] fasting capillary glucose values less than 110 mg/dl, and 2-hour postprandial levels less than 150 mg/dl.

Contraception

There is no evidence that diabetes mellitus impairs fertility. Family planning is thus an important consideration for the diabetic woman. Barrier methods continue to be a safe and inexpensive method of birth control. The intrauterine device may also be used by diabetic women without an increased risk of infection compared to nondiabetic controls.[163]

Combined oral contraceptives (OCs) are the most effective reversible method of contraception, with failure rates generally less than 1 percent. Low-dose OCs should probably be restricted to diabetic patients without vascular complications or additional risk factors such as a strong family history of myocardial disease. The lowest dose of estrogen and progesterone should be employed. Patients should have blood pressure monitoring after the first cycle and quarterly, with baseline and follow-up lipid levels. Although carbohydrate metabolism may be affected by the progestin component of the pill, disturbances in diabetic control are unusual.

Neither depomedroxyprogesterone acetate (Depo-Provera; DMPA) nor Norplant is recommended as a first-line method of contraception for women with diabetes. The progestin-only OC would be preferred, as it does not produce significant metabolic effects. For those choosing long-acting progestins, periodic lipid assessment in all diabetic women and glucose monitoring in former GDM is indicated. Sterilization should be considered in diabetic women who have completed their families or who have serious vasculopathy.

Postpartum, women who have had GDM should be evaluated to determine if they have persistent carbohydrate intolerance. A fasting plasma glucose level can be obtained at the 6-week postpartum visit. Values of 110 mg/dl or less are normal; values above 110 mg/dl but below 126 mg/dl indicate impaired fasting glucose requiring close follow-up; and values of 126 mg/dl or more, if confirmed on repeat testing, indicate diabetes mellitus. Women with a prior history of GDM who have a normal fasting glucose should be tested annually to detect the onset of type 2 diabetes mellitus.

Thyroid Disease

Thyroid Function During Pregnancy and Laboratory Assessment

Laboratory assessment of thyroid function is dramatically altered by the hormonal changes of pregnancy (Table 21-9).

Serum levels of free T_4, free (triiodothyronine (T_3), and thyroid-stimulating hormone (TSH) remain in the normal nonpregnant range during gestation.[185] Direct measurement of free levels of T_3 and T_4 is the most accurate method for assessing thyroid function in the

Table 21-9   Effects of Pregnancy and Hyperthyroidism on Tests Commonly Used to Evaluate Thyroid Status

Test	Normal Pregnancy	Hyperthyroidism
TSH	No change	Decreased[a]
TBG	Increased	No change
Total T_4	Increased	Increased
Free T_4	No change	Increased
Total T_3	Increased	Increased
Free T_3	No change	Increased
Radioiodine uptake	Increased	Increased
T_3RU	Decreased	Increased

[a] In rare cases may be increased from pituitary hypersecretion or tumor.

Adapted from American College of Obstetricians and Gynecologists: Thyroid Disease in Pregnancy (ACOG Technical Bulletin No. 181). Washington, DC, American College of Obstetricians and Gynecologists, 1993, with permission.

face of increased TBG concentrations. When assays for free T_3 and T_4 are not available, an estimate of free hormone activity is generally obtained by employing the T_3 resin uptake test (T_3RU).

It is useful to calculate the free thyroxine index (FT_4I) based on the results obtained by the T_3RU and total T_4. The use of this formula attempts to correct for states of altered TBG concentrations. In clinical practice, however, an elevated FT_4I is consistent with hyperthyroidism just as a low value reflects hypothyroidism:

$$FT_4I = \text{total } T_4 \times (\text{patient } T_3RU/\text{normal } T_3RU)$$

The most sensitive test for the detection of primary hypothyroidism is a measurement of serum TSH concentration.

Hyperthyroidism

Thyrotoxicosis is encountered in approximately 0.2 percent of pregnancies.[185] While menstrual irregularities have been observed in hyperthyroid women, fertility is generally not impaired. Most women with mild to moderate disease appear to tolerate pregnancy well. There is no clear evidence that pregnancy worsens the disease or makes it more difficult to treat. However, thyroid storm is a serious complication that can be encountered in undiagnosed or undertreated patients. Control of hyperthyroidism is essential for both fetal and maternal well-being. Uncontrolled disease is associated with an increased incidence of neonatal morbidity resulting from preterm birth and low birth weight.[190]

Graves disease is the most frequent cause of hyperthyroidism in pregnancy. Patients with Hashimoto disease may experience periods of hyperactive thyroid secretion before manifesting overt hypothyroidism.

The clinical diagnosis of hyperthyroidism in pregnancy may be difficult because of confusion with symptoms normally present during gestation. A resting tachycardia in excess of 100 bpm or weight loss despite good dietary intake should alert the physician to the possibility of hyperthyroidism. Ophthalmologic signs of Graves disease, including exophthalmos, and lid lag, are also helpful in making the diagnosis.

Patients with hyperemesis may also have underlying biochemical hyperthyroidism.[191] It is unusual for such women to have clinical signs of hyperthyroidism.[192] Elevated free T_4 associated with suppressed TSH levels may be present in up to 60 percent of women presenting with severe hyperemesis gravidarum.[192,193] These biochemical abnormalities generally return to normal by 18 weeks' gestation.

Treatment of hyperthyroidism during pregnancy involves either antithyroid medications or surgery. Radioactive ablation employing ^{131}I is contraindicated. By 10 weeks' gestation, the fetus may concentrate this radioisotope, resulting in hypothyroidism. A careful review of the patient's menstrual history and contraception practices should be undertaken before administering ^{131}I to any young woman.

Medical therapy for hyperthyroidism is generally preferred in the pregnant patient because it presents less risk than surgery. Propylthiouracil (PTU) and methimazole (Tapazole) are equally effective drugs that block thyroid hormone synthesis. Methimazole has been used less commonly because of a reported association with aplasia cutis of the scalp in newborns, although this concern has not been supported by recent studies. Some consider PTU the preferred thioamide for treatment of hyperthyroidism during pregnancy. It is recommended that the minimal amount of thioamide necessary to maintain the patient in a euthyroid state be used during pregnancy. The usual starting dose of PTU is approximately 300 mg/day in two or three divided doses. Patients must be closely followed for improvement in their symptoms, including weight gain and normalization of pulse, as well as a decline in serum

T_4 levels. These therapeutic effects do not usually occur until 2 to 4 weeks after the initiation of treatment. At that time, if the FT_4I is falling, the dose of PTU may be reduced. Subsequent determinations of thyroid activity are made every 2 weeks, and in one-third of cases the medication can be discontinued during the second half of pregnancy.[197] Because disease may flare in the postpartum period, it is important to determine thyroid hormone levels prior to discharge from the hospital.

Minor side effects are frequently noted in patients receiving antithyroid medications. Approximately 5 percent will develop a purpuric rash, pruritus, or drug fever. Agranulocytosis is the most serious complication. Patients taking antithyroid drugs are instructed to seek immediate medical attention if early signs of neutropenia such as a sore throat and fever develop. In this setting, a leukocyte count should be performed immediately.

A major concern when using antithyroid medications during gestation is transplacental passage of these drugs and their effects to the fetus. However, fetal goiter and neonatal hypothyroidism appear to be rare complications of maternal therapy.

Careful evaluation of the neonate for hyperthyroidism is equally important. It is estimated that 1 percent of pregnant women with Graves disease give birth to an infant with neonatal hyperthyroidism.[201]

Hypothyroidism

Hypothyroidism is rare in pregnancy because women with markedly reduced thyroid gland function are often infertile. Hypothyroidism is usually secondary to Hashimoto disease, thyroid gland ablation by [196]I, surgery, or antithyroid medications.

The rate of stillbirth and miscarriage appears to be increased in hypothyroid women, who also have an increased incidence of preeclampsia, abruption, and IUGR.

The diagnosis of maternal hypothyroidism is confirmed by the presence of a low FT_4I and an elevated serum TSH level. The clinical diagnosis of hypothyroidism may be extremely difficult. Nonspecific symptoms such as lethargy and weakness are often present.

The outcomes of these pregnancies generally appear to be good provided replacement therapy is instituted and patients are carefully followed. Therapy consists of sufficient replacement of thyroid medication to achieve a euthyroid state. The patient is generally begun on 0.05 to 0.1 mg daily of L-thyroxine (Synthroid), with the dose increased to a maximum of 0.2 mg daily over several weeks. Ideal replacement may be titrated by following the serum TSH concentration, which may take as long as 2 months to return to baseline.

Occasionally, a pregnant patient may present who is already taking thyroid replacement but does not have well-documented hypothyroidism. Because hypothyroidism may present a risk to mother and fetus, replacement therapy is generally not interrupted during pregnancy. In this setting, it is most appropriate to follow TSH and free thyroxine indices to determine the amount of medication required to keep the patient euthyroid.

Postpartum Thyroid Dysfunction

Postpartum exacerbations of subclinical thyroid disease have been reported. The usual pattern of postpartum thyroid dysfunction is hyperthyroidism followed by transient hypothyroidism with subsequent recovery.[215] During the first few postpartum months, transient thyrotoxicosis occurs abruptly in association with a small painless goiter. Fatigue and palpitations are often present. Thyrotoxicosis develops as a result of destructive thyroiditis and glandular release rather than stimulation. Treatment consists of peripheral β-blockade if symptoms are severe. Approximately two-thirds of women who develop transient hyperthyroidism return to a euthyroid state, whereas one-third develop hypothyroidism.[216]

Key Points

- During pregnancy in the insulin-dependent diabetic woman, periods of maternal hyperglycemia lead to fetal hyperglycemia and thus fetal pancreatic stimulation. The resulting fetal hyperinsulinemia is associated with excessive fetal growth and other morbidities.
- Congenital malformations are two to four times more common in the offspring of insulin-dependent diabetic women. Cardiac, central nervous system, and skeletal malformations are most commonly observed. Poor glycemic control during organogenesis is associated with an increased risk for malformations.
- Women with diabetic nephropathy are at increased risk for preeclampsia, fetal growth retardation, and early delivery. Management involves control of maternal hypertension and intensive fetal surveillance.
- Screening for gestational diabetes, a disorder of carbohydrate intolerance discovered during pregnancy,

should be undertaken at 24 to 28 weeks' gestation using a 1-hour 50-g oral glucose challenge.

- Delivery of the insulin-dependent diabetic should be delayed until fetal maturation has taken place, provided that the patient is well controlled and that antepartum fetal surveillance remains reassuring.
- Uncontrolled maternal hyperthyroidism is associated with an increased incidence of neonatal morbidity resulting from preterm birth and low birth weight.
- The rates of stillbirth, miscarriage, preeclampsia, and growth restriction appear to be increased in hypothyroid women.
- The usual pattern of postpartum thyroid dysfunction is hyperthyroidism followed by transient hypothyroidism with subsequent recovery.

Hematologic Complications of Pregnancy

Philip Samuels

Pregnancy-Associated Thrombocytopenia

Affecting approximately 4 percent of pregnancies, thrombocytopenia is the most frequent hematologic complication of pregnancy resulting in consultation. Hospital laboratories vary on their lower limit of a normal platelet count, but it is usually between 135,000 and 150,000/mm^3. Platelet counts generally fall slightly, due to hemodilution and increased turnover, as gestation progresses, but should not fall below the usual normal range. In pregnancy, the vast majority of cases of mild to moderate thrombocytopenia are caused by gestational thrombocytopenia.[1] This form of thrombocytopenia rarely causes maternal or neonatal problems.[2] The obstetrician, however, is obliged to rule out other forms of thrombocytopenia that are associated with severe maternal or perinatal morbidity. The common and rare causes of thrombocytopenia in the gravida at term are shown in Table 21-10.

Gestational Thrombocytopenia

Patients with gestational thrombocytopenia usually present with mild (platelet count = 100,000 to 149,000/mm^3) to moderate (platelet count = 50,000 to 99,000/mm^3) thrombocytopenia.[5] These patients usually require no therapy, and the fetus appears to be at little, if any, risk of being born with profound thrombocytopenia (platelet count less than 50,000/mm^3) or a bleeding diathesis.

The decrease in platelet count occurring in gestational thrombocytopenia is not merely due to dilution of platelets with increasing blood volume. It appears to be due to an acceleration of the normal increase in platelet destruction that occurs during pregnancy.[1]

Immune Thrombocytopenic Purpura

Although it only affects 1 to 3/1,000 pregnancies, immune thrombocytopenic purpura (ITP) has been asso-

Table 21-10   Pregnancy-Associated
Thrombocytopenia

Major causes
   Gestational thrombocytopenia
   Severe preeclampsia
     HELLP syndrome
   Immune thrombocytopenic purpura
   Disseminated intravascular coagulation
     Abruptio placenta
     Sepsis
     Following severe hemorrhage
     Retained dead fetus
Rare causes
   Human immunodeficiency virus infection
   Lupus anticoagulant/antiphospholipid antibody syndrome
   Systemic lupus erythematosus
   Thrombotic thrombocytopenic purpura
   Hemolytic–uremic syndrome
   Type IIB von Willebrand disease
   Other autoimmune diseases
   Folic acid deficiency

---

ciated with profound neonatal thrombocytopenia in infants born to mothers with this condition.

In general, pregnancy has not been determined to cause ITP or to change its severity. Approximately 90 percent of women with ITP will have platelet-associated immunoglobulin G (IgG).[21] Unfortunately, this is not specific for ITP, as studies have shown that these tests are also positive in women with gestational thrombocytopenia and preeclampsia.[3,4]

Table 21-11 lists several studies in which all patients had true ITP and delineates the rates of profound neonatal thrombocytopenia. These infants may suffer severe gastrointestinal bleeding, hemopericardium, intraventricular hemorrhage, and severe cutaneous manifestations of bleeding.

Evaluation of Thrombocytopenia During Pregnancy and the Puerperium

Before deciding on a course to follow in treating the patient with thrombocytopenia, the obstetrician must evaluate the patient and attempt to ascertain the etiology of her low platelet count. Important management decisions are dependent on arriving at an accurate diagnosis. A complete medical history is critically important. It is essential to learn whether the patient has previously had a depressed platelet count or bleeding diathesis. It is also important to know whether these clinical conditions occur coincidentally with pregnancy. A complete medication history should be elicited, as certain medications, such as heparin, can result in profound maternal thrombocytopenia. The obstetric history should focus on whether there have been any maternal or neonatal bleeding problems in the past. Excessive bleeding from an episiotomy site or cesarean delivery incision site, a need for blood component therapy, easy bruising, or bleeding from intravenous sites during labor should alert the physician to the possibility of thrombocytopenia in the previous pregnancy. The obstetrician should also question whether the infant had any bleeding diathesis or if there was any problem following a circumcision. The obstetrician should also ask pertinent questions to determine whether severe preeclampsia or HELLP syndrome is the cause of her thrombocytopenia. Importantly, all thrombocytopenic pregnant women should be carefully evaluated for the presence of risk factors for human immunodeficiency virus (HIV) infection, as this infection can cause an ITP-like syndrome.

A thorough physical examination of the patient should also be performed. The physician should look for the presence of ecchymoses or petechiae. Blood pressure should be determined to ascertain whether the

Table 21-11   Incidence of Profound Neonatal Thrombocytopenia in Mothers Known to Have Immune Thrombocytopenic Purpura

Reports	Total Patients with ITP	Infants with Platelet Count < 50,000/mm^3	95% Confidence Interval
Karapatkin et al.[15]	19	6 (31.6%)	20.9–52.5%
Burrows and Kelton[8]	60	3 (5%)	0–10.5%
Noriega-Guerra et al.[13]	21	8 (38.1%)	17.3–58.9%
Samuels et al.[3]	88	18 (20.5%)	12.0–28.9%
Pooled (crude)	*188*	*35 (18.6%)*	*13–24%*

patient has preeclampsia. If the patient is developing HELLP syndrome, scleral icterus may be present. The eye grounds should be examined for evidence of arteriolar spasm or hemorrhage.

It is imperative that a peripheral blood smear be examined by an experienced hematologist or pathologist whenever a case of pregnancy-associated thrombocytopenia is diagnosed to determine whether microangiopathic hemolysis is present. This specialist can also rule out platelet clumping, which will result in a factitious thrombocytopenia. Other laboratory evaluation should be performed as necessary to rule out preeclampsia and/or HELLP syndrome, as well as disseminated intravascular coagulopathy. If a diagnosis of ITP is entertained, appropriate platelet antibody testing should be performed.

Therapy of Thrombocytopenia During Pregnancy

Gestational Thrombocytopenia

Gestational thrombocytopenia, the most common form encountered in the third trimester, requires no special therapy. The most important therapeutic issue is to refrain from therapies and testing that may be harmful to the mother or fetus. If the maternal platelet count drops below 75,000/mm^3, the patient may still have gestational thrombocytopenia, but there are not enough data on mothers with counts this low to determine if there are any maternal or fetal risks. These patients therefore should be treated as if they have de novo ITP. Although approximately 4 percent of all pregnant patients have gestational thrombocytopenia, less than 1 percent of patients with gestational thrombocytopenia have platelet counts less than 100,000/mm^3.[8]

Immune Thrombocytopenic Purpura

Treatment of the gravida with ITP during pregnancy and the puerperium requires attention to both mother and fetus. Spontaneous bleeding does not usually occur unless the platelet count falls below 20,000/mm^3. Surgical bleeding does not usually occur until the platelet count is less than 50,000/mm^3. The conventional forms of therapy to raise the platelet count in the patient with ITP include glucocorticoid therapy, intravenous gammaglobulins, platelet transfusions, and splenectomy.

If the patient is bleeding or if the platelet count is below 20,000/mm^3, the platelet count must be increased in a relatively short period of time. Although oral glucocorticoids can be used, intravenous glucocorticoids may work more rapidly. Hematologists have the most experience with methylprednisolone. It can be given intravenously, and it has very little mineralocorticoid effect. The usual dose of methylprednisolone is 1.0 to 1.5 mg/kg of *total body weight* intravenously daily in divided doses. It usually takes about 2 days to see a response, but up to 10 days may be required to see a maximum response. Even though it does have very little mineralocorticoid effect, there is some present, and it is important to follow the patient's electrolytes. There is little chance methylprednisolone will cause neonatal adrenal suppression because little crosses the placenta. It is metabolized by placental 11-β-ol-dehydrogenase to an inactive 11-keto metabolite.

After the platelet count has risen satisfactorily using intravenous methylprednisolone, the patient can be switched to oral prednisone. The usual dose is 60 to 100 mg/day. It can be given in a single dose, but there is less gastrointestinal upset with divided doses. The physician can rapidly taper the dose to 30 or 40 mg/day, but the dose should be tapered slowly thereafter. The dose should be titrated to keep the platelet count around 100,000/mm^3. If the physician begins therapy with oral prednisone, the usual initial daily dose is 1 mg/kg total body weight. The response rate to glucocorticoids is about 70 percent. It is important to realize that, if the patient has been taking glucocorticoids for a period of at least 2 to 3 weeks, she may have adrenal suppression and should receive increased doses of steroids during labor and delivery to avoid an adrenal crisis.

Although glucocorticoids are the mainstays of treating maternal thrombocytopenia, up to 30 percent of patients will not respond to these medications. In this instance, the next medication to use is intravenous immunoglobulin. This agent probably works by binding to the Fc receptors on reticuloendothelial cells and preventing destruction of platelets. The usual dose is 0.4 g/kg/day for 3 to 5 days. However, it may be necessary to use as much as 1 g/kg/day. The response usually begins in 2 to 3 days and usually peaks in 5 days. The length of this response is variable, and the timing of the dose is extremely important. If the obstetrician wants a peak platelet count for delivery, he or she should institute therapy about 5 to 8 days before the planned delivery. Although intravenous immunoglobulin is very expensive, it should be used before contemplating splenectomy, as some patients with ITP will experience remission after delivery.[47]

In midtrimester, splenectomy can also be used to

raise the maternal platelet count. This procedure is reserved for those who do not respond to medical management, with the platelet count remaining below 20,000/mm³.

Platelet transfusions are indicated when there is clinically significant bleeding and while awaiting other therapies to become effective. Platelets can be given if the maternal platelet count is less than 50,000/mm³ before or during splenectomy, or before or during cesarean delivery. They can be used before a vaginal delivery if the mother's platelet count is less than 20,000/mm³. Each "pack" of platelets will increase the platelet count by approximately 10,000/mm³. The half-life of these platelets is extremely short because the same antibodies and reticuloendothelial cell clearance rates that affect the mother's endogenous platelets will also affect the transfused platelets. However, if these platelets are transfused at the time the skin incision is made, the hemostasis necessary to carry out the surgical procedure will be achieved.

There is no series large enough from which to draw adequate conclusions concerning mode of delivery of the profoundly thrombocytopenic fetus. Strong arguments have been made for both vaginal and cesarean delivery. In our series, 19.2 percent of ITP patients undergoing no therapy gave birth to profoundly thrombocytopenic infants, compared with 22.7 percent of those receiving prednisone alone, 23 percent of those who had undergone a splenectomy and received prednisone, and 17.8 percent of those having undergone only splenectomy.[3]

Even if there is no difference in perinatal morbidity between vaginal and cesarean delivery, there are advantages of knowing whether a fetus is at risk of being born with a platelet count less than 50,000/mm³. The use of scalp electrodes and vacuum extractors are examples of interventions that may be avoided in the profoundly thrombocytopenic fetus. The only method currently available to determine the fetal platelet count accurately before the onset of labor (cordocentesis) is both expensive and invasive. Cordocentesis should be reserved for those patients with true ITP and should be carried out in close proximity to the labor and delivery unit. Cordocentesis should be performed at term, prior to an elective delivery. If the fetal platelet count is below 50,000/mm³, the obstetrician should discuss potential ramifications with the patient. The patient and obstetrician should together decide upon an appropriate place and mode of delivery.

Summary

The treatment of thrombocytopenia during gestation is dependent on the etiology. The obstetrician need not act on the mother's platelet count unless it is below 20,000/mm^3 or, if it is below 50,000/mm^3 with evidence of clinical bleeding or if surgery is anticipated. In these cases, the treatment will depend upon the diagnosis. Furthermore, whether delivery needs to be expedited or can be delayed is also dependent on the etiology of thrombocytopenia. The fetal/neonatal platelet count need only be considered if the mother carries a true diagnosis of ITP or, in the case of presumed gestational thrombocytopenia, when the platelet count is less than 75,000/mm^3, as this may actually be de novo ITP. The key to managing these patients is to arrive at an accurate etiology for the thrombocytopenia and to approach the patient and her fetus rationally.

Neonatal Alloimmune Thrombocytopenia

In neonatal alloimmune thrombocytopenia, a rare disorder, the mother lacks a specific platelet antigen and develops antibodies to this antigen. The disease is somewhat analogous to Rh isoimmunization but involves platelets. If the fetus inherits this antigen from its father, maternal antibody can cross the placenta, resulting in severe neonatal thrombocytopenia. The mother, however, will have a normal platelet count. The most common antibodies noted in these patients are anti-PLA 1 and BAK antibodies.[57]

Iron Deficiency Anemia

The first pathologic change to occur in iron deficiency anemia is the depletion of bone marrow, liver, and spleen iron stores. The serum iron level falls, as does the percentage saturation of transferrin. The total iron-binding capacity rises, as this is a reflection of unbound transferrin. A fall in the hematocrit follows. Microcytic hypochromic RBCs are released into the circulation. Should iron deficiency be combined with folate deficiency, normocytic and normochromic RBCs will be observed on peripheral smear.

Care must be taken when using laboratory parameters to establish the diagnosis of iron deficiency anemia during gestation. A serum iron concentration less than 60 mg/dl with less than 16 percent saturation of transferrin is suggestive of iron deficiency. An increase in total iron-binding capacity, however, is not reliable, as 15 percent of pregnant women without iron deficiency will show an increase in this parameter.[66] Serum ferritin levels normally decrease mildly during pregnancy. A significantly reduced ferritin concentration is the best parameter to judge the degree of iron deficiency.

Iron prophylaxis is recommended. It is safe, and, with the exception of dyspepsia and constipation, side effects are few. One 325-mg tablet of ferrous sulfate daily provides adequate prophylaxis. It contains 60 mg of elemental iron, 10 percent of which is absorbed. If the iron is not needed, it will not be absorbed and will be excreted in the stool.

One iron tablet *three times daily* is recommended for the pregnant patient with iron deficiency anemia. To ensure maximum absorption, iron should be ingested about 30 minutes before meals. When taken in this manner, however, dyspepsia and nausea are more common. Therapy, therefore, must be individualized to maximize patient compliance. If isolated iron deficiency anemia is present, one should see a dramatic reticulocytosis approximately 2 weeks after the initiation of therapy. Because iron absorption is pH dependent, taking iron with ascorbic acid (vitamin C) may increase duodenal absorption. Conversely, taking iron with antacids will decrease absorption.

Folate Deficiency

During pregnancy, folate deficiency is the most common cause of megaloblastic anemia, as vitamin B_{12} deficiency is extremely rare. The daily folate requirement in the nonpregnant state is approximately 50 μg, but this rises three- to fourfold during gestation.[73] Fetal demands increase the requirement, as does the decrease in the gastrointestinal absorption of folate during pregnancy.[74]

Clinical megaloblastic anemia seldom occurs before the third trimester of pregnancy. If the patient is at risk for folate deficiency or has mild anemia, an attempt should be made to detect this disorder before megaloblastosis occurs. Serum folate and RBC folate levels are the best tests for folate deficiency.[75]

Prenatal vitamins that require physician prescription contain 1 mg of folic acid. Most nonprescription prenatal vitamins contain 0.8 mg of folic acid. These amounts are more than adequate to prevent and treat folate deficiency. Women with significant hemoglobinopathies, patients ingesting phenytoin or other anticonvulsants, women carrying a multiple gestation, and women with frequent conception may require more than 1 mg supplemental folate daily. If the patient is folic acid deficient, her reticulocyte count will be depressed. Within 3 days after the administration of sufficient folic acid, reticulocytosis usually occurs. Folic acid deficiency should be considered when a patient has unexplained thrombocytopenia. The hematocrit level may rise as much as 1 percent per day after 1 week of folate replacement.

Iron deficiency is frequently concomitant with folic acid deficiency. If a patient with folate deficiency does not develop a significant reticulocytosis within 1 week after administration of sufficient replacement therapy, appropriate tests for iron deficiency should be performed.

Hemoglobinopathies

The prevalences of the most common hemoglobinopathies are listed in Table 21-12.

Hemoglobin S

Hemoglobin S, an aberrant hemoglobin, is present in patients with sickle cell disease (hemoglobin SS) and sickle cell trait (hemoglobin AS). At low oxygen tensions, RBCs containing hemoglobin S assume a sickle shape. Sludging in small vessels occurs, resulting in microinfarction of the affected organs. Sickle cells have a life span of 5 to 10 days, compared with 120 days for a normal RBC. Sickling is triggered by hypoxia, acidosis, or dehydration.

Approximately 1/12 adult blacks in the United States is heterozygous for hemoglobin S and, therefore, has sickle cell trait (hemoglobin AS) and carries the affected gene. These individuals generally have 35 to 45 percent hemoglobin S and are asymptomatic. The child of two individuals with sickle cell trait has a 50 percent proba-

Table 21-12 Hemoglobinopathies

Hemoglobinopathy	Frequency in Adult Blacks
Sickle cell trait	1/12
Sickle cell disease	1/708
Hemoglobin C trait	1/41
Hemoglobin C disease	1/4,790
Hemoglobin SC disease	1/757
Hemoglobin S/β-thalassemia	1/1,672

bility of inheriting the trait and a 25 percent probability of actually having sickle cell disease. One of every 625 black children born in the United States is homozygous for hemoglobin S, and the frequency of sickle cell disease among adult blacks is 1/708.[77] All at-risk patients should be screened for hemoglobin S at their first prenatal visit. Patients with a positive screen should undergo hemoglobin electrophoresis. Women identified as having sickle cell trait (hemoglobin AS) are not at increased risk for poor perinatal outcome. The spouse, however, should be tested, and, if both are carriers of a hemoglobinopathy, prenatal diagnosis should be offered. Prenatal diagnosis can be performed by DNA analysis with the polymerase chain reaction (PCR) and Southern blotting.[78,79]

Painful vaso-occlusive episodes involving multiple organs are the clinical hallmark of sickle cell anemia. The most common sites for these episodes are the extremities, joints, and abdomen. Vaso-occlusive episodes can also occur in the lung, resulting in pulmonary infarction. Analgesia, oxygen, and hydration are the clinical foundations for treating these painful crises.

Many pregnancies complicated by sickle cell anemia are associated with poor perinatal outcomes. The rate of spontaneous abortion may be as high as 25 percent.[84–86] Perinatal mortality rates of up to 40 percent were reported in the past, but the current estimate is approximately 15 percent.[85–90] Much of this poor perinatal outcome is related to preterm birth. Approximately 30 percent of infants born to mothers with sickle cell disease have birth weights below 2,500 g.[85] Stillbirth rates of 8 to 10 percent have been described. These fetal deaths happen not only during crises but also unexpectedly. Careful antepartum fetal testing must therefore be utilized, including serial ultrasonography to assess fetal growth.

Although maternal mortality is rare in patients with sickle cell anemia, maternal morbidity is great. Infections are common, occurring in 50 to 67 percent of women with hemoglobin SS. Most are urinary tract infections (UTIs), which can be detected by frequent urine cultures. Patients with hemoglobin AS are also at greater risk for a UTI and should be screened as well. Pulmonary infection and infarction are also common. Patients with sickle cell anemia should receive pneumococcal vaccine before pregnancy. Any infection demands prompt attention, because fever, dehydration, and acidosis will result in further sickling and painful crises. The incidence of pregnancy-induced hypertension is increased in patients with sickle cell anemia and may complicate almost one-third of pregnancies in these patients.[88,93]

The care of the pregnant patient with sickle cell anemia must be individualized and meticulous. A folate supplement of at least 1 mg/day should be administered as soon as pregnancy is confirmed. Although hemoglobin and hematocrit levels are decreased, iron supplements need not be routinely given.

The role of prophylactic transfusions in the gravida with sickle cell anemia is controversial. This therapy, which replaces the patient's sickle cells with normal RBCs, can both improve oxygen-carrying capacity and suppress the synthesis of sickle hemoglobin. If one chooses to perform prophylactic transfusion, the goal is to maintain the percentage of hemoglobin A above 20 percent at all times and preferably above 40 percent, as well as to maintain the hematocrit above 25 percent. It has been recommended that prophylactic transfusion begin at 28 weeks' gestation. Buffy-coat-poor washed RBCs are used to reduce the risk of isosensitization.

Vaginal delivery is preferred for patients with sickle cell disease. Cesarean delivery should be reserved for obstetric indications. Patients should labor in the left lateral recumbent position and receive supplemental oxygen. While adequate hydration should be maintained, fluid overload must be avoided. Conduction anesthesia is recommended, as it provides excellent pain relief and can be used for cesarean delivery, if necessary.

Key Points

- Four percent of pregnancies will be complicated by maternal platelet counts of less than 150,000/mm^3. The vast majority of these patients will have gestational thrombocytopenia with a benign course and will need no intervention.
- Surgical bleeding occurs if the platelet count falls below 50,000/mm^3 and spontaneous bleeding occurs if the platelet count falls below 20,000/mm^3.
- If the platelet count falls below 75,000/mm^3, the patient still may have gestational thrombocytopenia, but it is the physician's responsibility to rule out other serious causes of thrombocytopenia before making this diagnosis.
- Glucocorticoids are the first-line medication used to raise a low platelet count.
- Iron deficiency anemia is the most common cause of anemia in pregnancy, and serum ferritin is the single best test to diagnose it.
- If a patient with presumed iron deficiency does not

increase her reticulocyte count with iron therapy, she may also have a concomitant folic acid deficiency.

- Patients pregnant with twins, those on anticonvulsant therapy, those with a hemoglobinopathy, and those who conceive frequently need supplemental folic acid during gestation.
- Most hereditary hemoglobinopathies can be detected in utero and prenatal diagnosis should be offered to the patient early in pregnancy.
- As in the nonpregnant patient, analgesia, hydration, and oxygen are the key factors in treating pregnant women with sickle cell crisis.
- Patients with sickle cell disease are at high risk of having a fetus with growth restriction and adverse fetal outcomes. Therefore, they warrant frequent sonography and antepartum fetal evaluation.

Collagen Vascular Diseases

Philip Samuels

With the exception of rheumatoid arthritis, autoimmune diseases are associated with an increased risk of poor pregnancy outcome. Many of these diseases have a predisposition for women in their childbearing years. These diseases are characterized by the production of autoantibodies. Increasingly sensitive and specific laboratory tests have been developed to aid in the diagnosis of these disorders.

Systemic Lupus Erythematosus

The course of systemic lupus erythematosus (SLE) is characterized by chronic exacerbations and remissions. The prevalence of the disease in women 15 to 64 years of age is estimated to be 1/700,[1] but in black women of the same age group the prevalence is 1/245.[2] The diagnosis of SLE is based on a patient meeting at least four of the diagnostic criteria accepted by the American Rheumatism Association.

Laboratory Diagnosis

More than 90 percent of patients with SLE will exhibit significant titers of antinuclear antibodies. In 80 to 90 percent of patients, an autoantibody directed against double-stranded DNA will be detected. Extractable nuclear antibodies can be subdivided into antibodies against ribonuclear protein (anti-RNP, anti-SM), anti-SSA (Ro), and anti-SSB (La). Anti-SSA and anti-SSB antibodies, which are found in 25 and 12 percent of patients with SLE, respectively, have been associated with fetal and neonatal heart block. Anti-SSA antibodies are generally associated with manifestations of neonatal lupus.

The Effects of Pregnancy on SLE

Pregnancy does not appear to affect or alter the long-term prognosis of patients with SLE.[3] Several studies, however, have documented increased flares of SLE during pregnancy and particularly during the puerperium.[3,4]

Although it remains debatable whether SLE is exacerbated by pregnancy, there is no dispute that there is a risk of major maternal morbidity and potentially of mortality in the gravida with SLE. Most maternal deaths occur during the puerperium as a result of pulmonary hemorrhage or lupus pneumonitis.[12,13] Most perinatologists advise their patients not to conceive during a time of increased lupus activity, as this is associated with flares during pregnancy. In general, a patient's disease should be quiescent for 5 to 7 months before conception. Women with lupus nephritis must be aware that there is a small but significant risk of permanent deterioration of renal function during pregnancy.

The Effects of SLE on Pregnancy

Although fertility is not impaired, SLE can have an adverse effect on pregnancy outcome in each trimester.[26] There is an increase in the spontaneous abortion rate, with the estimated incidence between 16 and 40 percent.[10,17,26–29] The risk of miscarriage is not necessarily related to disease activity.

Preterm birth, intrauterine growth restriction (IUGR), and fetal death are all increased in the pregnancy complicated by SLE. Hypertension increases the risk of these adverse outcomes.

The lupus inhibitor antibody and anti-cardiolipin antibodies have been associated with recurrent miscarriage. The diagnosis of the lupus inhibitor is often confusing. Some clinicians rely solely on a prolongation of the activated partial thromboplastin time (APTT) using platelet-poor plasma. A sensitive reagent must be used, or there will be many false-negative results. Other commonly used tests include the tissue thromboplastin inhibition test, kaolin clotting time, dilute Russell viper venom time, and platelet neutralization procedure.

There is also confusion concerning the difference between anti-cardiolipin antibodies and anti-phospholipid antibodies. Anti-phospholipid antibodies encompass many phospholipids, of which cardiolipin is only one. Nonetheless, these terms are often used interchangeably in the obstetrics literature.

The presence of the lupus inhibitor antibody and anti-cardiolipin antibodies has been related to poor pregnancy outcome and recurrent spontaneous abortions. In the absence of SLE, anti-cardiolipin antibodies can be associated with an increased risk for early preeclampsia, IUGR and fetal death.[42,44] Patients with elevated anti-cardiolipin antibodies who have SLE are at significant risk to develop fetal distress in the second trimester with subsequent fetal death.

Anti-cardiolipin antibodies and the lupus inhibitor are associated with in vitro anticoagulation, but in vivo they are associated with thrombosis. Because infarctions are often found in the placentas of patients with anti-cardiolipin antibodies, clinicians have begun using heparin therapy in this group.

I currently individualize therapy of patients with lupus inhibitor and anti-phospholipid antibodies. The patient's history and laboratory results are taken into account when making decisions regarding therapy. For the patient truly thought to have this syndrome, I usually prescribe low-dose aspirin and heparin. Heparin dosing is started at 5,000 units twice daily and increased to 10,000 units twice daily by term. If the patient has an aversion to administering injections or carries the diagnosis of a collagen vascular disease, prednisone and low-dose aspirin may be used. The prednisone is usually administered in a dose of 15 mg daily. This dose is adequate to cause immunosuppression and may cause fewer side effects than higher doses. There appears to be no advantage to administering all three medications, and such therapy may truly increase adverse side effects. The true key in treating these patients is to make certain they understand the potential side effects of the prescribed medication regimen and that they undergo the proper fetal and maternal surveillance throughout pregnancy.

Neonatal Manifestations of SLE

Complete congenital heart block, an infrequent complication of SLE, can be diagnosed prenatally. In the midtrimester, a fetal heart rate of about 60 bpm with no baseline variability is indicative of congenital heart block. The patient should immediately undergo fetal echocardiography to rule out associated congenital cardiac malformations. Affected fetuses usually show no evidence of congestive heart failure or hydrops. Nonetheless, they should be followed with serial ultrasonography every 1 to 2 weeks to ascertain if any evidence of hydrops has developed.

Infants born to mothers with SLE may exhibit erythematous skin lesions of the face, scalp, and upper thorax.[11,75,76] These lesions usually disappear by 12 months of age.

Surveillance

Because of the increased risk of miscarriage, stillbirth, preterm delivery, and IUGR, the obstetrician caring for the patient with SLE should maintain close maternal and fetal surveillance. Any patient with a history of SLE should undergo preconceptual counseling and should have tests performed for the presence of the lupus inhibitor, anti-cardiolipin antibodies, anti-SSA (Ro) antibodies, and anti-SSB (La) antibodies. As previously described, these findings are associated with a poorer pregnancy outcome. If indicated, therapy should be initiated after fully informing the patient of risks and benefits to both her and the fetus. If anti-SSA or anti-SSB antibodies are present, fetal echocardiography should be performed in the second trimester to rule out complete congenital heart block. Because of the risks of IUGR and preterm birth, accurate gestational dating is imperative in the patient with SLE. Patients should also have an examination of their urine sediment and a 24-hour urine collection for creatinine clearance and total protein excretion in early pregnancy to determine if there is any renal involvement of their SLE.

At 28 weeks' gestation, weekly antepartum fetal heart rate testing should be initiated using the nonstress test. Antepartum fetal heart rate testing has been shown to improve fetal outcome in patients with SLE.[78] At 34 weeks, the frequency of testing should be increased to twice weekly.

Despite the sophisticated array of laboratory studies that are available to follow patients with SLE, the patient's clinical status remains of prime importance. There is no substitute for careful monitoring of maternal blood pressure and weight gain. Twenty-four-hour urine collections for creatinine clearance and total protein excretion should be carried out monthly. Serum creatinine, blood urea nitrogen, and uric acid levels should be determined whenever these urine collections are performed. A rise in serum uric acid can be a sign of impending preeclampsia.

The timing of delivery is important and should be individualized. Steroids should be tapered slowly and with great care in the postpartum period to prevent an exacerbation of SLE.[21,82]

Key Points

- Systemic lupus erythematosus is associated with an increase in poor pregnancy outcome (i.e., from IUGR, stillbirth, and spontaneous abortion).

- The rate of pregnancy complications is decreased if patients with SLE have quiescent disease for 6 months prior to conception.
- Glucocorticoids are safe to use in pregnancy for treating patients with SLE.
- The lupus inhibitor and anti-cardiolipin antibodies are found in 50 percent of patients with SLE. They are associated with an increased risk of pregnancy loss, including second- and third-trimester losses.
- Anti-SSA (Ro) and anti-SSA (La) antibodies are associated with complete congenital heart block and other manifestations of neonatal lupus.
- Low-dose heparin and low-dose aspirin are the therapies of choice for patients with lupus inhibitor/antiphospholipid antibodies who do not have active SLE.

Hepatic and Gastrointestinal Disorders

Philip Samuels and Mark B. Landon

Hepatic Disease

Philip Samuels

Acute Fatty Liver

Acute fatty liver is a rare condition of unknown etiology with an incidence of between 1/6,692 and 1/15,900 pregnancies.[1-3] Before 1970, the published mortality rate for both mother and infant was approximately 85 percent.[4] Since 1975, maternal survival has increased to 72 percent, with neonatal survival slightly lower. These improved outcomes have been attributed to early recognition of the disorder followed by prompt delivery.[1,5-7] Usually beginning late in the third trimester, acute fatty liver often presents with nausea and vomiting[1,7,8] followed by severe abdominal pain and headache. The right upper quadrant is generally tender, but the liver is not enlarged to palpation. Within a few days jaundice appears, and the patient becomes somnolent and eventually comatose. Hematemesis and spontaneous bleeding result when the patient develops hypoprothrombinemia and disseminated intravascular coagulation (DIC). Oliguria, metabolic acidosis, and eventually anuria occur in approximately 50 percent of patients with acute fatty liver of pregnancy.[9] If the disease is allowed to progress, labor begins and the patient delivers a stillborn infant. During the immediate postpartum period, the mother becomes febrile and comatose and, without therapy, dies within a few days.

The primary differential diagnoses in cases of acute fatty liver include fulminant hepatitis and the liver dysfunction associated with the HELLP syndrome (hemolysis, elevated liver enzymes, and low platelet count) or preeclampsia (Table 21-13).[13-15]

Laboratory Diagnosis

In acute fatty liver of pregnancy, serum transaminase levels are elevated but usually remain below 500 IU/L.[5] In acute hepatitis, however, these levels are frequently

Table 21-13 Differential Diagnosis of Liver Disease in Pregnancy

	Serum Transaminase Levels (IU/L)	Bilirubin Level (mg/dl)	Coagulopathy	Histology	Other Features
Acute hepatitis B	>1,000	>5	–	Hepatocellular necrosis	Potential for perinatal transmission
Acute fatty liver	<500	<5	+	Fatty infiltration	Coma, renal failure, hypoglycemia
Intrahepatic cholestasis	<300	<5, mostly direct	–	Dilated bile canaliculi	Pruritus, increased bile acids
HELLP	>500	<5	+	Variable periportal necrosis	Hypertension, edema, thrombocytopenia

Abbreviations: HELLP, hemolysis, elevated liver enzymes, low platelets; –, absent; +, present.

above 1,000 IU/L. In liver dysfunction associated with preeclampsia or the HELLP syndrome, the transaminases are often in the same range as in acute fatty liver of pregnancy but are occasionally higher. As a result of DIC, the prothrombin time and activated partial thromboplastin times (APTT) are often prolonged. The prothrombin time is usually increased before the APTT because it reflects the vitamin K–dependent clotting factors synthesized in the liver. A decreased fibrinogen level is accompanied by an elevation in fibrin degradation products, the D-dimer, and prothrombin. Although the serum bilirubin level is elevated, it usually remains below 5 mg/dl and rarely rises as high as 10 mg/dl, a level lower than one would expect in acute hepatitis. A liver biopsy specimen will reveal pericentral microvesicular fatty change.

Management

Once the diagnosis has been established, delivery should be accomplished as quickly as is safely possible.[29] Important supportive measures must first be undertaken to ensure maternal well-being. The patient's coagulopathy must be corrected with fresh frozen plasma. If more concentrated fibrinogen is needed, cryoprecipitate can be administered. Intravenous fluids containing adequate glucose should be given. This will prevent hypoglycemia, which can be fatal in this disorder. If there is not a severe coagulopathy or the coagulopathy has been corrected, invasive hemodynamic monitoring may be instituted if necessary before delivery. Delivery soon after diagnosis is paramount. Vaginal delivery is preferable. Cesarean delivery, however, is warranted if it appears that delivery cannot be effected in a timely fashion, and the patient is deteriorating. If the patient's coagulopathy has been corrected, epidural anesthesia is the best choice. Spinal anesthesia can also be used. Regional anesthesia is preferable, because it allows adequate assessment of the patient's level of consciousness. General anesthesia should be avoided if possible because of the hepatotoxicity of some anesthetic agents. Narcotic doses must be adjusted, as these drugs are metabolized by the liver.

Intrahepatic Cholestasis of Pregnancy

Intrahepatic cholestasis is characterized by pruritus and mild jaundice during the last trimester of pregnancy. It can, however, occur earlier in gestation.[31,32] Intrahepatic cholestasis tends to recur in subsequent pregnancies, but the severity may vary from one pregnancy to the next.

Clinical Manifestations

Patients with intrahepatic cholestasis usually begin having pruritus at night. It progresses, and the patient is soon experiencing bothersome pruritus continuously. Approximately 2 weeks later, clinical jaundice will develop in 50 percent of cases. The jaundice is usually mild, soon plateaus, and remains constant until delivery. The pruritus worsens with the onset of jaundice, and the patient's skin can become excoriated. The symptoms usually abate within 2 days after delivery. The differential diagnosis must include viral hepatitis and gallbladder disease.

Laboratory Diagnosis

Serum alkaline phosphatase levels are increased 5- to 10-fold in intrahepatic cholestasis of pregnancy. Alkaline phosphatase, however, is normally increased in pregnancy due to placental production of this enzyme. Upon fractionation, most of the alkaline phosphatase is hepatic in origin rather than placental. Serum 5'-nucleotidase levels are also increased. Bilirubin is elevated, but usually not above 5 mg/dl. Most is the direct, conjugated form. If intrahepatic cholestasis lasts for several weeks, liver dysfunction may result in decreased vitamin K reabsorption or decreased prothrombin production, leading to a prolongation of the prothrombin time. Serum transaminase levels are usually normal or moderately elevated, remaining well below the levels associated with viral hepatitis. Serum cholesterol and triglyceride levels may also be markedly elevated.

The serum bile acids (chenodeoxycholic acid, deoxycholic acid, and cholic acid) are increased. The levels are often more than 10 times the normal concentration. These acids are deposited in the skin and probably cause the extreme pruritus.[38] The degree of pruritus, however, is not always related to the serum level of bile acids.[39] To make the diagnosis of intrahepatic cholestasis of pregnancy, the fasting levels of serum bile acids should be at least three times the upper limit of normal. Elevation of serum bile acids alone cannot be used to make the diagnosis. The patient must also have clinical symptoms.

Perinatal Outcome

The risk of preterm birth and fetal death may be increased in patients suffering from intrahepatic cholestasis of pregnancy.[31,42] Antepartum fetal heart rate testing and intense surveillance should be undertaken in gravidas with intrahepatic cholestasis of pregnancy. It may also be prudent to induce labor at term or when amniotic fluid studies indicate fetal lung maturity.[44]

Management

Treatment is aimed at reducing the intense pruritus. Diphenhydramine, hydroxyzine, and other antihistamines are of little use, but cholestyramine resin has proven highly effective. Cholestyramine is an anion-binding resin that interrupts the enterohepatic circulation, reducing the reabsorption of bile acids. A total of 8 to 16 g/day in three to four divided doses is often helpful in relieving pruritus. It is most effective if started as soon as the pruritus is noted, before it becomes severe. It often takes up to 2 weeks to work. Because cholestyramine also interferes with vitamin K absorption, the prothrombin time should be checked at least weekly. If prolonged, parenteral vitamin K should be administered. When the prothrombin time returns to normal, the frequency of injections can be decreased. Cholestyramine causes a sensation of bloating and often results in constipation. If the patient cannot tolerate cholestyramine, antacids containing aluminum may be used to bind bile acids. These medications are usually not as effective as cholestyramine. An occasional patient may not respond to cholestyramine therapy. In those cases, phenobarbital, in a dose of 90 mg daily given at bedtime, can be helpful.

When pruritus is intolerable, delivery may be undertaken as soon as fetal lung maturity has been documented. Jaundice usually disappears within 2 days after delivery. The patient should be counseled that the condition may recur during subsequent pregnancies.[34] It is also important to note that some patients may manifest symptoms of intrahepatic cholestasis when taking oral contraceptives.[36]

Key Points

- Acute fatty liver of pregnancy is a medical emergency requiring stabilization of the patient and timely delivery. Almost all cases will be complicated by DIC.
- Liver transaminase levels in acute fatty liver of pregnancy are lower than what one would see in acute hepatitis.
- Profound hypoglycemia is a frequent concomitant of acute fatty liver and can cause death if untreated.

- Pregnancy-induced cholestasis usually occurs in the third trimester, causing intense pruritus and jaundice. Elevated serum bile acids are the best laboratory test for making the diagnosis in symptomatic patients.

Gastrointestinal Disease

Mark B. Landon

Acute Pancreatitis

There is a greater association of gallstones with the development of pancreatitis during gestation. Other causes for pancreatitis include idiopathic factors, infection, previous surgery, preeclampsia, hyperparathyroidism, thiazide ingestion, and penetrating duodenal ulcer. The normal hypertriglyceridemia of pregnancy may be exaggerated in patients with hyperlipidemia, thereby inducing acute pancreatitis.[14] The clinical presentation of pancreatitis is not significantly altered in pregnancy.

In most cases, acute pancreatitis resolves spontaneously within several days. However, in some 10 percent of cases the illness is complicated, and such patients are best managed in an intensive care environment.

Percutaneous aspiration of pancreatic exudate is important in refractory cases. This CT-guided procedure may be necessary to distinguish between sterile and infected pancreatic necrosis. For infected cases, surgical drainage of the pancreatic exudate is necessary.

Inflammatory Bowel Disease

The inflammatory bowel diseases ulcerative colitis (UC) and Crohn disease (CD) or regional enteritis are idiopathic disorders that have their peak incidence in the reproductive age group. UC is a disease of the colon or rectum, marked by acute attacks of bloody stools, diarrhea, cramping, abdominal pain, weight loss, and dehydration. The prevalence of UC in the female population under 40 years of age is 40 to 100/100,000.[18] CD is considerably less common than UC, with an incidence of 2 to 4/100,000. The average age of onset is between 20 and 30 years. CD, in contrast to UC, tends to run a more subacute and chronic course, with symptoms including fever, diarrhea, and cramping abdominal pain.[19] CD may be found anywhere from mouth to anus, including the perineum. However, the distal ileum, colon, and anorectal region are most frequently involved.

Ulcerative Colitis

Patients with inactive UC at the start of pregnancy have the best prognosis in terms of perinatal and maternal outcome, while those whose UC has its onset in pregnancy or is active have the highest rate of complications. Overall, pregnancy outcome is good for most women with UC.

Crohn Disease

Studies describing the effect of CD on pregnancy suggest minimal if any increased risk to both mother and fetus, although the rate of spontaneous abortion may be increased. Term delivery rates of 73 to 83 percent have been observed.

The effect of pregnancy on CD is similar to that reported for patients with UC. Overall, the risk of exacerbation during pregnancy is not higher than that in the nonpregnant population.[31]

Treatment of Inflammatory Bowel Disease During Pregnancy

The medical treatment of inflammatory bowel disease is not altered greatly by pregnancy. All patients should be followed closely so that the activity of their disease may be assessed and psychologic support can be provided. Dietary counseling for patients with UC should emphasize proper nutritional intake. Patients with mild disease may respond to a low-roughage diet or to the exclusion of milk products if they are lactose intolerant. In contrast, patients with CD often benefit from low-residue diets, presumably because the caliber of their small bowel may be limited by inflammation.

The initial therapy for episodes of diarrhea generally includes narcotics such as codeine and diphenoxylate. Chronic use of narcotics should be avoided as it may incite toxic megacolon in patients with UC. When simple measures are unsuccessful in quieting an attack, sulfasalazine and steroid therapy should be strongly considered. The safety of both of these drugs has been well established in pregnancy. Sulfasalazine and 5-aminosalicylic acid can be given safely to nursing mothers.[36] Steroids are indicated in patients who fail to respond to simple supportive measures.

Key Points

- Most cases of pancreatitis during pregnancy are associated with gallstones. Conservative supportive care aimed at decreasing pancreatic secretion is generally successful therapy.
- Women with active ulcerative colitis in early pregnancy usually have recurrent flare-ups during gestation and postpartum.
- The onset of ulcerative colitis or Crohn disease during pregnancy may be associated with increased miscarriage and fetal loss rates.
- Sulfasalazine (Azulfidine) may be safely used to treat inflammatory bowel disease during pregnancy and in lactating women.

Neurologic Disorders

Philip Samuels

Seizure Disorders

Affecting approximately 1 percent of the general population, seizure disorders are the most frequent major neurologic complication encountered in pregnancy. Seizure disorders may be divided into those that are acquired and those that are idiopathic.

In general, initial therapy is based on the type of seizure disorder experienced by the patient. Patients may be placed on a certain medication because they did not tolerate the side effect profile of another anticonvulsant (Table 21-14). The obstetrician and neurologist must work closely together to guide the patient through her pregnancy and find the safest and most effective medical therapy for the patient. Through this cooperation, the vast majority of pregnant women with seizure disorders can have a successful pregnancy with minimal risk to mother and fetus.

Effects of Epilepsy on Reproductive Function

Contraception may present a challenge to women with epilepsy. The use of oral contraceptives may require special adjustments because certain antiepileptic medications have been associated with contraceptive failure. Carbamazepine, phenobarbital, and phenytoin enhance the activities of hepatic microsomal oxidative enzymes.[1] This increased enzymatic activity may lead to rapid clearance of these hormones, which may allow ovulation to occur. Therefore, medicated patients taking low-dose oral contraceptives may have more breakthrough bleeding[2] and may be at increased risk for unplanned pregnancy.[3,4] This rapid clearance does not appear to be induced by valproate or benzodiazepines.[1]

Effect of Pregnancy on Epilepsy

Between 30 percent and 50 percent of patients will show an increase in seizure frequency during pregnancy. Patients with more frequent seizures tend to have exacerbations during pregnancy.[8]

Table 21-14 Common Side Effects of Anticonvulsants

Drug	Maternal Effects	Fetal Effects
Phenytoin	Nystagmus, ataxia, hirsutism, gingival hyperplasia, megaloblastic anemia	Possible teratogenesis and carcinogenesis, coagulopathy, hypocalcemia
Phenobarbital	Drowsiness, ataxia	Possible teratogenesis, coagulopathy, neonatal depression, withdrawal
Primidone	Drowsines, ataxia, nausea	Possible teratogenesis, coagulopathy, neonatal depression
Carbamazepine	Drowsiness, leukopenia, ataxia, mild hepatotoxicity	Possible craniofacial and neural tube defects
Valproic acid	Ataxia, drowsiness, alopecia, hepatotoxicity, thrombocytopenia	Neural tube defects and possible craniofacial and skeletal defects
Trimethadione	Drowsiness, nausea	Strong teratogenic potential
Ethosuximide	Nausea, hepatotoxicity, leukopenia, thrombocytopenia	Possible teratogenesis

Effects of Pregnancy on the Disposition of Anticonvulsant Medications (Table 21-15)

Levels of anticonvulsant medications can change dramatically during pregnancy, usually decreasing in total concentration as pregnancy progresses. Altered protein binding, delayed gastric emptying, nausea and vomiting, changes in plasma volume, and changes in the volume of distribution affect the levels of anticonvulsant medications. Free levels of phenobarbital, carbamazepine, and phenytoin rise significantly throughout pregnancy while total levels fall. The nonpregnant relationship between total drug and free (active) drug is not maintained. Free phenytoin levels should preferably be measured. If free levels are unavailable, drug doses should be adjusted according to the total serum level and the clinical picture. If the patient has increased seizure activity, medication doses should be increased as long as the patient is not showing signs of toxicity. Likewise, if the medication level is low but the patient is seizure free, no adjustment in dosing is necessary.

All anticonvulsants interfere with folic acid metabolism. Patients on anticonvulsants may actually become folic acid deficient and develop macrocytic anemia. Given that folic acid deficiency has been associated with neural tube defects, folic acid supplementation should be begun before pregnancy if possible. A dose of 4 mg daily is recommended.

Neonatal hemorrhage due to decreased vitamin K–dependent clotting factors (II, VII, IX, X) has been seen in infants born to mothers taking phenobarbital, phenytoin, and primidone.[17] Therefore, infants should be given 1 mg of vitamin K intramuscularly at birth.

Effect of Epilepsy on Pregnancy

The majority of women with seizure disorders who become pregnant will have an uneventful pregnancy with an excellent outcome. There appears to be an increased risk of stillbirths in women with seizure disorders. The cause is not readily apparent but may be due to factors that are detectable, such as intrauterine growth restriction (IUGR). Infants born to mothers with seizure disorders, on average, are smaller than their control counterparts.

Effects of Anticonvulsant Medications on the Fetus

Anticonvulsant medications are associated with an increase in congenital malformations, but the magnitude of this risk and the association of certain anomalies with specific drugs remain debatable.

A specific fetal hydantoin syndrome exists. The characteristics are growth and performance delays, cranio-

Table 21-15 Anticonvulsants Commonly Used During Pregnancy

Drug	Therapeutic Level (mg/L)	Usual Nonpregnant Dosage	Half-Life
Carbamazepine	4–10	600–1,200 mg/day in three divided doses	Initially 36 hr; chronic therapy 16 hr
Phenobarbital	15–40	90–180 mg/day in two or three divided doses	100 hr
Phenytoin	10–20, total; 1–2, free	300–500 mg/day in single or divided doses[a]	Average 24 hr
Primidone	5–15	750–1,500 mg/day in three divided doses	8 hr
Valproic acid	50–100	550–2,000 mg/day in three divided doses	Average 13 hr

[a] If a total dose of more than 300 mg is needed, dividing the dose will result in a more stable serum concentration.

facial abnormalities (including clefting), and limb anomalies (including hypoplasia of nails and distal phalanges). Approximately 7 to 11 percent of infants exposed to phenytoin exhibit this recognizable pattern of malformations, while 31 percent of exposed fetuses have some aspects of the syndrome.

It remains of prime importance to treat the patient with the medication that best controls her seizures. Patients treated with a single anticonvulsant have infants with a lower rate of anomalies than women taking multiple drug regimens.

Carbamazepine was once considered safer than the other anticonvulsant medications for use in pregnancy, but a pattern of minor craniofacial defects, fingernail hypoplasia, and developmental delay is now accepted in infants exposed in utero to carbamazepine. There is also a 1 percent risk of spina bifida in infants of mothers taking carbamazepine. The use of valproic acid in the first trimester has been associated with a 1.5 percent risk of neural tube defects, especially lumbosacral spina bifida.

Preconceptual Counseling for the Reproductive-Age Woman with a Seizure Disorder

Although not always possible, it is preferable to counsel the patient with epilepsy before she becomes pregnant. Overall, the obstetrician can reassure the patient that she has greater than a 90 percent chance of having a successful pregnancy resulting in a normal newborn. The patient must be informed that, if she has frequent seizures before conception, this pattern will probably continue. If she has frequent seizures, she should delay conception until control is better, even if this entails a change of medication. The patient will need to take whatever medication(s) are necessary to control her seizure throughout her pregnancy. If the patient has had no seizures during the past 2 to 5 years, an attempt may be made to withdraw her from anticonvulsant medications.

Labor and Delivery

Vaginal delivery is the route of choice for the mother with a seizure disorder. If the mother has frequent seizures brought on by the stress of labor, she may undergo cesarean delivery after stabilization. Seizures during labor may cause transient fetal bradycardia.[22]

New Onset of Seizures in Pregnancy and the Puerperium

Occasionally, seizures will be diagnosed for the first time during pregnancy. This may present a diagnostic dilemma (Table 21-16).

Table 21-16 Differential Diagnosis of Peripartum Seizures

	Blood Pressure	Proteinuria	Seizures	Timing	CSF	Other Features
Eclampsia	+++	+++	+++	Third trimester	Early: RBC, 0–1,000; protein, 50–150 mg/dl Late: grossly bloody	Platelets normal or ↓ RBC normal
Epilepsy	Normal	Normal to +	+++	Any trimester	Normal	Low anticonvulsant levels
Subarachnoid hemorrhage	+ to +++ (labile)	0 to +	+	Any trimester	Grossly bloody	
Thrombotic thrombocytopenic purpura	Normal to +++	++	++	Third trimester	RBC 0–100	Platelets ↓↓ RBC fragmented
Amniotic fluid embolus	Shock	−	+	Intrapartum	Normal	Hypoxia, cyanosis Platelets ↓↓ RBC normal

Cerebral vein thrombosis	+	–	++	Postpartum	Normal (early)	Headache Occasional pelvic phlebitis
Water intoxication	Normal	–	++	Intrapartum	Normal	Oxytocin infusion rate >45 mU/min Serum Na <124 mEq/L
Pheochromocytoma	+++ (labile)	+	+	Any trimester	Normal	Neurofibromatosis
Autonomic stress syndrome of high paraplegics	+++ with labor pains	–	–	Intrapartum	Normal	Cardiac arrhythmia
Toxicity of local anesthetics	Variable	–	++	Intrapartum	Normal	

Modified from Donaldson JO: Peripartum convulsions. In Donaldson JO (ed): Neurology of Pregnancy. Philadelphia, WB Saunders Company, 1989, p 312, with permission.

Postpartum Period

The levels of anticonvulsant medications must be monitored frequently during the first few weeks postpartum, as they can rapidly rise. If the patient's medication dosages were increased during pregnancy, levels need to be decreased rapidly after delivery to pre-pregnancy levels.

All of the major anticonvulsant medications cross into breast milk.[55,58] These medications are not a contraindication to breast-feeding.

All methods of contraception are available to women with idiopathic seizure disorders. Oral contraceptive failures are more common in women taking anticonvulsants.

Migraine

Headaches are extremely common in women, and the majority of migraine headaches occur in women of childbearing age. Migraine symptoms tend to improve during pregnancy.[62–64] Approximately two-thirds of patients report improvement of migraine symptoms, with some experiencing no headache at all during pregnancy.

Supportive therapy is recommended for patients who experience migraine attacks during gestation. Both narcotic and non-narcotic analgesics can be used as necessary.

Ergotamine is best avoided during pregnancy.

Carpal Tunnel Syndrome

The median nerve and flexor tendons pass through this carpal tunnel, which has little room for expansion. If the wrist is extremely flexed or extended, the volume of the carpal tunnel is reduced. In pregnancy, weight gain and edema further restrict the tunnel and predispose to the carpal tunnel syndrome, which leads to compression of the median nerve. The syndrome is characterized by pain, numbness, and/or tingling in the distribution of the median nerve in the hand and wrist (thumb, index finger, long finger, and radial side of the ring finger on the palmar aspect). In severe cases, weakness and decreased motor function can occur.

Supportive and conservative therapies are usually adequate for the treatment of carpal tunnel syndrome. Symptoms usually subside in the postpartum period as total body water returns to normal.[110] Conservative therapy with splinting of the wrist at night completely relieves symptoms in 80 percent of cases. Splints placed on the dorsum of the hand keep the wrist in a neutral position and maximize the capacity of the carpal tunnel. Local injections of glucocorticoids may also be used in severe cases.

Surgical correction of this syndrome should not be delayed in patients with deteriorating muscle tone and motor function.

Key Points

- Idiopathic seizures affect approximately 1 percent of the general population and are the most frequent neurologic complication of pregnancy.
- Pre-pregnancy counseling is imperative in the patient with a seizure disorder; preconceptual folic acid therapy (4 mg daily) should be implemented.
- Those with seizures occurring less than once each month will have the best control during pregnancy.
- The anticonvulsant medication that best controls the patient's seizures should be used during pregnancy.
- Because of the changes in plasma volume, drug distribution, and metabolism that occur during pregnancy, anticonvulsant levels should be checked frequently and dosages increased accordingly.
- Patients taking anticonvulsants have an increased risk of giving birth to an infant with both major and minor anomalies, but this risk is probably less than 10 percent. Therefore, 90% of patients with epilepsy will give birth to healthy infants. The risk seems lower if only a single agent is administered.
- Carbamazepine and valproate are associated with neural tube defects. All epileptic women and especially patients taking these drugs should receive folic acid daily before and during early pregnancy.
- The vasoconstrictor drugs used to treat migraines should be avoided during pregnancy and lactation.
- Carpal tunnel syndrome is common in pregnancy, but usually responds to conservative splinting. Surgery can be safely undertaken if indicated during pregnancy.

Malignant Diseases and Pregnancy

Larry J. Copeland and Mark B. Landon

While cancer is the second most common cause of death for women in their reproductive years, only about 1/1,000 pregnancies[1] is complicated by cancer. A successful outcome is dependent on a cooperative multidisciplinary approach. The malignancies most commonly encountered in the pregnant patient are, in descending order, breast cancer, cervical cancer, melanoma, ovarian cancer, thyroid cancer, leukemia, lymphoma, and colorectal cancer (see box p 554).[3]

Chemotherapy During Pregnancy

Drug Effects on the Fetus

Teratogenicity

In summary, the risks of exposing a fetus to chemotherapy correlate highly with the gestational age at the time of the exposure. Most organogenesis occurs between 3 and 8 weeks of embryonic life, and it is during this time that major morphologic abnormalities are most likely to occur from exposure to any chemotherapeutic agent. Second- and third-trimester chemotherapy exposure does not appear to carry a significantly increased risk of major fetal anomalies. Since antineoplastic agents can be found in breast milk, breast-feeding is contraindicated.[5]

Pregnancy Following Cancer Treatment

With improved survival rates for many childhood and adolescent malignancies, one must be prepared to offer prenatal counseling to the young woman who presents with a personal cancer history. Issues worthy of review and in need of clarification for the obstetrician and the patient are listed in the box on p 554.

Cancer During Pregnancy

General Considerations

Approximately one-third of recorded maternal deaths are secondary to a coexisting malignancy. Delays in di-

Factors Impacting Management of the Pregnant Patient With a Malignancy

1. The gestation of the pregnancy—fetal viability
2. The stage of the cancer and associated prognosis
3. The potential for the cancer treatment to have adverse effects on the fetus, including the potential for long-term occult problems
4. The risk to the mother of delaying therapy to permit fetal viability
5. The risk to the fetus of early delivery to allow more timely cancer therapy
6. The possible need to terminate an early pregnancy to allow an optimal opportunity to treat and cure the malignancy

agnosis of the cancer during pregnancy are common for a number of reasons: (1) many of the presenting symptoms of cancer are often attributed to the pregnancy; (2) many of the physiologic and anatomic alterations of pregnancy can compromise the physical examination; (3) many serum tumor markers (β-hCG, α-fetoprotein, CA 125, and others) are increased during pregnancy; and (4) our ability to perform either imag-

Counseling Issues for Pregnancy Following Cancer Treatment

1. What is the risk of recurrence of the malignancy?
2. If a recurrence were diagnosed, depending on the most likely sites, what would be the nature of the probable treatment? How would such treatment compromise both the patient and the fetus?
3. Will prior treatments—pelvic surgery, radiation to pelvis or abdomen, or chemotherapy—affect fertility or reproductive outcome?
4. Will the hormonal milieu of pregnancy adversely affect an estrogen-receptor-positive tumor?

ing studies or invasive diagnostic procedures is often altered during pregnancy.

Since the gestational age is significant when evaluating the risks of treatments, it is important to determine gestational age accurately.

Breast Cancer

The predicted number of breast cancer cases in women in the United States for 1996 is 184,300, and the predicted number of related deaths is 44,300.[31] Approximately 2 to 3 percent of all breast cancers in women under age 40 occur concurrent with pregnancy or lactation, and approximately 1/1,360 to 3,330 pregnancies is complicated by breast cancer.[32]

Diagnosis and Staging

Breast abnormalities should be evaluated in the same manner as if the patient were not pregnant. The most common presentation of breast cancer in pregnancy is a painless lump discovered by the patient. Despite the striking physiologic breast changes of pregnancy, including nipple enlargement and increases in glandular tissue resulting in engorgement and tenderness, breast cancer should be screened for during pregnancy. Since the breast changes become more pronounced in later pregnancy, it is important to perform a thorough breast examination at the initial visit. Diagnostic delays are often attributed to physician reluctance to evaluate breast complaints or abnormal findings in pregnancy.[35] While bilateral serosanguinous discharge may be normal in late pregnancy, masses require prompt and definitive evaluation.

Mammography in pregnancy is controversial. While the radiation exposure to the fetus is negligible,[38,39] the hyperplastic breast of pregnancy is characterized by increased tissue density, making interpretation more difficult.[40]

Fine-needle aspiration (FNA) of a mass for cytologic study is recommended. FNA is reliable for a diagnosis of carcinoma (false-positive results are rare), but if a solid mass is negative for tumor it should be evaluated by excisional biopsy. Similar to the nonpregnant patient, approximately 20 percent of breast biopsies performed in pregnancy reveal cancer.[35] Tissue biopsies should be submitted for estrogen receptor (ER) and progesterone receptor (PR) analyses. Consistent with the fact that these patients are young, the majority are receptor negative.[41]

Prior to proceeding with treatment, the patient requires staging. All draining lymph nodes areas should be evaluated. The contralateral breast must be carefully assessed. Laboratory tests should include baseline liver function tests and serum tumor markers, carcinoembryonic antigen (CEA), and CA 15-3. A chest x-ray is indicated, and, if the liver function tests are abnormal, the liver can be evaluated by ultrasound. In a symptomatic patient, radiographs of the specific symptomatic bones are advised.

Breast cancers in pregnancy are histologically identical to those in the nonpregnant patient of the same age. Because inflammatory breast cancer can be mistaken for mastitis, a biopsy of breast tissue should be performed when a breast suspected of being infected is incised and drained.

Treatment

Local Therapy

The usual criteria for breast-preserving therapy versus modified radical mastectomy pertain to the patient with breast cancer stages I to III.[44] However, the option of lumpectomy, axillary node dissection, and irradiation is complicated by the presence of the pregnancy. Consideration should be given to the delay of irradiation until after delivery.

Pregnancy Termination

At present, a harmful effect of continuing pregnancy has not been demonstrated in most published series.

Prognosis

As with any malignant disease, the prognosis best correlates with the anatomic extent of disease at the time of diagnosis. In the pregnant patient, the 5-year survival rate is 82 percent for patients with three or fewer positive nodes and 27 percent if greater than three nodes contain tumor.[43] Pregnancy, probably due to the associated delays in diagnosis, appears to increase the frequency of nodal disease, with 60 to 85 percent of patients exhibiting axillary nodal disease at diagnosis.[43,56]

When controlled for age and stage, pregnancy does not seem to affect prognosis adversely.[37,55,57,58] Some have suggested a worse prognosis if the cancer is diagnosed in the second trimester.[57]

Subsequent Pregnancy

While the general consensus is that subsequent pregnancies do not adversely affect survival, there are recommendations regarding the timing of a subsequent pregnancy.[59] It is generally advised that women with node-negative disease wait for 2 to 3 years, and this interval should be extended to 5 years for patients with positive nodes. It has been advised that patients should undergo a complete metastatic work-up prior to a subsequent pregnancy.

Cervical Cancer

Approximately 3 percent of all invasive cervical cancers occur during pregnancy. Cervical cancer is the most common gynecologic malignancy associated with pregnancy, occurring in approximately 1/2,200 pregnancies.[115-117]

All pregnant patients should be evaluated on their initial obstetric visit with visualization of the cervix and cervical cytology, including an endocervical brush. The general principles of screening for cervical neoplasia apply to the pregnant patient. The Papanicolaou smear is used to screen the normal-appearing cervix. If the cervix appears friable, cervical cytology alone may not be sufficient to detect a malignant tumor. False-negative cervical cytology is an increased risk in pregnancy due to excess mucous and bleeding from cervical eversion. Therefore it is necessary to obtain a biopsy to ensure that tissue friability is not secondary to tumor. Also, an ulcerative or exophytic lesion must have histologic sampling performed. While approximately one-third of pregnant patients with cervical cancer are asymptomatic at the time of diagnosis, the most common symptoms are vaginal bleeding or discharge.

The diagnosis of cervical cancer is commonly made postpartum rather than during pregnancy and, while stage IB disease is the most commonly diagnosed stage, all stages are represented in significant numbers. Both patient and physician factors, including lack of prenatal care, failure to obtain cervical cytology or to biopsy gross cervical abnormalities, false-negative cytology, and failure to evaluate abnormal cytology or vaginal bleeding properly, contribute to the delays in diagnosis.

Cervical cytology suggestive of a squamous intraepithelial lesion or a report of atypical glandular cells during pregnancy requires appropriate clinical evaluation (Fig. 21-4). The colposcopic evaluation of the pregnant cervix is altered by the physiologic changes of pregnancy, and, since most practicing physicians will diagnose invasive cervical cancer associated with pregnancy only once or twice in their careers, it may be prudent to consult a gynecologic oncologist. While colposcopy

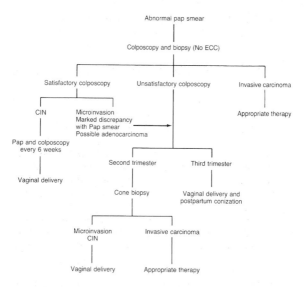

Fig. 21-4 Suggested protocol for evaluation of abnormal cervical cytology in pregnancy. ECC, endocervical curettage; CIN, cervical intraepithelial neoplasia. (From Hacker NF, Berek JS, Lagasse LD et al: Carcinoma of the cervix associated with pregnancy. Obstet Gynecol 59: 735, 1982, with permission.)

during pregnancy is usually enhanced by the physiologic eversion of the lower endocervical canal, vascular changes and redundant vagina may alter or obscure normal visualization. During pregnancy, failure to visualize the entire transformation zone and squamocolumnar junction is uncommon. While endocervical curettage is not generally recommended during pregnancy, lesions involving the lower endocervical canal can often be directly visualized and biopsied. Serious hemorrhage from an outpatient biopsy is uncommon, and the risk of bleeding is offset by the risk of missing an early invasive cancer. Following a colposcopic evaluation with appropriate tissue sampling, most patients with preinvasive lesions can be followed with repeat colposcopy at 6- to 8-week intervals to delivery.[118,119]

Patients then require a careful and complete colposcopic evaluation 6 weeks' postpartum. Cone biopsy during pregnancy, when necessary, should ideally be performed during the second trimester to reduce the risks of first-trimester abortion and rupture of membranes or premature labor in the third trimester.[120–122] Complications from conization of the pregnant cervix are common. Therapeutic conization for intraepithelial squamous lesions is contraindicated during pregnancy. Diagnostic cone biopsy in pregnancy is reserved for patients whose colposcopic-directed biopsy has shown superficial invasion (suspect microinvasion) or in other situations where an invasive lesion is suspected but cannot be confirmed by biopsy. When a cone biopsy is necessary during pregnancy, one should keep in mind the anatomic alteration of the cervix secondary to pregnancy. A shallow disk-like cone is usually satisfactory to clarify the diagnosis with a minimum of morbidity. It should be kept in mind that patients who have had a conization during pregnancy are at higher risk for residual disease. Therefore close follow-up is essential.

Following the diagnosis of invasive cervical cancer, a staging evaluation is indicated. The standard cervical staging is clinical and usually based on the results of physical examination, cystoscopy, proctoscopy, chest x-ray, and intravenous pyelogram. CT or, in some centers, lymphangiography is often performed to identify lymph node metastasis. In the pregnant patient the standard staging evaluation is modified. The chest radiograph is performed with abdominal shielding. Sonography is used to detect hydronephrosis, and, if additional retroperitoneal imaging is desired for the evaluation of lymphadenopathy, consideration should be given to using MRI.

Ovarian Cancer

While adnexal masses are frequently encountered in pregnancy, only 2 to 5 percent are malignant ovarian tumors.[136,137] Ovarian cancer occurs in approximately 1/18,000 to 1/47,000 pregnancies.[138,139]

While the three major categories of ovarian tumors—epithelial, germ cell, and stromal—occur during pregnancy, there is a disproportionate number of patients with germ cell tumors compared with nonpregnant patients. Germ cell tumors account for 45 percent; 37.5 percent are epithelial tumors, 10 percent are stromal tumors, and 7.5 percent are categorized as miscellaneous. This distribution is undoubtedly skewed by the reporting bias associated with rare tumors. The majority of epithelial ovarian tumors complicating pregnancy are of low grade (grade 1 or low malignant potential) or early stage, not uncommonly both low grade and stage I.

Management of the adnexal mass in pregnancy is the subject of some controversy. The risks of surgical intervention may favor a conservative approach.[140] Serial sonograms may be of some value in determining the nature and biologic potential of the tumor. If the clinical presentation is consistent with torsion, rupture, or hemorrhage, immediate surgical intervention is indicated. Prompt surgical exploration is also performed for the mass associated with ascites or when there is evidence of metastatic disease. Since surgical exploration during pregnancy is associated with an increase in pregnancy loss and neonatal morbidity, it is ideal to delay surgical intervention until term or after delivery. A number of opposing risks require consideration prior to following a conservative approach. The risk of greatest concern is that a delay of surgical intervention could permit a malignant ovarian tumor to spread, resulting in a decreased opportunity for cure. However, considering the rarity of advanced-stage poorly differentiated epithelial tumors in this age group, this risk is relatively small. There does appear to be an increased probability that an adnexal mass during pregnancy will undergo torsion or rupture,[141,142] and surgical intervention for these events is associated with higher fetal loss than an elective procedure.[136,143] While ovarian tumors may be the cause of obstructed labor,[136] this is uncommon. Serial sonographic evaluations will identify the rare tumor that remains pelvic as the gestation progresses. Since most ovarian masses relocate to the abdomen as the pregnancy advances, other explanations should be considered for persistent pelvic masses, including pelvic kidney, uterine fibroids, and colorectal or bladder tumors.

When a malignant ovarian tumor is encountered at laparotomy, surgical intervention should be similar to that for the nonpregnant patient. If the patient is preterm and the tumor appears confined to one ovary, consideration should be given to limiting the staging to removal of the ovary, cytologic washings, and a thorough manual exploration of the abdomen and pelvis. The potential benefit of more extensive staging, including aortic node sampling, may be offset by higher pregnancy loss or neonatal morbidity. Prior to surgery, a comprehensive discussion with the patient should guide the extent of surgery if metastatic disease, especially a high-grade epithelial lesion, is encountered. Depending on the gestational age and the patient's desires, limited surgery followed by chemotherapy and additional extirpative surgery following delivery must be offered in select cases. Preoperative serum tumor markers are of limited value during pregnancy secondary to the physiologic increases in human chorionic gonadotropin (hCG), α-fetoprotein, and CA 125.

Virilizing ovarian tumors during pregnancy are most commonly secondary to theca–lutein cysts, and their evaluation and management should be conservative.[145]

Fetal-Placental Metastasis

Metastatic spread of a maternal primary tumor to the placenta or fetus is rare. Malignant melanoma is the most frequently reported tumor metastatic to the placenta. Hematologic malignancies are the second most common tumor to spread to the placenta. Placental and fetal dissemination of lymphomas have been reported.[182–185]

Gestational Trophoblastic Disease and Pregnancy-Related Issues

Hydatidiform Mole (Complete Mole)

In the United States hydatidiform mole occurs in approximately 1 in 1/000 to 1 in 1/500 pregnancies. The two clinical risk factors that carry the highest risk of a molar pregnancy are (1) the extremes of the reproductive years (age 50 or older carries a relative risk of over 500)[188] and (2) the history of a prior hydatidiform mole (the risk for development of a second molar pregnancy is 1 to 2 percent,[189–191] and the risk of a third after two is approximately 25 percent[192]). Patients with these risk factors should have an ultrasound evaluation of uterine contents in the first trimester. Most patients are diagnosed either by ultrasound while asymptomatic or by ultrasound for the evaluation of vaginal spotting or cramping symptoms.

The safest technique of evacuating a hydatidiform mole is with the suction aspiration technique. Oxytocin should not be initiated until the patient is in the operating room and evacuation is imminent in order to minimize the risk of embolization of trophoblastic tissue. The alternative management for the older patient who requests concurrent sterilization is hysterectomy. Following either evacuation or hysterectomy, weekly β-hCG is drawn until the hCG titer is within normal limits for 3 weeks. The titers are then observed at monthly intervals for 6 to 12 months. Figure 21-5 illustrates an algorithm for molar pregnancy management.[193]

For the patient with a complete molar pregnancy, the risk of requiring chemotherapy for persistent gestational trophoblastic disease (GTD) is approximately 20 percent. Clinical features that increase this risk include delayed hemorrhage, excessive uterine enlargement, theca–lutein cysts, serum hCG greater than 100,000 mIU/ml, and maternal age over 40. It is obviously particularly important not to misinterpret a rising β-hCG due to a new intervening pregnancy as persistent GTD. Intervention with chemotherapy would be a significant

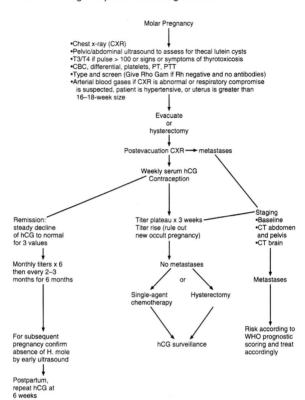

Fig. 21-5 Algorithm for the management of molar pregnancy. (From Copeland LJ: Gestational trophoblastic neoplasia. In Copeland LJ [ed]: Textbook of Gynecology. Philadelphia, WB Saunders Company, 1993, p 1137, with permission.)

risk to a new gestation, inducing either abortion or possible teratogenic defects.

Key Points

- Since many of the common complaints of pregnancy are also early symptoms of metastatic cancer, pregnant women with cancer are at risk for delays in diagnosis and therapeutic intervention.
- The safest interval for most cancer therapies in pregnancy is the second trimester, thereby avoiding induction of teratogenic risks or miscarriage in the first trimester and avoiding neonatal morbidity associated with preterm delivery in the third trimester.

- Antimetabolites and alkylating agents present the greatest hazard to the developing fetus.
- Diagnostic delays of breast cancer in pregnancy are often attributed to physician reluctance to properly evaluate breast complaints or abnormal findings in pregnancy.
- After stratifying for stage and age, patients with pregnancy-associated cervical carcinoma have survival rates similar to nonpregnant patients.
- Since most malignant ovarian tumors found in pregnancy are either germ cell tumors or low-grade, early-stage epithelial tumors, the therapeutic plan will usually permit continuation of the pregnancy and preservation of fertility.

Dermatologic Disorders

Michael C. Gordon and Mark B. Landon

Specific Dermatologic Conditions Associated With Pregnancy
(Table 21-17)

Pruritus

Pruritus is a common symptom in pregnancy, occurring in 3 to 14 percent of all women.[9] Cholestasis of pregnancy is one of the most common causes of pruritus. It is caused by intrahepatic cholestasis leading to increased levels of serum bile salts.[9,10] Itching, a result of the increased deposition of bile salts found in the skin, occurs in the third trimester of pregnancy.

The differential diagnosis of dermatologic disorders specific to pregnancy that present with pruritus as a common symptom include herpes gestationis, pruritic urticarial papules and plaques of pregnancy (PUPPP), prurigo gestationis, and pruritic folliculitis of pregnancy.

Herpes Gestationis

Herpes (pemphigoid) gestationis is a pruritic, autoimmune, bullous disease of the skin that occurs during pregnancy and the puerperium.[14]

Clinically, the disease presents with lesions that initially may closely resemble PUPPP and later, when bullae or vesicles develop, may closely resemble dermatitis herpetiformis and pemphigus vulgaris (Fig. 21-6).[18,19] The initial symptom is pruritus, characteristically extreme, followed by erythema and edema of the subcutaneous tissue. Within days or weeks, papules and plaques form that have been described as having urticarial quality. The lesions are often present on the trunk, back, buttocks, forearms, palms, and soles and initially develop around the umbilicus in 50 percent of patients. Vesicles and tense, serum-filled bullae develop at the margins of the edematous, erythematous plaques or can appear de novo in otherwise clinically uninvolved skin within 2 to 4 weeks of the initial onset of the disease. This represents the final stage of the disease and does not always develop.[14] The lesions tend to heal without scarring if secondary

Table 21-17   Pruritic Dermatoses of Pregnancy

Disease	Onset	Degree of Pruritus	Types of Lesions	Distribution	Increased Incidence of Fetal Morbidity or Mortality
Herpes gestationis	1st month to postpartum	Moderate to severe	Erythematous papules, vesicles, bullae	Abdomen, extremities, generalized	Unresolved
Prurigo gestationis	4th to 9th month	Moderate	Excoriated papules	Extensor surfaces of extremities	No
Impetigo herpetiformis	1st to 9th month	Minimal	Pustules	Genitalia, medial thighs, umbilicus, breasts, axillae	Yes
Pruritic urticarial papules and plaques of pregnancy	3rd trimester	Severe	Erythematous urticarial papules and plaques	Abdomen, thighs, buttocks, occasionally arms and legs	No
Cholestasis of pregnancy	3rd trimester	Moderate to severe	None or excoriations	Generalized	Unresolved

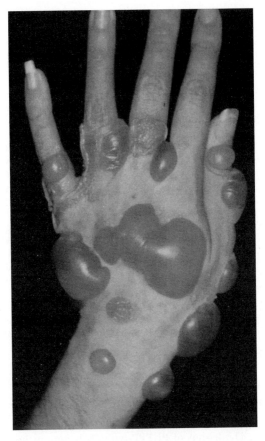

Fig. 21-6 Herpes gestationis during the third trimester. This patient developed erythematous macules on the chest and hands that progressed to bullae formation. Biopsy revealed a heavy linear complement deposition at the basement membrane zone, consistent with herpes gestationis. (Courtesy of Dr. Steven Wolverton, Division of Dermatology, Department of Medicine, The Ohio State University.)

infection is prevented. The onset is usually during the second or third trimester, with a mean onset of 21 weeks' gestation, although patients may present with recurring crops of blisters at any time during pregnancy. Herpes gestationis occurs for the first time during the early postpartum period (less than 4 days) in about 20 percent of cases.[14] The puerperium is often marked by exacerbation of this condition within 24 to 48 hours of delivery. The duration postpartum is variable. Herpes gestationis may be recurrent and is usually more severe with an earlier onset in subsequent pregnancies.

The diagnosis of herpes gestationis can be made with reasonable assurance if there is a typical clinical presentation and recurrence with pregnancy, as well as peripheral eosinophilia. Absolute confirmation is made by biopsy and immunopathologic studies that reveal complement C_3 in a band-like distribution along the basement membrane between the epidermis and dermis.[20]

The treatment for herpes gestationis is aimed at controlling pruritus, suppressing the formation of new vesicles and bullae and preventing secondary infection of skin lesions. Topical steroids and antihistamines may be used initially if the symptoms are mild. Most patients will, however, require systemic corticosteroid therapy. Prednisone is often begun in doses of 40 to 60 mg/day. The dose of steroid can be tapered to 10 to 20 mg/day if clinical improvement is noted. Azathioprine, dapsone, and, rarely, plasmapheresis have been employed in cases that fail to respond to corticosteroids.[14] Herpes gestationis does not increase the risk of maternal mortality. However, it appears that the risk for intrauterine growth restriction, IUGR, preterm birth, and possibly fetal death are increased. For this reason, antepartum testing is currently recommended.

PUPPP Syndrome

With an incidence of 1/200 women, PUPPP is the most common dermatosis of pregnancy. The etiology and pathogenesis are unknown.[19]

The lesions of PUPPP typically begin on the abdomen and initially consist of 1- to 2-mm erythematous papules surrounded by a narrow pale halo that coalesce into urticarial plaques.[31] Small vesicles can also develop on the plaques. They usually spread to the thighs and possibly the buttocks and arms within 2 to 3 days. In contrast to herpes gestationis, the periumbilical area is uninvolved in PUPPP. The face is not affected. Most patients complain of intense pruritus that improves rapidly following delivery, with resolution in 1 to 2 weeks. The average onset of the skin lesions is 36 weeks' gestation, and PUPPP rarely develops postpartum.[31] PUPPP is thought not to recur.

Therapy employing topical steroids is generally successful in the vast majority of women, but some will require systemic steroids.[31] Antipruritic drugs such as hydroxyzine or diphenhydramine may be helpful. The response to treatment may be difficult to evaluate, as abatement of cutaneous lesions and pruritus typically accompanies delivery.[28] The main goal of therapy is symptomatic relief of the intense pruritus.[31] In some women, the pruritus will be significant enough to warrant induction of labor once fetal lung maturity is ensured.

Prurigo Gestationis (Papular Dermatitis)

This disorder consists of pruritic excoriated papules usually limited to the extensor surfaces of the extremities. The disease is said to occur in 1/50 to 200 pregnancies.[32] Lesions generally appear during the second half of gestation. They are small, 1- to 2-mm papules that are distributed symmetrically. Vesicle or bullae formation does not occur. The disease usually resolves following delivery. Maternal and fetal conditions are not affected, and recurrence during subsequent gestations is uncommon. Papular dermatitis probably represents a more severe and widespread form of this condition.

The pruritus responds to calamine lotion and oral antipruritics. Corticosteroid therapy is rarely necessary for the treatment of prurigo gestationis.

KEY POINTS

- Pruritus is a relatively common symptom in pregnancy (3 to 14 percent) but infrequently is due to a serious dermatologic disease and usually resolves postpartum. In addition to evaluating the pregnant woman for dermatologic diseases that occur unassociated with pregnancy, the health care provider must evaluate for pregnancy-specific dermatologic diseases.
- Herpes (pemphigoid) gestationis is a pruritic, autoimmune, bullous disease of the skin that occurs during pregnancy and the puerperium. Clinically, the disease presents with lesions that initially may closely resemble PUPPP and later, when bullae or vesicles develop, may closely resemble dermatitis herpetiformis and pemphigus vulgaris.
- In the majority of cases PUPPP and herpes gestationis can be diagnosed by the appearance of the rash, but occasionally a skin biopsy with immunofluorescence studies will be needed to differentiate the two disorders.
- The treatment for herpes gestationis is aimed at controlling pruritus, suppressing the formation of new vesicles and bullae, and preventing secondary infection of skin lesions. Topical steroids and antihista-

mines may be used initially if the symptoms are mild. Most patients will, however, require systemic corticosteroid therapy.

- Therapy employing topical steroids is generally successful in the vast majority of women with PUPPP, but some will require systemic steroids. Antipruritic drugs such as hydroxyzine or diphenhydramine may be helpful. The main goal of therapy is symptomatic relief of the intense pruritus. In some women, the pruritus will be significant enough to warrant induction of labor once fetal lung maturity is ensured.

Critical Care Obstetrics

William C. Mabie

Indications for Invasive Hemodynamic Monitoring

The mainstay of intensive obstetric care is pulmonary artery catheterization, common indications for which are listed below. Invasive monitoring is not necessary in every patient with one of these conditions, nor is this an all-inclusive list. Swan-Ganz monitoring should be considered for any critically ill patient whose volume status must be known. The standards and criteria for invasive monitoring should be the same for pregnant as for nonpregnant patients.[2]

The Swan-Ganz catheter is useful in:

1. Differentiating cardiogenic from noncardiogenic forms of pulmonary edema. It may also be used to guide diuretic therapy and manipulations of cardiac output such as preload and afterload reduction or inotropic therapy. In patients with oliguria, the catheter may be used to assess volume status. In preeclampsia it has been shown that central venous pressure is not adequate for assessing volume status.[3,4] The change in wedge pressure and cardiac output in response to a fluid challenge is the most important guide to intravascular volume.

2. While invasive hemodynamic monitoring is not necessary for acute resuscitation from hemorrhagic shock, it is useful in the subsequent 24 to 72 hours to guide fluid therapy in complex cases in which it is not clear if internal bleeding is continuing or if oliguria, pulmonary edema, liver dysfunction, or severe coagulopathy is present.

3. In septic shock, invasive monitoring allows manipulation of cardiovascular parameters with fluid and inotropic therapy as well as assessment of response to therapy through such parameters as oxygen delivery and consumption.

Indications for Pulmonary Artery Catheterization in Obstetrics

Refractory or unexplained pulmonary edema

Refractory or unexplained oliguria

Massive hemorrhage

Septic shock

Adult respiratory distress syndrome

Class 3 and 4 cardiac disease

Intraoperative or intrapartum cardiovascular decompensation

Respiratory distress of unknown cause

4. In the adult respiratory distress syndrome, the catheter is used to exclude cardiogenic pulmonary edema and to guide supportive therapy with mechanical ventilation, positive end-expiratory pressure, intravenous fluids, diuretics, and inotropic agents.
5. New York Heart Association class 3 and 4 cardiac patients require invasive monitoring to guide fluid and drug therapy, as well as for anesthesia management during labor and delivery. The cause of sudden intraoperative or intrapartum cardiovascular decompensation may be clarified by obtaining wedge pressure and cardiac output.
6. The final indication includes patients in whom the contribution of cardiac or pulmonary disease to respiratory distress is unclear by clinical examination. The pulmonary artery catheter can help to differentiate heart failure from pneumonia, pulmonary emboli, adult respiratory distress syndrome, or chronic pulmonary disorders.

Risks Versus Benefits in Catheter Insertion

Complications associated with invasive hemodynamic monitoring include pneumothorax, ventricular arrhythmias, air embolism, pulmonary infarction, pulmonary artery rupture, sepsis, local vascular thrombosis, intracardiac knotting, and valvular damage.[5] Complications have decreased over the years at least partially due to better physician and nurse awareness.

The main benefit of pulmonary artery catheterization is its ability to provide information that clinical examination alone cannot supply.[7] The technique is more accurate than clinical assessment in determining the cause of shock or for assessing the etiology of pulmonary edema.

Determining the Hemodynamic Profile

The following measured hemodynamic variables are used to calculate the rest of the hemodynamic profile: heart rate, blood pressure, pulmonary artery pressure, pulmonary capillary wedge pressure, central venous pressure, cardiac output, and patient height and weight. The derived variables include cardiac index, stroke volume and index, systemic vascular resistance and index, pulmonary vascular resistance and index, and left and right ventricular stroke work and indices. Table 21-18 summarizes the mean values for several of the hemodynamic studies in normal third-trimester pregnancy.

Table 21-18   Normal Hemodynamic Values for the Third Trimester of Pregnancy

Parameter	Value
Heart rate	60–100 beats/min
Mean arterial pressure	70–100 mm Hg
Pulmonary capillary wedge pressure	6–12 mm Hg
Central venous pressure	1–7 mm Hg
Cardiac output	5.0–7.5 L/min
Cardiac index	3.0–4.6 L/min/m^2
Stroke volume	60–90 ml/beat
Systemic vascular resistance	800–1,500 dynes/sec/cm^{-5}
Systemic vascular resistance index	1,360–2,550 dynes/sec/cm^{-5}/m^2
Pulmonary vascular resistance	50–150 dynes/sec/cm^{-5}
Pulmonary vascular resistance index	85–255 dynes/sec/cm^{-5}/m^2

Definitions of Hemodynamic Terms

Wedge pressure—a measure of left ventricular preload. The pulmonary artery wedge pressure is obtained with a balloon-tipped catheter advanced into a branch of a pulmonary artery until the vessel is occluded, forming a free communication through the pulmonary capillaries and veins to the left atrium. A true wedge position is in a lung zone where both pulmonary artery and pulmonary venous pressures exceed alveolar pressure

Preload—initial stretch of the myocardial fiber at end-diastole. Clinically, the right and left ventricular end-diastolic pressures are assessed by the central venous pressure and wedge pressure, respectively

Afterload—wall tension of the ventricle during ejection. Best reflected by systolic blood pressure

Contractility—the force of myocardial contraction when preload and afterload are held constant

Hemodynamic Support

Cardiac output is determined by four factors: preload, afterload, rate, and contractility. According to the Frank-Starling principle, the force of striated muscle contraction varies directly with the initial muscle length. Fiber length can best be equated with preload or filling volume of the ventricle. To allow clinical estimation of preload, the pressure correlate of the filling volume is used (i.e., right or left ventricular end-diastolic pressure). Varying compliance will alter the pressure–volume relationship. For example, a poorly compliant left ventricle resulting from myocardial hypertrophy or ischemia requires higher intracavitary pressure to achieve a specific end-diastolic volume or fiber stretch.[18]

Afterload is defined as the wall tension of the ventricle during ejection. This is best reflected by the systolic blood pressure. In the absence of aortic or pulmonary stenosis, vascular resistance in the appropriate bed—systemic or pulmonary—will determine the afterload for that side of the heart.

Heart rate has a marked effect on cardiac output (i.e.,

cardiac output = heart rate × stroke volume). Increases in heart rate are accomplished at the expense of diastolic filling time, systolic emptying time being rate independent. Marked increases in heart rate may lead to circulatory depression when they cause myocardial ischemia or when reduced diastolic filling or loss of atrial "kick" prevents adequate ventricular preload. As a general rule, heart rates exceeding 220 − age/min reduce cardiac output and myocardial perfusion.[19]

Contractility is defined as the force of ventricular contraction when preload and afterload are held constant. An increase in contractility is associated with an increase in stroke volume despite no change in preload. Factors that affect contractility include sympathetic impulses, catecholamines, acid–base and electrolyte disturbances, ischemia, loss of myocardium, hypoxia, and drugs or toxins. A third heart sound, distant heart sounds, and a narrow pulse pressure suggest impaired contractility.

The agents used to treat hemodynamic instability are grouped in Table 21-19. The primary adjustment to improve low cardiac output is to optimize preload using

Table 21-19   Hemodynamic Therapy

Preload	Afterload	Contractility
Decreased	Decreased	Dopamine
Crystalloid	Volume	Dobutamine
Colloid	Inotropic support	Epinephrine
Blood	Vasopressors	Calcium[a]
	Norepinephrine	Digitalis[b]
	Phenylephrine	
	Metaraminol	
Increased	Increased	
Diuretics	Arterial dilators	
Furosemide	Hydralazine	
Ethacrynic	Diazoxide	
acid	Mixed arterial–	
Mannitol	venous dilators	
Venodilators	Nitroprusside	
Furosemide	Trimethaphan	
	Venous dilators	
Nitroglycerin	Nitroglycerin	
Morphine		

[a] May produce marked increase in systemic vascular resistance.

[b] Of questionable value and safety for acute management.

Adapted from Rosenthal MH: Intrapartum intensive care management of the cardiac patient. Clin Obstet Gynecol 24: 789, 1981, with permission.

volume administration. Because of the lack of correlation between measurements on the right and left sides of the heart in patients with significant cardiopulmonary disease, pulmonary capillary wedge pressure is monitored to optimize left ventricular preload and to avoid pulmonary edema. If blood pressure and cardiac output do not respond to fluids (e.g., pulmonary capillary wedge pressure of approximately 15 mm Hg), then a positive inotropic agent may be needed to increase myocardial contractility. Dopamine is the drug of choice in most situations. It is utilized because its activity is modified at different doses. At 2 to 3 μg/kg/min, renal and splanchnic vasodilatation occur. Positive inotropy occurs up to 10 μg/kg/min. Vasoconstriction predominates over 10 μg/kg/min. These dose ranges reflect a predominance of action only. There is a great deal of overlap and individuality of response. The usual therapeutic range for dopamine in clinical practice is 1 to 10 μg/kg/min. When the requirement exceeds this, a more potent vasopressor such as norepinephrine is added and the dopamine is decreased to renotonic doses in the hope that renal blood flow will be preserved.

Afterload may be manipulated with vasodilators in cardiac failure or in low cardiac output states secondary to severe hypertension. Vasodilators have varying effects on arterial and venous resistances. Nitroglycerin, which is predominantly a venodilator, may cause a greater reduction in preload than in afterload. Nitroprusside, an equal arterial and venular vasodilator, may be preferred; however, marked decreases in systemic vascular resistance result in hypotension, poor perfusion, and myocardial ischemia. The use of a vasodilator requires careful observation of the adequacy of intravascular volume and the net effect on cardiac output.[18]

Key Points

- The mainstay of intensive obstetric care is pulmonary artery catheterization.
- Supportive care guided by invasive monitoring includes determining the hemodynamic profile and manipulating preload, afterload, heart rate, and myocardial contractility.

Chapter 22

Maternal and Perinatal Infection

Patrick Duff

This chapter reviews the major maternal and perinatal infections that the obstetrician confronts in clinical practice. The first portion of the chapter focuses primarily on bacterial infections of the lower and upper genital tract. The second portion considers the infections that pose special risks to the fetus. The principal features of these infections are summarized in Tables 22-1 and 22-2.

Vaginal Infections

Bacterial Vaginosis

Epidemiology

Bacterial vaginosis (BV) is responsible for approximately 45 percent of cases of vaginitis. It is a polymicrobial infection, and the predominant pathogens are anaerobes, *Gardnerella vaginalis, Mobiluncus* species, and genital mycoplasmas.[1] BV usually results from disturbances in the normal vaginal ecosystem caused by hormonal changes, pregnancy, or antibiotic administration. The principal feature of this alteration in vaginal flora is a marked decrease in the lactobacilli species that produce hydrogen peroxide and a corresponding increase in anaerobic organisms. In some instances, BV can result from sexual contact with an infected partner. In contrast to trichomoniasis and candidiasis, symptomatic BV in pregnancy has been associated with several serious maternal complications, including preterm labor, preterm premature rupture of membranes, chorioamnionitis, and puerperal endometritis.[2–4]

Diagnosis

The most prominent clinical manifestation of BV is a thin, gray, homogeneous, malodorous vaginal dis-

Table 22-1 Etiology, Diagnosis, and Management of Major Obstetric Infections

Condition	Microbiology	Confirmatory Diagnostic Test	Treatment[a]
Vaginal infection			
Bacterial vaginosis	*Gardnerella vaginalis, Mobiluncus* species, anaerobes, mycoplasmas	Saline preparation	Oral metronidazole
Candidiasis	*Candida albicans, C. tropicalis, C. glabrata*	KOH preparation	Topical antifungal cream
Trichomoniasis	*Trichomonas vaginalis*	Saline preparation	Oral metronidazole
Endocervical infection			
Gonorrhea	*Neisseria gonorrhoeae*	Endocervical culture	Oral cefixime or intramuscular ceftriaxone
Chlamydia	*Chlamydia trachomatis*	Endocervical culture, antigen detection	Oral erythromycin, azithromycin, or amoxicillin
Urinary tract infection			
Urethritis	*N. gonorrhoeae*	Culture of urethral discharge	Oral cefixime or intramuscular ceftriaxone
	C. trachomatis	Culture of urethral discharge or antigen detection	Oral erythromycin, azithromycin, or amoxicillin

Asymptomatic bacteriuria or cystitis	*Escherichia coli, Klebsiella pneumoniae, Proteus* species	Urinalysis, culture	Sulfisoxazole, nitrofurantoin macrocrystals, trimethoprim–sulfamethoxazole
Pyelonephritis	As above	As above	Intravenous cefazolin and/or gentamicin or aztreonam
Chorioamnionitis	Group B streptococci, coliforms, anaerobes	Clinical examination; amniotic fluid leukocyte esterase, glucose, Gram stain, and culture	Intravenous ampicillin or penicillin plus gentamicin; add clindamycin or metronidazole if cesarean delivery is required
Puerperal endometritis	Group B streptococci, coliforms, anaerobes	Clinical examination	Intravenous clindamycin plus gentamicin or extended-spectrum cephalosporin or penicillin

[a] See text for detailed prescribing information.

Table 22-2 Summary of Etiology, Diagnosis, and Management of Major Perinatal Infections

Condition	Complications		Diagnosis		Management[a]	
	Maternal	Fetal/Neonatal	Maternal	Fetal/Neonatal	Maternal	Fetal/Neonatal
CMV	Chorioretinitis, pneumonia in immunocompromised patient	Congenital infection	Detection of antibody	Amniocentesis—culture of amniotic fluid, ultrasound	Ganciclovir for severe infection	Consider pregnancy termination when mother has primary infection
Group B streptococci	UTI, chorioamnionitis, endometritis, wound infection, preterm labor, PROM	Sepsis, pneumonia, meningitis	Culture	Culture	Intrapartum antibiotic prophylaxis	Treatment with antibiotics
Hepatitis B	Chronic liver disease	Neonatal infection	Detection of surface antigen	NA	HBIG + HBV for susceptible household contacts	HBIG + HBV immediately after delivery
C	Chronic liver disease	Neonatal infection	Detection of antibody	NA	Supportive care	No immunoprophylaxis available

Disease		Neonatal infection				
Herpes simplex	Disseminated infection in immunocompromised patient	Neonatal infection	Clinical examination, culture, PCR	Clinical examination, culture	Acyclovir for severe primary infection	Cesarean delivery when mother has overt infection
HIV infection	Opportunistic infection, malignancy	Congenital or perinatal infection	Detection of antibody or antigen	Same	Zidovudine for prevention of vertical transmission	Zidovudine
Parvovirus infection	Rare	Anemia → hydrops	Detection of antibody	Ultrasound	Supportive care	Intrauterine transfusion for severe anemia
Rubella	Rare	Congenital infection	Detection of antibody	Ultrasound	Supportive care	Pregnancy termination for affected fetus
Syphilis	Aortitis, neurosyphilis	Congenital infection	Darkfield examination or serology	Ultrasound	Penicillin	Penicillin
Toxoplasmosis	Chorioretinitis, CNS infection	Congenital infection	Detection of antibody	Cordocentesis, detection of fetal antibody	Sulfadiazine, pyrimethamine, spiramycin	Treatment of mother prior to delivery prevents fetal infection
Varicella	Pneumonia, encephalitis	Congenital infection	Clinical examination, detection of antibody	Amniocentesis, detection of organism with PCR; Ultrasound	VZIG, acyclovir for prophylaxis or treatment	VZIG, acyclovir for prophylaxis or treatment of neonate

Abbreviations: CMV, cytomegalovirus; CNS, central nervous system; HBIG, hepatitis B immune globulin; HBV, hepatitis B vaccine; HIV, human immunodeficiency virus; PCR, polymerase chain reaction; PROM, premature rupture of membranes; UTI, urinary tract infection; VZIG, varicella-zoster immune globulin.

[a] See text for detailed discussion of patient management.

charge. Vulvar or vaginal pruritus is uncommon, and the vaginal pH is characteristically more than 4.5. When vaginal secretions are mixed with several drops of a 10 percent potassium hydroxide (KOH) solution, a pungent fishy odor is produced ("whiff test" or amine test). On microscopic examination of a saline preparation, the normal lactobacilli flora are largely replaced by multiple small bacilli and cocci. Motile, comma-shaped *Mobiluncus* species and clue cells are present.

Treatment

Because of the potential serious sequelae associated with BV, *pregnant* patients should be screened for this condition and treated once the diagnosis is established. Concurrent treatment of the woman's sexual partner(s) has not been shown to improve outcome or prevent recurrences. The most cost-effective treatment for BV in pregnancy is oral metronidazole, 250 mg three times daily for 7 days.[6–8]

Candidiasis

Epidemiology

Candidiasis is responsible for approximately 25 to 30 percent of all cases of vaginitis. Several conditions predispose to symptomatic moniliasis, including recent antibiotic or corticosteroid therapy, diabetes, use of oral contraceptives, pregnancy, and immunodeficiency states.

Diagnosis

Infected patients usually report vaginal and vulvar pruritus and a white, curd-like vaginal discharge. The vaginal mucosa and vulva may be erythematous and edematous, and punctate, erythematous satellite lesions may be present on the lateral aspect of the vulva and medial aspect of the thighs.[9]

The simplest test for confirmation of diagnosis is microscopic examination of a KOH preparation for hyphae, pseudohyphae, and budding yeast.

Treatment

For uncomplicated *Candida* infections, topical therapy for 3 to 7 days with agents such as miconazole, terconazole, clotrimazole, and butoconazole is usually highly effective. Treatment of women with persistent or recurrent infection is more problematic. These patients should be counseled about preventive measures such as avoidance of bubble baths, use of cotton undergarments, and close attention to perineal hygiene.[9,10] In particularly refractory cases, administration of systemic antimicrobials such as ketoconazole or fluconazole should be considered because of their greater activity against reservoirs of yeast in the gastrointestinal tract.[11-13] In pregnancy, fluconazole appears to have a more favorable toxicity profile. The appropriate treatment for a refractory infection is a single oral dose of 150 mg.

Trichomoniasis

Epidemiology

Trichomoniasis is a sexually transmitted disease caused by the protozoan *Trichomonas vaginalis*. Trichomonas is responsible for approximately 25 percent of cases of vaginitis. It is an extremely contagious infection. Trichomoniasis has not been *conclusively* associated with serious maternal or neonatal complications.

Diagnosis

The usual symptoms of trichomoniasis are vaginal pruritus, superficial dyspareunia, frequency, dysuria, and a malodorous, yellow-green, frothy vaginal discharge. On physical examination, the vaginal mucosa is typically erythematous, and punctate hemorrhages may be present on the cervix ("strawberry cervix").

The most useful test for rapid confirmation of infection is direct visualization of the flagellated organisms in a saline preparation (wet mount). The sensitivity of this test is 60 to 80 percent.

Treatment

Metronidazole is the only antibiotic with uniform activity against *T. vaginalis*. Treatment efficacy is at least 95 percent if the patient is compliant and her sexual partner is treated concurrently.

Metronidazole can be given in three oral dosage regimens: a single dose of 2 g; 250 mg three times daily for 7 days; or 500 mg twice daily for 7 days. The former dosage schedule improves compliance and reduces expense.

Endocervical Infections

Chlamydia

Epidemiology

Chlamydia trachomatis is the most common sexually transmitted pathogen in Western nations. The organism can cause localized infection of the urethra, endocervix, and rectum. Infants delivered to infected women may develop conjunctivitis or pneumonia. The former complication occurs in up to 50 percent of infants delivered to infected mothers; the latter complication affects 3 to 18 percent of infants.[17,18]

Diagnosis and Clinical Management

Rapid identification tests such as the monoclonal antibody test (Microtrak), enzyme-linked immunosorbent assay (ELISA, Chlamydiazyme), and DNA probe are used in clinical practice to identify chlamydial infection. In high-risk populations, the sensitivity and specificity of these tests is approximately 90 and 95 percent, respectively.[17,19]

Although tetracycline and doxycycline have the greatest activity against *C. trachomatis,* these drugs should not be used in pregnancy because of their harmful effects on fetal teeth. The agent of choice in pregnancy is erythromycin base 500 mg orally four times daily for 7 days. Erythromycin estolate should not be used in pregnancy because of possible hepatotoxicity.[20] For patients who cannot tolerate erythromycin, azithromycin, 1,000 mg orally in a single dose,[21] and amoxicillin, 500 mg orally three times a day for 7 days,[22] are acceptable alternatives. Azithromycin should be prescribed in the powder formulation because it is less expensive than the capsules.

A culture for test of cure should be performed approximately 2 weeks after therapy is completed. In addition, infected patients should be screened for other sexually transmitted diseases such as gonorrhea, syphilis, hepatitis B, and human immunodeficiency virus (HIV) infection. Neonates delivered to infected mothers should receive prophylaxis with tetracycline or erythromycin ophthalmic preparations and be observed for evidence of an ensuing respiratory tract infection.

Gonorrhea

Epidemiology

Gonorrhea is caused by the gram-negative, intracellular diplococcus *Neisseria gonorrhoeae.* The infection is transmitted primarily by sexual contact. Gonorrhea also may be transmitted perinatally from mother to infant and cause serious ophthalmic injury.

In pregnant women, gonorrhea may be manifested as an asymptomatic to mildly symptomatic localized infection of the urethra, endocervix, or rectum. Local infection may increase the risk of preterm labor and preterm premature rupture of membranes and predispose to intrapartum and postpartum infection. Gonorrhea also may present as a disseminated infection.[17]

Diagnosis and Management

The most reliable test for confirmation of gonococcal infection is culture of the organism on selective agar such as Thayer-Martin medium.

The drugs of choice for treating *localized* gonococcal infections in pregnancy are ceftriaxone (125 to 250 mg IM in a single dose) and cefixime (400 mg PO once). The former drug is the preferred agent for treatment of *disseminated* infection and should be administered in a dose of 1 g IV or IM every 24 hours until a clinical response has been achieved.[17] Tests of cure are *not* routinely indicated when patients are treated with ceftriaxone and cefixime. Patients who are allergic to β-lactam antibiotics may be treated with a single 2-g intramuscular dose of spectinomycin.[17] Treatment of the neonate with either silver nitrate or tetracycline ophthalmic preparations is effective in preventing most cases of ophthalmia neonatorum.

Patients who test positive for gonorrhea should be screened for other sexually transmitted diseases.

Urinary Tract Infections

Acute Urethritis

Acute urethritis (acute urethral syndrome) is usually caused by one of three organisms: coliforms (principally *Escherichia coli*), *N. gonorrhoeae*, and *C. trachomatis.*

Affected patients typically experience frequency, urgency, and dysuria. On microscopic examination the urine usually has white blood cells, but bacteria are not consistently present. Urine cultures may have low colony counts of coliform organisms, and cultures of the urethral discharge may be positive for gonorrhea and chlamydia.

Most patients with acute urethritis warrant empiric treatment before the results of urine or urethral cultures are available. Infections caused by coliforms will usually respond to the antibiotics described below for treatment of asymptomatic bacteriuria and cystitis. If chlamydial or gonococcal infection is suspected, the patient should be treated as described above.

Asymptomatic Bacteriuria and Acute Cystitis

The prevalence of asymptomatic bacteriuria in pregnancy is 5 to 10 percent, and the vast majority of cases antedate the onset of pregnancy. The frequency of acute cystitis in pregnancy is 1 to 3 percent.

E. coli is responsible for 80 to 90 percent of cases of *initial* infections and 70 to 80 percent of recurrent cases. *Klebsiella pneumoniae* and *Proteus* species also are important pathogens, particularly in patients who have a history of recurrent infection. Approximately 3 to 7 percent of infections will be caused by gram-positive organisms such as group B streptococci, enterococci, and staphylococci.[24,25]

All pregnant women should have a urine culture at their first prenatal appointment to detect preexisting asymptomatic bacteriuria. If the culture is negative, the likelihood of the patient subsequently developing an *asymptomatic* infection is 5 percent or less. If the culture is positive (defined as at least 10^5 colonies/ml urine from a midstream, clean-catch specimen), prompt treatment is necessary to prevent ascending infection.[25]

Patients with acute cystitis usually have symptoms of frequency, dysuria, urgency, suprapubic pain, hesitancy, and dribbling. Gross hematuria may be present, but fever and systemic symptoms are uncommon. In symptomatic patients, microscopic examination of the urine shows white cells and bacteria. The leukocyte esterase and nitrate tests will usually be positive if urine has been incubating in the bladder for several hours. When a urine culture is obtained, a catheterized sample is preferred because it minimizes the probability that urine will be contaminated by vaginal flora. With a catheterized specimen, a colony count of at least 10^2/ml is considered indicative of infection.[26]

Asymptomatic bacteriuria and acute cystitis characteristically respond well to short courses of oral antibiotics. Single-dose therapy is not as effective in pregnant women as in nonpregnant patients. However, a 3-day course of treatment appears to be comparable to a 7- to 10-day regimen for an initial infection.[24] The longer courses of therapy are most appropriate for patients with recurrent infections. Table 22-3 lists several antibiotics of value for treatment of asymptomatic bacteriuria and cystitis. When sensitivity tests are available (e.g., in patients with asymptomatic bacteriuria), they may be

Table 22-3 Antibiotics for Treatment of Asymptomatic Bacteriuria and Acute Cystitis

Drug	Strength of Activity	Oral Dose × 3 Days	Relative Cost
Amoxicillin	Some *E. coli*, most *Proteus* species, group B streptococci, enterococci, some staphylococci	250 mg tid	Low
Amoxicillin–clavulanic acid (Augmentin)	Most gram-negative aerobic bacilli and gram-positive cocci	875 mg bid	High
Ampicillin	Some *E. coli*, most *Proteus* species, group B streptococci, enterococci, some staphylococci	250–500 mg qid	Low
Cephalexin (Keflex)	Most *E. coli*, most *Klebsiella* and *Proteus* species, group B streptococci, staphylococci	250 mg qid	Low
Nitrofurantoin macrocrystals—sustained-release preparation (Macrobid)	Most gram-negative aerobic bacilli	100 mg bid	Moderate
Sulfisoxazole (Gantrisin)	Most gram-negative aerobic bacilli	2 g × 1 dose, then 1 g qid	Low
Trimethoprim–sulfamethoxazole DS (Bactrim, Septra)	Most gram-negative aerobic bacilli	800 mg/160 mg bid	Low

Abbreviations: bid, twice daily; tid, three times daily; qid, four times daily.
Modified from Duff P: Urinary tract infections. Prim Care Update Ob/Gyn 1:12, 1994, with permission.

used to guide antibiotic selection. Because of theoretical concerns about their effect on protein binding of bilirubin, sulfonamide drugs should probably be avoided near the time of delivery.

For patients who have an initial infection and experience a prompt response to treatment, a urine culture for test of cure is probably unnecessary.[29] Cultures during, or immediately after, treatment are indicated for patients who have a poor response to therapy or who have a history of recurrent infection. During subsequent clinic appointments, the patient's urine should be screened for nitrites and leukocyte esterase. If either of these tests is positive, repeat urine culture and retreatment are indicated.[30]

Acute Pyelonephritis

The incidence of pyelonephritis in pregnancy is 1 to 2 percent.[25] The vast majority of cases develop as a consequence of undiagnosed or inadequately treated lower urinary tract infection.

Approximately 75 to 80 percent of cases of pyelonephritis occur on the right side. *E. coli* is again the principal pathogen.[25,27] *K. pneumoniae* and *Proteus* species also are important causes of infection, particularly in women with recurrent episodes of pyelonephritis.[27] Highly virulent gram-negative bacilli, such as *Pseudomonas, Enterobacter,* and *Serratia,* are unusual isolates except in immunocompromised patients.

The usual clinical manifestations of acute pyelonephritis in pregnancy are fever, chills, flank pain and tenderness, frequency, urgency, hematuria, and dysuria. Patients also may have signs of preterm labor, septic shock, and adult respiratory distress syndrome (ARDS). Urinalysis is usually positive for white cell casts, red blood cells, and bacteria.

Pregnant patients with pyelonephritis may be considered for outpatient therapy if their disease manifestations are mild, they are hemodynamically stable, and they have no evidence of preterm labor. If an outpatient approach is adopted, the patient should be treated with agents that have a high level of activity against the common uropathogens. Acceptable oral agents include amoxicillin–clavulanic acid, 875 mg twice daily, or trimethoprim–sulfamethoxazole-DS, one twice daily for 7 to 10 days. Alternatively, a visiting home nurse may be contracted to administer a parenteral agent, such as ceftriaxone, 2 g IM or IV, once daily.

Pregnant patients who appear to be moderately to severely ill or who show any signs of preterm labor should be hospitalized for intravenous antibiotic therapy. They should receive appropriate supportive treatment and be monitored closely for complications, such as sepsis, ARDS, and preterm labor. One of the best choices for empiric intravenous antibiotic therapy is cefazolin, 1 to 2 g every 8 hours.[27] If the patient is critically ill or is at high risk for a resistant organism, a second antibiotic, such as gentamicin (1.5 mg/kg every 8 hours) or aztreonam (500 mg to 1 g every 8 to 12 hours) should be administered along with cefazolin until the results of susceptibility tests are available.

Approximately 75 percent of patients defervesce within 48 hours after antibiotic treatment has been started. The two most likely causes of treatment failure are a resistant microorganism or obstruction.

Once the patient has begun to defervesce and her clinical examination has improved, she may be discharged from the hospital. Oral antibiotics should be prescribed to complete a total of 7 to 10 days of therapy.

Approximately 20 to 30 percent of pregnant patients with acute pyelonephritis will develop a recurrent urinary tract infection later in pregnancy.[25] The most cost-effective way to reduce the frequency of recurrence is to administer a daily prophylactic dose of an antibiotic, such as sulfisoxazole, 1 g, or nitrofurantoin macrocrystals, 100 mg. Patients receiving prophylaxis should have their urine screened for bacteria at each subsequent clinic appointment.

Chorioamnionitis

Epidemiology

Chorioamnionitis (amnionitis, intra-amniotic infection) occurs in approximately 1 to 5 percent of term pregnancies.[32] In patients with preterm delivery, the frequency of clinical or subclinical infection may approach 25 percent.[33] Chorioamnionitis is usually an ascending infection caused by organisms that are part of the normal vaginal flora. The principal pathogens are *Bacteroides* and *Prevotella* species, *E. coli*, anaerobic streptococci, and group B streptococci.[34] The most important clinical risk factors for chorioamnionitis are young age, low socioeconomic status, nulliparity, extended duration of labor and ruptured membranes, multiple vaginal examinations, and preexisting infections of the lower genital tract.[32]

Diagnosis

The diagnosis of chorioamnionitis can be established on the basis of the clinical findings of maternal fever and maternal and fetal tachycardia, in the absence of other localizing signs of infection. In more severely ill patients, uterine tenderness and purulent amniotic fluid may be present.[32] The differential diagnosis of chorioamnionitis includes upper respiratory infection, bronchitis, pneumonia, pyelonephritis, viral syndrome, and appendicitis.

Laboratory confirmation of the diagnosis of chorioamnionitis is not routinely necessary in term patients who are progressing to delivery. However, in preterm patients who are being evaluated for tocolysis or corticosteroids, laboratory assessment may be of value. In this clinical context, amniotic fluid should be obtained by amniocentesis. Table 22-4 summarizes the abnormal laboratory findings that may be present in infected patients.[32,35-40]

Management

Both the mother and infant may experience serious complications when chorioamnionitis is present. Bacteremia occurs in 3 to 12 percent of infected women. When cesarean delivery is required, up to 8 percent of women develop a wound infection and approximately 1 percent develop a pelvic abscess. Maternal death due to infection is exceedingly rare.[32]

Five to 10 percent of neonates delivered to mothers with chorioamnionitis have pneumonia or bacteremia. The predominant organisms responsible for these infections are group B streptococci and *E. coli*. Mortality due to infection ranges from 1 to 4 percent in term neonates but may approach 15 percent in preterm infants.

To prevent maternal and neonatal complications, parenteral antibiotic therapy should be initiated as soon as the diagnosis of chorioamnionitis is made, unless delivery is imminent. The most extensively tested intravenous antibiotic regimen for treatment of chorioamnionitis is the combination of ampicillin (2 g every 6 hours) or penicillin (5 million units every 6 hours) plus gentamicin (1.5 mg/kg every 8 hours).[15,32] In patients who are allergic to β-lactam antibiotics, vancomycin (500 mg every 6 hours or 1 g every 12 hours), erythromycin (1 g every 6 hours), or clindamycin (900 mg every 8 hours) can be substituted for ampicillin.

If a patient with chorioamnionitis requires cesarean delivery, a drug with activity against anaerobic organisms should be added to the antibiotic regimen, either clindamycin (900 mg every 8 hours) or metronidazole (500 mg every 12 hours).

Extended-spectrum cephalosporins, penicillins, and

Table 22-4 Diagnostic Tests for Chorioamnionitis

Test	Abnormal Finding	Comment
Maternal white blood cell count (WBC)[32]	$\geq 15,000$ cells/mm^3 with preponderance of leukocytes	Labor and/or corticosteroids may result in elevation of WBC
Amniotic fluid glucose[35–37]	≤ 10–15 mg/dl	Excellent correlation with positive amniotic fluid culture and clinical infection
Amniotic fluid interleukin-6[38]	≥ 7.9 ng/ml	Excellent correlation with positive amniotic fluid culture and clinical infection
Amniotic fluid leukocyte esterase[39]	$\geq 1^+$ reaction	Good correlation with positive amniotic fluid culture and clinical infection
Amniotic fluid Gram stain[32]	Any organism in an oil immersion field	Allows identification of particularly virulent organism such as group B streptococci. However, the test is very sensitive to inoculum effect. In addition, it cannot identify pathogens such as mycoplasmas
Amniotic fluid culture[32]	Growth of aerobic or anaerobic microorganism	Results are not immediately available for clinical management
Blood cultures[32,40]	Growth of aerobic or anaerobic microorganism	Will be positive in 5–10% of patients. However, will usually not be of value in making clinical decisions unless patient is at increased risk for bacterial endocarditis, is immunocompromised, or has a poor response to initial treatment

carbapenems also provide excellent coverage against the bacteria that cause chorioamnionitis.[44]

Parenteral antibiotics should be continued until the patient has been afebrile and asymptomatic for approximately 24 hours. Once an adequate clinical response has been achieved, antibiotics may be discontinued and the patient discharged. A course of oral antibiotics administered on an outpatient basis is rarely indicated.[15,32,44]

There are two principal exceptions to the above rule. First, a patient with a documented staphylococcal bacteremia may require a longer period of intravenous therapy and, subsequently, an extended course of oral antibiotics. Second, the patient who has a vaginal delivery and then experiences a rapid defervescence may be a suitable candidate for a short course of oral antibiotics administered on an outpatient basis. In this situation, amoxicillin–clavulanic acid (875 mg twice daily) provides effective coverage.

Patients with chorioamnionitis are at increased risk for dysfunctional labor. Affected patients need close monitoring during labor to ensure that uterine contractility is optimized. In addition, the fetus also needs close surveillance. Fetal heart rate abnormalities such as tachycardia and decreased variability occur in many cases.

Puerperal Endometritis

Epidemiology

The frequency of puerperal endometritis in women having a vaginal delivery is approximately 1 to 3 percent; in women having a scheduled cesarean prior to the onset of labor and rupture of membranes, 5 to 15 percent; and in woman having a cesarean delivery performed after an extended period of labor and ruptured membranes, 30 to 35 percent without antibiotic prophylaxis and 15 to 20 percent with prophylaxis.

Endometritis is a polymicrobial infection caused by microorganisms that are part of the normal vaginal flora. These bacteria gain access to the upper genital tract, peritoneal cavity, and, occasionally, the bloodstream as a result of vaginal examinations during labor and manipulations during surgery. The most common pathogenic bacteria are group B streptococci, anaerobic streptococci, aerobic gram-negative bacilli (predominantly *E. coli, K. pneumoniae,* and *Proteus* species), and anaerobic gram-negative bacilli (principally *Bacteroides* and *Prevotella* species).

The principal risk factors for endometritis are cesarean delivery, young age, low socioeconomic status, extended duration of labor and ruptured membranes, and multiple vaginal examinations. In addition, preexisting infection or colonization of the lower genital tract (gonorrhea, group B streptococci, BV) also predisposes to ascending infection.[46]

Clinical Presentation and Diagnosis

Affected patients typically have a fever of 38°C or higher within 36 hours of delivery. Associated findings include malaise, tachycardia, lower abdominal pain and tenderness, uterine tenderness, and discolored, malodorous lochia.

The initial differential diagnosis of puerperal fever should include endometritis, atelectasis, pneumonia, viral syndrome, pyelonephritis, and appendicitis. Endometrial cultures are of primary value in evaluating patients who have a poor initial response to antibiotic treatment. When these cultures are obtained, they should be collected with a double-lumen instrument to prevent contamination by lower genital tract flora.[47] Blood cultures also are indicated in such patients and in those who are immunocompromised or at increased risk for bacterial endocarditis.[46]

Management

Patients who have mild to moderately severe infections, particularly after vaginal delivery, can be treated with short intravenous courses of single agents such as the extended-spectrum cephalosporins and penicillins or imipenem–cilastatin. Combination antibiotic regimens should be considered for more severely ill patients, particularly those who are indigent and in poor general health and those who have had cesarean deliveries.

Once antibiotics are begun, approximately 90 percent of patients will defervesce within 48 to 72 hours. When the patient has been afebrile and asymptomatic for approximately 24 hours, parenteral antibiotics should be discontinued and the patient should be discharged. An extended course of oral antibiotics is not necessary following discharge.[18]

Patients who fail to respond to the antibiotic therapy outlined above usually have one of two problems, a resistant organism or a wound infection. Table 22-5 lists possible weaknesses in coverage of selected antibiotics and indicates the appropriate change in treatment. When changes in antibiotic therapy do not result in clinical improvement and no evidence of wound infec-

Table 22-5   Treatment of Resistant Microorganisms in Patients with Puerperal Endometritis

Initial Antibiotic(s)	Principal Weakness in Coverage	Modification of Therapy
Extended-spectrum cephalosporins	Some aerobic and anaerobic gram-negative bacilli Enterococci	Change treatment to clindamycin or metronidazole plus penicillin or ampicillin plus gentamicin
Extended-spectrum penicillins	Some aerobic and anaerobic gram-negative bacilli	As above
Clindamycin plus gentamicin or aztreonam	Enterococci Some anaerobic gram-negative	Add ampicillin or penicillin Consider substitution of metronidazole for clindamycin

From Duff P: Antibiotic selections for infections in obstetric patients. Semin Perinatol 17:367, 1993, with permission.

tion is present, several unusual disorders should be considered (Table 22-6).[46]

Prevention of Puerperal Endometritis

Prophylactic antibiotics are clearly of value in reducing the frequency of postcesarean endometritis, particularly in women having surgery after an extended period of labor and ruptured membranes.[50] The most appropriate agent for prophylaxis is a limited-spectrum (first-generation) cephalosporin, such as cefazolin, administered in an intravenous dose of 1 to 2 g immediately after the neonate's umbilical cord is clamped. A second dose is indicated approximately 4 to 8 hours after the first dose in high-risk patients, especially when operating time is prolonged beyond 1 hour.

Patients who have an immediate hypersensitivity to β-lactam antibiotics pose a special problem. One alternative is to administer metronidazole, 500 mg IV. Another alternative is to administer a single dose of clindamycin (900 mg) plus gentamicin (1.5 mg/kg). Although these antibiotics are commonly used for treatment of overt infections, their administration is still warranted in penicillin-allergic patients who are at high risk for postoperative infection.

Serious Sequelae of Puerperal Infection

Wound Infection

Wound infection after cesarean delivery occurs in approximately 3 to 5 percent of patients with endometritis. The major risk factors for wound infection are listed below. The principal causative organisms are *Staphylococcus aureus,* aerobic streptococci, and aerobic and anaerobic bacilli.[51]

The diagnosis of wound infection should always be considered in patients with endometritis who have a poor clinical response to antibiotic therapy.[46] Clinical examination characteristically shows erythema, induration, and tenderness at the margins of the abdominal incision. When the wound is probed with either a cotton-tipped applicator or a fine needle, pus usually exudes. Some patients, however, may have an extensive cellulitis without harboring frank pus in the incision. Clinical examination should be sufficient to establish the correct diagnosis. Gram stain and culture of the wound exudate are not routinely needed.

When pus is present in the incision, the wound must be opened and drained completely. Antibiotic therapy

Table 22-6 Differential Diagnosis of Persistent Puerperal Fever

Condition	Diagnostic Test(s)	Treatment
Resistant microorganism	Endometrial culture, blood culture	Modify antibiotic therapy
Wound infection	Physical examination, needle aspiration, ultrasound	Incision and drainage, antibiotics
Pelvic abscess	Physical examination, ultrasound, CT, MRI	Drainage, antibiotics
Septic pelvic vein thrombophlebitis	Ultrasound, CT, MRI	Heparin anticoagulation, antibiotics
Recrudescence of connective tissue disease	Serology	Corticosteroids
Drug fever	Inspection of temperature graph, WBC—identify eosinophilia	Discontinue antibiotics
Mastitis	Physical examination	Modify antibiotic treatment to provide coverage of staphylococcal organisms

Abbreviations: CT, computer tomography; MRI, magnetic resonance imaging.
From Duff P: Antibiotic selections for infections in obstetric patients. Semin Perinatol 17:367, 1993, with permission.

Principal Risk Factors for Postcesarean Wound Infection

Poor surgical technique

Low socioeconomic status

Extended duration of labor and ruptured membranes

Preexisting infection such as chorioamnionitis

Obesity

Type 1 diabetes

Immunodeficiency disorder

Corticosteroid therapy

Immunosuppressive therapy

should be modified to provide coverage against staphylococci. Nafcillin, 2 g IV every 6 hours, would be a suitable drug. In a patient who is allergic to β-lactam antibiotics, vancomycin, 1 g IV every 12 hours, is an acceptable alternative.[44]

Once the wound is opened, a careful inspection should be made to be certain that the fascial layer is intact. If it is disrupted, surgical intervention will be necessary to reapproximate the fascia. Otherwise, the wound should be irrigated two to three times daily with a solution such as warm saline, a clean dressing should be maintained, and the incision should be allowed to heal by secondary intention. Antibiotics should be continued until the base of the wound is clean and all signs of cellulitis have resolved. Patients usually can be treated at home once the acute signs of infection have subsided.

Necrotizing fasciitis is an uncommon, but extremely serious, complication of abdominal wound infection.[52] This condition is most likely to occur in patients with type 1 or type 2 diabetes, cancer, or an immunosuppressive disorder. Multiple bacterial pathogens, particularly anaerobes, have been isolated from patients with necrotizing fasciitis.

Necrotizing fasciitis should be suspected when the margins of the wound become discolored, cyanotic, and devoid of sensation. When the wound is opened, the subcutaneous tissue is easily dissected free of the underlying fascia, but muscle tissue is not affected. If the diagnosis is uncertain, a tissue biopsy should be performed and examined by frozen section.

Necrotizing fasciitis is a life-threatening condition and requires aggressive medical and surgical management. Broad-spectrum antibiotics with activity against all potential aerobic and anaerobic pathogens should be administered. Intravascular volume should be maintained with infusions of crystalloid, and electrolyte abnormalities should be corrected. Finally, and most importantly, the wound must be debrided and all necrotic tissue removed. In many instances, the dissection must be quite extensive and may be best managed in conjunction with an experienced surgeon.[52]

Pelvic Abscess

With the advent of modern antibiotics, pelvic abscesses after cesarean or vaginal delivery have become extremely rare. When present, abscess collections are typically located in the anterior or posterior cul de sac, most commonly the latter, or the broad ligament. The usual bacteria isolated from abscess cavities are coliforms and anaerobic gram-negative bacilli, particularly *Bacteroides* and *Prevotella* species.[54]

Patients with an abscess typically experience a persistent fever despite initial therapy for endometritis. In addition, they usually have malaise, tachycardia, lower abdominal pain and tenderness, and a palpable pelvic mass anterior, posterior, or lateral to the uterus. The peripheral white blood cell (WBC) count is usually elevated, and there is a shift toward immature cell forms. Ultrasound, computed tomographic (CT) scan, and magnetic resonance imaging (MRI) may be used to confirm the diagnosis of pelvic abscess.[55]

Patients with a pelvic abscess require surgical intervention to drain the purulent collection and antibiotics with excellent activity against coliform organisms and anaerobes.[54] One regimen that has been tested extensively in obstetric patients with serious infections is the combination of penicillin (5 million units IV every 6 hours) or ampicillin (2 g IV every 6 hours) plus gentamicin (1.5 mg/kg IV every 8 hours) or 7 mg/kg ideal body weight in a single daily dose plus clindamycin (900 mg IV every 8 hours) or metronidazole (500 mg IV every 12 hours). If a patient is allergic to β-lactam antibiotics, vancomycin (500 mg IV every 6 hours or 1 g IV every 12 hours) can be substituted for penicillin or ampicillin. Antibiotics should be continued until the patient has been afebrile and asymptomatic for a minimum of 24 to 48 hours.[46]

Septic Pelvic Vein Thrombophlebitis

Like pelvic abscess, septic pelvic vein thrombophlebitis is extremely rare. Septic pelvic vein thrombophlebitis occurs in two distinct forms.[57] The most commonly described disorder is acute thrombosis of one (usually the right), or both, ovarian veins (*ovarian vein syndrome*).[58] Affected patients typically develop a moderate temperature elevation in association with lower abdominal pain in the first 48 to 96 hours postpartum.

On physical examination, the patient's pulse is usually elevated. The principal conditions that should be considered in the differential diagnosis of ovarian vein syndrome are pyelonephritis, nephrolithiasis, appendicitis, broad ligament hematoma, adnexal torsion, and pelvic abscess.

The second presentation of septic pelvic vein thrombophlebitis is termed *enigmatic fever*.[59] Initially, affected patients have clinical findings of endometritis and receive systemic antibiotics. Subsequently, they experience subjective improvement, with the exception of temperature instability. They do not appear to be seriously ill, and positive findings are limited to persistent fever and tachycardia. Disorders that should be considered in the differential diagnosis of enigmatic fever are drug fever, viral syndrome, collagen vascular disease, and pelvic abscess.

The diagnostic tests of greatest value in evaluating patients with suspected septic pelvic vein thrombophlebitis are CT scan and MRI. These tests are most sensitive in detecting large thrombi in the major pelvic vessels. In some cases, the ultimate diagnosis may depend on the patient's response to an empiric trial of heparin.[60,61]

Patients with septic pelvic vein thrombophlebitis should be treated with therapeutic doses of intravenous heparin.[57,60] The dose of heparin should be adjusted to maintain the activated partial thromboplastin time (APTT) at two times normal or to achieve a serum heparin concentration of 0.2 to 0.7 IU/ml. Therapy should be continued for 7 to 10 days. Long-term anticoagulation with oral agents in probably unnecessary. Patients should be maintained on broad-spectrum antibiotics throughout the period of heparin administration.

Once medical therapy is initiated, the patient should have objective evidence of a response within 48 to 72 hours. If no improvement is noted, surgical intervention may be necessary.[57,60]

Cytomegalovirus Infection

Epidemiology

Cytomegalovirus (CMV) is not highly contagious, and, therefore, close personal contact is required for infection to occur. *Horizontal transmission* may result from sexual contact or from contact with contaminated saliva or urine. *Vertical transmission* may occur as a result of transplacental infection, exposure to contaminated genital tract secretions during delivery, or breast-feeding. The incubation period of the virus ranges from 28 to 60 days, with a mean of 40 days.[70–72]

In addition to acquiring infection from young children, adolescents and adults may develop infection as a result of sexual contact.

Clinical Manifestations

Most adults with either primary or recurrent CMV are asymptomatic. Symptomatic patients typically have findings suggestive of mononucleosis.

Diagnosis of Infection

The diagnosis of CMV infection can be confirmed by isolation of virus in tissue culture. The highest concentration of CMV is usually present in urine, seminal fluid, saliva, and breast milk.

Serologic methods also are helpful in establishing the diagnosis of CMV infection provided that the reference laboratory is skilled in performing such tests. In the acute phase of infection, viral-specific immunoglobulin M (IgM) antibody is present in serum. IgM titers usually decline rapidly over a period of 30 to 60 days but can remain elevated for several months. There is no absolute IgG titer that clearly will differentiate acute from recurrent infection. However, a fourfold or greater change in the IgG titer is consistent with recent acute infection.[70]

Congenital and Perinatal Infection

Approximately 50 to 80 percent of adult women in the United States have serologic evidence of past CMV infection. Unfortunately, the presence of antibody is not perfectly protective against vertical transmission, and, thus, pregnant women with both recurrent and primary infection pose a special risk to their fetus. Fetal and neonatal CMV infection may occur at three distinct times: antepartum, intrapartum, and postpartum. Antepartum or congenital infection is the greatest risk to the fetus.

Congenital (Antepartum) Infection

Congenital CMV infection results from hematogenous dissemination of virus across the placenta. Dissemination may occur with both primary and recurrent (reactivated) infection but is much more likely in the former setting. In women who acquire primary infection, 40 to 50 percent of the fetuses will be infected. The overall risk of congenital infection is greatest when maternal infection occurs in the third trimester, but the probability of severe fetal injury is highest when maternal infection occurs in the first trimester.

Of fetuses with congenital infection, 5 to 18 percent will be overtly symptomatic at birth. The most common clinical manifestations are hepatosplenomegaly, intracranial calcifications, jaundice, growth restriction, microcephaly, chorioretinitis, and hearing loss. Approximately 30 percent of severely infected infants die. Eighty percent of the survivors have severe neurologic morbidity, ocular abnormalities, or sensorineural hearing loss.[86,87] Approximately 85 to 90 percent of infants delivered to mothers with primary infection will be asymptomatic at birth. Ten to 15 percent subsequently develop hearing loss, chorioretinitis, or dental defects within the first 2 years of life.

Overall, approximately 1 percent of infants (40,000) born in the United States each year have congenital CMV infection. Approximately 3,000 to 4,000 infants are symptomatic at birth, and an additional 4,000 to 6,000 subsequently have neurologic or developmental problems in the first years of life. CMV infection is now the principal cause of hearing deficits in children.

Perinatal (Intrapartum and Postpartum) Infection

Perinatal infection may occur *during delivery* as a result of exposure to infected genital tract secretions. Infants rarely have serious sequelae if infection is acquired during delivery.[86,89]

Perinatal infection also may develop as a *result of breast-feeding*. Fortunately, serious sequelae do not occur in infected infants.

Diagnosis of Fetal Infection

In recent years, much attention has focused on analysis of amniotic fluid and fetal serum as a means to diagnose congenital infection. Amniotic fluid culture is superior in confirming the diagnosis of congenital CMV infection.

Although identification of virus in amniotic fluid appears to be the most sensitive and specific test for diagnosing congenital infection, it does not necessarily identify the *severity* of fetal injury. Detailed sonography can be invaluable in providing information about severity of fetal impairment. The principal sonographic findings suggestive of serious fetal injury include microcephaly, ventriculomegaly, intracerebral calcifications, hydrops, growth restriction, and oligohydramnios.[92]

Treatment and Prevention

At the present time, a vaccine for CMV is not available. Antiviral agents have moderate activity against CMV, but their use is limited to treatment of severe infections in immunocompromised patients. Accordingly, obstetrician/gynecologists should focus most of their attention on educating patients about preventive measures.

One of the most important interventions is helping patients understand that CMV infection can be a sexually transmitted disease. Another important intervention is educating health care workers, day care workers, elementary school teachers, and mothers of young children about the importance of simple infection control measures such as handwashing and proper cleansing of environmental surfaces. Obstetricians must be aware of the importance of transfusing only CMV-free blood products to pregnant women. Finally, health care workers must adhere to the principles of universal precautions when treating patients and handling potentially infected body fluids.[84]

Routine prenatal screening for CMV infection is not recommended.

Group B Streptococcal Infection

Epidemiology

Group B streptococcus is one of the most important causes of early-onset neonatal infection. The prevalence of neonatal group B streptococcal infection is 1 to 2/1,000 live births, with approximately 10,000 to 12,000 cases of neonatal streptococcal septicemia in the United States each year.[97,98]

Neonatal group B streptococcal infection can be divided into *early-onset* and *late-onset* infection. Approximately 80 to 85 percent of cases of neonatal group B streptococcal infection are early in onset and result almost exclusively from vertical transmission from a colonized mother. Early-onset infection presents primarily as a severe pneumonia or overwhelming septicemia. In preterm infants, the mortality from early-onset group B streptococcal infection approaches 25 percent. In term infants, the mortality is approximately 5 percent. Late-onset neonatal group B streptococcal infection occurs as a result of both vertical and horizontal transmission. It is manifested by bacteremia, meningitis, and pneumonia. The mortality from late-onset infection is approximately 5 to 10 percent.[97,98]

Major risk factors for early-onset infection include preterm labor, especially when complicated by preterm premature rupture of membranes (PROM); intrapartum maternal fever (chorioamnionitis); prolonged rupture of membranes, defined as more than 12 to 18 hours; and previous delivery of an infected infant.[97,99,100] Approximately 25 percent of pregnant women have at least one risk factor for group B streptococcal infection. The neonatal attack rate in colonized patients is 40 to 50 percent in the presence of a risk factor and 5 percent or less in the absence of a risk factor. In infected infants, neonatal mortality approaches 30 to 35 percent when a maternal risk factor is present but is 5 percent or less when a risk factor is absent.[97–99]

Maternal Complications

Group B streptococcus is a major cause of chorioamnionitis and postpartum endometritis. It also may cause postcesarean wound infection. Group B streptococci are responsible for approximately 2 to 3 percent of lower urinary tract infections in pregnancy, a risk factor for preterm labor. Investigations have confirmed the association between group B streptococcal colonization, preterm labor, and preterm PROM.

Diagnosis

The gold standard for the diagnosis of group B streptococcal infection is bacteriologic culture. Todd-Hewitt broth or selective blood agar is the preferred medium. Specimens for culture should be obtained from the lower vagina, perineum, and perianal area, using a simple cotton swab. Although rapid diagnostic tests have reasonable sensitivity in identifying heavily colonized

Table 22-7   Antibiotics with Activity Against
            Group B Streptococci

Drug	Dose for Intrapartum Prophylaxis
Ampicillin	2 g initally, then 1 g q4h
Penicillin	5 million units initially, then 2.5 million units q4h
Erythromycin	500 mg q6h
Clindamycin	900 mg q8h
Vancomycin	500 mg q6h or 1,000 mg q12h

patients, they have poor sensitivity in identifying lightly and moderately colonized patients, limiting their usefulness in clinical practice.

Prevention of Group B Streptococcal Infection

Several strategies have been proposed for the prevention of neonatal group B streptococcal infection. No strategy is perfectly applicable in all clinical situations, and no strategy can prevent all cases of neonatal infection. However, the recent guidelines recommended by the Centers for Disease Control (CDC) represent a reasonable approach to this difficult clinical problem (Prevention of perinatal group B streptococcal disease: a public health perspective. MMWR [suppl] 1996;45:1).

The CDC guidelines recommend universal culturing for group B streptococcal infection at 35–37 weeks' gestation. All patients with a positive culture should be treated with prophylactic antibiotics intrapartum (Table 22-7). If the colonization status of a patient is unknown, intrapartum prophylaxis should be administered if any of the above-mentioned risk factors are present.

Hepatitis

Hepatitis B

Approximately 40 to 45 percent of all cases of hepatitis in the United States are caused by hepatitis B virus. The virus has three major structural antigens: surface antigen (HB_sAg), core antigen (HB_cAg), and e antigen (HB_eAg). Transmission of hepatitis B occurs primarily as a result of parenteral injection, sexual contact, and perinatal exposure.[114]

Following an acute infection caused by hepatitis B virus, less than 1 percent of patients develop fulminant hepatitis and die. Eighty-five to 90 percent experience complete resolution of their physical findings and develop protective levels of antibody. Ten to 15 percent of patients become chronically infected. Of these, 15 to 30 percent subsequently develop chronic active or persistent hepatitis or cirrhosis.

The diagnosis of *acute* hepatitis B is confirmed by detection of the surface antigen and IgM antibody to the core antigen. Identification of HB_eAg is indicative of an exceptionally high viral inoculum and active viral replication. Patients who have *chronic* hepatitis B infection have persistence of the surface antigen, with or without the e antigen, in the serum and liver tissue.

Infected women may transmit infection to their fetuses. Perinatal transmission occurs primarily as a result of the infant's exposure to infected blood and genital secretions during delivery. In the absence of immunoprophylaxis for the neonate, perinatal transmission occurs in 10 to 20 percent of women who are seropositive for HB_sAg. The frequency of perinatal transmission increases to almost 90 percent in women who are seropositive for both HB_sAg and HB_eAg.[114,115,119]

A combination of passive and active immunization is highly effective in preventing both horizontal and vertical transmission of hepatitis B infection. All individuals who have had household or sexual exposure to another person with hepatitis B infection should be tested to determine if they have antibody to the virus. If they are seronegative, they should immediately receive immunoprophylaxis with hepatitis B immune globulin (HBIG), 0.06 ml/kg IM. They then should receive the hepatitis B vaccination series. Similarly, infants who are delivered to seropositive mothers should receive HBIG, 0.5 ml IM, immediately after birth. They then should begin the hepatitis B vaccination series within 12 hours of birth.

In view of the extremely favorable results of immunoprophylaxis, the Centers for Disease Control and Prevention (CDC) recently recommended universal hepatitis B vaccination for all infants.[120] Dosage recommendations vary depending on the mother's serostatus. Infants born to seronegative mothers require only the vaccine. Infants born to seropositive mothers should receive both the vaccine and HBIG. Therefore, obstetricians must continue to screen *all* of their patients for hepatitis B at some point during pregnancy.

Hepatitis C

The principal risk factors for hepatitis C are intravenous drug abuse, transfusion, and sexual intercourse.[122] Its incubation period is 5 to 10 weeks. Hepatitis C is particularly likely to result in chronic liver disease. Approximately 50 percent of infected patients develop biochemical evidence of hepatic dysfunction. Of these, about 20 percent subsequently develop chronic active hepatitis or cirrhosis.[114] Approximately 75 percent of patients with hepatitis C are asymptomatic. The diagnosis of hepatitis C infection is confirmed by identification of anti-C antibody.

In a general obstetric population, the prevalence of hepatitis C is 1 to 3 percent. The principal risk factors that identify an obstetric patient at high risk for hepatitis C include concurrent sexually transmitted diseases (STDs), multiple sexual partners, history of recent multiple transfusions, and history of intravenous drug abuse.[125] The frequency of perinatal transmission of hepatitis C infection has ranged from 10 to 44 percent, and transmission is partially likely to occur when the patient is coinfected with HIV.[122,126]

At the present time, a vaccine for hepatitis C is not available. Passive immunization with immunoglobulin (0.06 ml/kg IM) should be administered following percutaneous exposure to a person with hepatitis C.

Herpes Simplex Virus Infection

Epidemiology

Herpes simplex virus (HSV), is transmitted by direct, intimate contact. Following the initial infection, the virus remains dormant in neuronal ganglia and may reactivate at later times. Two strains of the virus have been identified: HSV-1 and HSV-2. The former causes primarily oropharyngeal infection and the latter, genital tract infection. Approximately 0.5 to 1.0 percent of women have an overt herpetic infection during pregnancy. About 400 cases of neonatal herpes occur annually in the United States.

HSV infections are classified as primary, nonprimary–first episode, and recurrent on the basis of historical and clinical findings and serologic testing.[137–140] Table 22-8 summarizes the criteria for each diagnosis. Approximately 20 to 40 percent of Americans are seropositive for HSV. Up to 80 percent of these individuals do not have a history of an overt primary infection.

Clinical Manifestations

The onset of HSV infection is usually heralded by a prodrome of neuralgias, paresthesias, and hypesthesias, followed by an eruption of painful vesicles in either

Table 22-8   Classification of Herpes Simplex
            Virus Infection

Classification	Criteria
Primary	First clinical infection No preexisting antibody
Nonprimary, first episode	No history of genital tract infection Positive antibody for HSV-1 or HSV-2
Recurrent	Prior history of clinical infection Positive antibody for HSV-2

the orolabial area or genitalia. The vesicles typically rupture, forming a shallow-based ulcer, and then form a dry crust. Some vesicles become secondarily infected and evolve into frank pustules. Ultimately, the vesicles heal without scarring.[137,138]

In patients experiencing a primary HSV infection, vesicles may be present for up to 3 weeks. Systemic symptoms may be moderately severe, and local complications such as urinary retention may occur. In recurrent infections, overt vesicles are fewer in number and less painful and typically persist for 14 days or less. Table 22-9 compares the incubation period and clinical features of primary and recurrent HSV infection.[137]

Diagnosis

Serology is useful in classifying the initial herpetic episode as *primary* versus *nonprimary–first episode*.[137,138] However, serologic testing is rarely indicated in patients who experience recurrent HSV infection.

Viral isolation is usually possible within 72 to 96

Table 22-9   Comparison of Primary Versus Recurrent
            Herpes Simplex Virus Infection

Stage of Illness	Type of Infection	
	Primary	Recurrent
Incubation period and/or prodrome (days)	2–10	1–2
Vesicle, pustule (days)	6	2
Wet ulcer (days)	6	3
Dry crust (days)	8	7
Total	22–30	13–14

hours of inoculation of the tissue culture. The highest rate of isolation is achieved when clinical specimens are obtained from fresh vesicles or pustules. Vesicular fluid should be aspirated with a fine needle into a tuberculin syringe. Ulcers should be scraped vigorously with a wooden spatula or cotton-tipped applicator.[137,138]

Obstetric and Perinatal Complications

Severe primary HSV infection has been associated with spontaneous abortion, preterm delivery, and intrauterine growth restriction (IUGR). The greatest risk to the fetus occurs when overt HSV infection is present at the time of labor. In this situation, the principal mechanism of infection is direct contact with infected vesicles during the process of vaginal birth. The frequency of neonatal infection clearly is dependent on whether the mother has a primary or recurrent HSV infection. In the setting of a primary infection, the viral inoculum in the genital tract is high, and maternal antibody is not present. Approximately 40 percent of neonates delivered vaginally to such women will become infected. In the absence of antiviral chemotherapy, almost half of these infants die and 35 to 40 percent experience severe neurologic morbidity such as chorioretinitis, microcephaly, seizures, and mental retardation. In women who have recurrent *symptomatic* HSV infection, the risk of neonatal infection following vaginal delivery is 5 percent or less. In women who have a history of recurrent HSV infection but no prodromal symptoms or overt lesions, the risk of neonatal infection with vaginal delivery is 1/1,000 or less.[137,138,140,143–145]

Neonatal HSV infection may appear as a localized abscess at the site of attachment of a scalp electrode or as isolated mucocutaneous lesions. In its more severe forms, neonatal HSV infection may present as widely disseminated mucocutaneous lesions, visceral infection, meningitis, and encephalitis. In such instances, mortality may approach 50 to 60 percent, and up to half of the survivors may have persistent morbidity.[137,138,140,142,143,146]

Management During Pregnancy

At the time of the patient's initial prenatal appointment, she should be questioned about a prior history of HSV infection. If her history is positive, she should be screened for other STDs such as gonorrhea, chlamydia, syphilis, hepatitis B, and HIV infection. When the patient ultimately is admitted for delivery, she should be asked about prodromal symptoms and examined thoroughly for cervical, vaginal, and vulvar lesions. If no prodromal symptoms or overt lesions are present, vaginal delivery should be anticipated. If symptoms or lesions are present, cesarean delivery should be performed. Cesarean delivery is indicated even in the presence of ruptured membranes of extended duration since operative delivery significantly decreases the size of the viral inoculum to which the infant is exposed.

Mothers with symptomatic infection do not need to be isolated from their infants or other patients. They should wash their hands carefully before handling the infant and shield the baby from any contact with vesicular lesions. Breast-feeding is permissible as long as no skin lesions are present on the breast.

Prophylactic treatment with acyclovir, 400 mg twice daily, may be appropriate in women with frequent recurrent infections in pregnancy, particularly near term.[151] Acyclovir is classified by the Food and Drug Administration (FDA) as a category C drug. To date, the Acyclovir Registry has reported no increase in the frequency of adverse effects in infants exposed in utero to this antiviral agent.[153,154]

Human Immunodeficiency Virus Infection

Epidemiology

At the present time, almost half a million Americans have acquired immunodeficiency syndrome (AIDS) or have died from AIDS. An additional 1 million are infected with the virus but are not yet in the terminal stage of their illness. In the United States, approximately 15 to 20 percent of all cases of HIV infection occur in women. Almost 75 percent of infected women are black or Hispanic. In women, the two most important mechanisms of HIV infection are intravenous drug abuse and heterosexual contact with a high-risk male. Heterosexual transmission is increasing in importance as a mechanism of spread of HIV infection.[161] In the general obstetric population in the United States, the frequency of HIV infection is approximately 1/1,000. However, in some inner city populations, the prevalence of infection is as high as 1 to 1.5 percent.[158–160]

Clinical Manifestations

Symptomatic patients with HIV infection typically have fever, malaise, fatigue, anorexia, nausea, vomiting, diarrhea, weight loss, and generalized lymphadenopathy. Opportunistic infections, of course, are the hall-

mark of HIV infection.[162] Among the most common are
Pneumocystis carinii pneumonia, mycobacterium avium
complex (MAC), tuberculosis, toxoplasmosis, candidiasis, and CMV infection. Genital herpes, hepatitis B, C,
and D, and syphilis are common concurrent STDs.

Diagnosis

The diagnosis of HIV infection can be confirmed by
direct culture of virus from peripheral blood lympho-
cytes and monocytes. The diagnosis also can be established by detection of viral antigen by the polymerase
chain reaction. Infected patients usually have a decreased number of CD4 cells and an inverted CD4/CD8
ratio. Serum immunoglobulin levels also are elevated.[164]

The principal diagnostic test at present is identification of viral-specific antibody.[164] The initial serologic
screening test should be an ELISA or enzyme immuno-
assay (EIA). If the initial ELISA or EIA test is positive,
the test should be repeated. If the second test is positive,
a confirmatory Western blot assay should be performed. This test detects specific viral antigens, and it
is considered positive when any two of the following
three antigens are identified: p24 (viral core), gp-41
(envelope), and gp-120/160 (envelope). If a patient has
two positive ELISAs or EIAs, followed by a confirmatory
Western blot, the likelihood of a false-positive test is
less than 1/10,000.[165,166]

Perinatal Transmission

Approximately 90 percent of all cases of HIV infection
in children are due to perinatal transmission. Perinatal
transmission occurs as a result of hematogenous dissemination and as a result of intrapartum exposure to
infected maternal blood and genital tract secretions.
The relative importance of each mechanism has not
been precisely delineated.[157,159]

The frequency of vertical transmission of HIV infection varies from a low of 5 to 10 percent to a high
of 50 to 60 percent. The average in most investigations has been 20 to 30 percent.[167,168]

Obstetric Complications

Infected women appear to be at increased risk for several major complications: preterm delivery, preterm
PROM, IUGR, increased perinatal mortality, and postpartum endometritis. Pregnancy per se probably does

not significantly accelerate the progression of HIV infection.[157,159]

Management

All obstetric patients should be offered voluntary screening for HIV infection at the time of their first prenatal appointment. Selective screening only in patients presumed to be high risk will fail to identify approximately 50 percent of seropositive women.[169] Infected women should be counseled about the risk of perinatal transmission of infection and about potential obstetric complications. They should then be offered the option of pregnancy termination. In addition, arrangements should be made for patients to obtain assistance from appropriate support personnel such as social workers, nutritionists, and psychologists.

Infected patients should be screened for other sexually transmitted diseases such as gonorrhea, chlamydia, herpes, hepatitis B, C, and D, and syphilis. They should be tested for antibody to CMV and toxoplasmosis and have a tuberculin skin test. Patients should receive vaccinations for hepatitis B, pneumococcal infection, hemophilus B influenza, and viral influenza. Finally, a Papanicolaou smear should be done to determine if cervical intraepithelial neoplasia is present.

Patients with HIV infection also should receive antiviral chemotherapy. The rationale for treatment is twofold: prevention of perinatal transmission of infection and improvement in the course of the mother's disease. Recently, several treatment trials in nonpregnant patients have demonstrated a clear advantage for multiagent regimens compared to monotherapy with respect to suppression of viral load, elevation of CD4 count, improvement in quality of life, and prolongation of disease-free interval. Pending new information from ongoing trials, a reasonable approach to pregnant women with HIV infection is treatment with two nucleoside reverse transcriptase inhibitors and a protease inhibitor (Carpenter CCJ, Fischel M, Harmer SM, et al: Antiretroviral therapy for HIV infection in 1997. Updated recommendations of the International AIDS Society—USA Panel. JAMA 277:1962, 1997).

From the perspective of cost effectiveness and maternal/fetal safety, the combination of zidovudine (300 mg PO twice daily) plus lamivudine (150 mg PO twice daily) plus nelfinavir (750 mg three times daily) seems particularly well suited for pregnant women.

When the physician is caring for the HIV-positive patient intrapartum, every effort must be made to avoid instrumentation that would increase the neonate's exposure to infected maternal blood and secretions. Specifically, whenever feasible, the fetal membranes should be left intact until delivery. In addition, application of the fetal scalp electrode and scalp pH sampling should be avoided. In the postpartum period, the mother should be advised to avoid any contact between her body fluids and an open area on the skin or mucous membranes of the neonate. She also should be cautioned against breast-feeding. Finally, infected patients should be urged to use secure contraception and adopt responsible sexual practices to prevent spread of infection to their partners.

Parvovirus Infection

Epidemiology

Human parvovirus B19 is transmitted by respiratory droplets and infected blood components. The incubation period is 4 to 20 days. Serum and respiratory secretions become positive for the virus several days before clinical symptoms develop. Once symptoms appear, respiratory secretions and serum are usually free of the virus.[174,175] Prevalence of antibody to parvovirus increases with age. In adolescents and adults the seroprevalence exceeds 60 percent.[174,175]

Clinical Manifestations

The most common clinical presentation of parvovirus infection is erythema infectiosum or fifth disease. This illness typically occurs in elementary school and day care populations in the late winter and early spring. Patients usually have low-grade fever, malaise, adenopathy, and polyarthritis affecting the hands, wrists, and knees. In addition, they have a characteristic pruritic, erythematous "slapped cheek" rash on the face and a finely reticulated erythematous rash on the trunk and extremities. Erythema infectiosum is a self-limited illness, and serious long-term sequelae rarely occur.[174,175]

The second major clinical presentation of parvovirus infection is transient aplastic crisis, resulting from viral infection of the bone marrow, with resultant destruction of red blood cell precursors. Full recovery without sequelae is the usual outcome.

Fetal Infection

The risk that a susceptible mother will acquire infection from an infected household member is 50 to 90 per-

Table 22-10   Association Between Gestational Age at Time of Exposure and Risk of Fetal Parvovirus Infection

Time of Exposure (Weeks' Gestation)	Frequency of Severely Affected Fetuses (%)
1–12	19
13–20	15
>20	6

cent.[174–176] The risk of transmission in a day care setting or classroom is lower, ranging from 20 to 30 percent.[176–178] Published information regarding subsequent risk of transmission to the fetus is based on one principal endpoint, namely, fetal hydrops. Hydrops appears to result primarily from viral infection of fetal erythroid stem cells, leading to an aplastic anemia and high-output congestive heart failure. The risk of fetal infection is greatest when maternal illness occurs in the first trimester, as noted in Table 22-10.[176]

Diagnosis of Maternal Infection

The mainstay of laboratory diagnosis is serologic testing. IgM-specific antibody is usually positive by the third day after symptoms develop. It typically disappears within 30 to 60 days but may persist for up to 120 days. IgG antibody is detectable by the seventh day of illness and persists for life[174–176] (Table 22-11).

Diagnosis of Fetal Infection

The most valuable test for diagnosis of fetal parvovirus infection is ultrasound. Severely affected fetuses typi-

Table 22-11   Interpretation of Serologic Tests for Maternal Parvovirus Infection

	Maternal Antibody	
Condition	IgM	IgG
Susceptible	−	−
Immune—infection >120 days ago	−	+
Infection within 7 days	+	−
Infection within 7–120 days	+	+

cally have evidence of hydrops. Since the incubation period of the virus may be longer in the fetus than in the child or adult, the patient should be followed with serial ultrasound examinations for up to 10 weeks after her acute illness. If the fetus shows no signs of hydrops, additional diagnostic studies are unnecessary. If hydropic changes appear and the fetus is at an appropriate gestational age, cordocentesis is indicated (see below).[174–176,182]

Maternal Management

Following a documented exposure to parvovirus, the mother should immediately have a serologic test to determine if she is immune or susceptible to the virus. If preexisting IgG antibody is present, the patient can be reassured that second infections are extremely unlikely and that her fetus is not at risk. If the patient is susceptible, she should have a repeat serologic test in approximately 3 weeks to determine if she has seroconverted. If seroconversion is detected, serial ultrasound examinations should be performed over the ensuing 10 weeks to evaluate fetal well-being.

No antiviral agent or vaccine is presently available for treatment of parvovirus infection, but patients with erythema infectiosum rarely need more than simple supportive care. Isolation of patients with erythema infectiosum is not of value in reducing transmission of infection since spread by respiratory droplets has already occurred by the time the patient has clear signs of clinical disease.

Fetal Management

If fetal hydrops is documented by ultrasound, cordocentesis should be performed. Fetal blood should be collected for determination of hematocrit and detection of IgM-specific antibody.[182] If severe anemia is present, intrauterine transfusion should be performed.[185,186] Although the long-term prognosis for the neonate is excellent, there are case reports of infants who have had neurologic injury and/or prolonged anemia as a result of congenital parvovirus infection.

Rubella

Epidemiology

Rubella occurs primarily in young children and adolescents. The disease is most common in the springtime. With licensure of an effective rubella vaccine in 1969, the frequency of rubella has declined by almost 99 percent.[190] The persistence of rubella appears to be due to failure to vaccinate susceptible individuals rather than to lack of immunogenicity of the vaccine.

The rubella virus enters the host through the upper respiratory tract. The incubation period is approximately 2 to 3 weeks. The virus is present in blood and nasopharyngeal secretions for several days before appearance of the characteristic rash. The virus is also shed from the nasopharynx for several days after appearance of the exanthem. Therefore, the patient can be contagious for an extended period of time.[189,192]

Antibody against rubella does not normally appear in the serum until after the rash has developed. Acquired immunity to rubella is usually lifelong. Second infections have occurred after both natural primary infections and vaccination. However, recurrent infections generally are not associated with serious illness, viremia, or congenital infection.

Clinical Manifestations

Most children and adults with rubella have mild constitutional symptoms such as malaise, headache, myalgias, and arthralgias. The principal clinical manifestation of this illness, of course, is a widely disseminated, nonpruritic, erythematous, maculopapular rash. Postauricular adenopathy and mild conjunctivitis also are common. These clinical manifestations usually are short lived and typically resolve within 3 to 5 days.

Diagnosis

The diagnosis of rubella can usually be established on the basis of the patient's physical examination. If necessary, serologic tests can be used to confirm the diagnosis. IgM antibody usually reaches a peak 7 to 10 days after the onset of illness and then declines over a period of 4 weeks. The serum concentration of IgG antibody usually rises more slowly, but antibody levels persist throughout the lifetime of the individual. EIA and latex agglutination tests are the most rapid and convenient methods for screening for antibody to rubella.

Congenital Rubella Syndrome

Approximately 10 to 20 percent of women in the United States remain susceptible to rubella and, hence, their fetuses are at risk for serious injury should the mother become infected during pregnancy.

The rubella virus crosses the placenta by hematogenous dissemination, and the frequency of congenital infection is critically dependent on the time of exposure to the virus.[189,194,195] Approximately 50 percent of infants exposed to the virus within 4 weeks of conception will manifest signs of congenital infection. When maternal infection occurs in the second 4-week period after conception, approximately 25 percent of fetuses will be infected. When infection develops in the third month, approximately 10 percent of fetuses will be infected. Beyond this point in time, less than 1 percent of fetuses will be infected.

Of anomalies associated with congenital rubella syndrome, the four most common are deafness (affecting 60 to 75 percent of fetuses), eye defects (10 to 30 percent), central nervous system defects (10 to 25 percent), and cardiac malformations (10 to 20 percent). The most common cardiac abnormality associated with congenital rubella is patent ductus arteriosus, although supravalvular pulmonic stenosis is perhaps the most pathognomonic. Other possible abnormalities include microcephaly, mental retardation, pneumonia, IUGR, hepatosplenomegaly, hemolytic anemia, and thrombocytopenia.[194,195] Detailed ultrasound examination is the best test to determine if serious fetal injury has occurred. Abnormalities that can be identified accurately by ultrasound include IUGR, microcephaly, and cardiac malformations.

The prognosis for infants with congenital rubella syndrome is guarded.[194–196] Approximately 50 percent of affected individuals have to attend schools for the hearing impaired. An additional 25 percent of infected children require at least some special schooling because of hearing impairment, and only 25 percent are able to attend mainstream regular schools.

Obstetric Management

If preconception serologic testing demonstrates they are susceptible, women should be vaccinated with rubella vaccine.[189] When preconception counseling is not possible, all obstetric patients should have a test for rubella at their first prenatal appointment. Women who are susceptible should be counseled to avoid exposure to other individuals who may have viral exanthems.

If a susceptible patient is subsequently exposed to rubella, serologic tests should be obtained to determine whether acute infection has occurred. If acute infection is documented, patients should be counseled about the risk of congenital rubella syndrome. Obviously, specific counseling should be based on the time in gestation when maternal infection occurred. The detection of in utero infection should be reviewed. Patients should be offered the option of pregnancy termination based on the assessed risk of serious fetal injury.[192]

Approximately 95 percent of patients who receive rubella vaccine seroconvert. Antibody levels persist for at least 18 years in more than 90 percent of vaccinees. There are few adverse effects of vaccination, even in adults. Breast-feeding is not a contraindication to vaccination. In addition, the vaccine can be administered in conjunction with other immunoglobulin preparations such as Rh immune globulin.

Women who receive rubella vaccine should practice secure contraception for a minimum of 3 months after vaccination. The maximum theoretical risk of congenital rubella resulting from rubella vaccine in early pregnancy is 1 to 2 percent.

Syphilis

Epidemiology

Syphilis is caused by the spirochete *Treponema pallidum*. Infection occurs primarily as a result of sexual contact. The organism penetrates mucosal barriers and is highly contagious. Infection develops in 10 percent of contacts after a single exposure and in 70 percent after multiple exposures.[208,209] Syphilis may also be transmitted perinatally, with devastating consequences for the fetus.

The prevalence of syphilis in the United States has increased dramatically in recent years, coincident with the upsurge in cases of HIV infection and the growing epidemic of drug abuse. The greatest increase has been in females ages 15 to 24 years, and a disproportionate number of cases have occurred in blacks and Hispanics living in urban areas.[208,209]

Clinical Manifestations and Staging

Syphilis can be divided into four *clinical* categories: primary, secondary, tertiary, and neurosyphilis. In addition, syphilis can present as a latent infection. Latent syphilis is subdivided into early latent (<1 year duration) and late latent (>1 year) infection.[208–210] The incubation period of syphilis ranges from 10 to 90 days. At the end of this period, the characteristic raised, painless chancre appears. In women, the chancre is usually on the cervix or vaginal wall and may not be apparent except on close inspection. The chancre usually heals in 3 to 6 weeks even without specific antimicrobial treatment. The principal disorders that must be considered in the differential diagnosis of primary syphilis are HSV infection, chancroid, trauma, scabies, and carcinoma.

Patients who receive either no treatment or inadequate treatment may develop secondary syphilis 2 to 6 months after their primary infection. The principal clinical manifestation of this stage of the infection is a generalized maculopapular rash that is most obvious on the palms of the hands and soles of the feet. This rash may be confused with disseminated gonococcal infection, measles, rubella, scabies, psoriasis, and drug eruption. Other findings associated with secondary syphilis include mucous patches of the oropharynx and condylomata lata, which are gray, raised papules that appear on the vulva and near the anus. In addition, bone tenderness, iritis, alopecia, and generalized lymphadenopathy also may be present. The lesions of secondary syphilis usually resolve spontaneously in 3 to 6 weeks, even without treatment. Untreated patients then enter a latent phase of their illness. In this phase, infected women pose only a small risk of horizontal transmission of infection to their sexual partner. However, vertical transmission to the fetus still can occur.[208–210]

Approximately one-third of patients with untreated secondary disease ultimately develop tertiary syphilis after an interval of several years. Tertiary syphilis is distinguished by three principal findings: gumma formation, cardiac lesions, and central nervous system abnormalities (neurosyphilis).

Diagnosis

T. pallidum cannot be cultured. It can be identified from overt lesions such as the chancre by darkfield microscopy and fluorescent antibody staining. However, most cases of infection, particularly those in the latent stage, are diagnosed by serology. The initial screening test for syphilis should be a nontreponemal assay such as the Venereal Disease Research Laboratory (VDRL) test or Rapid Plasma Reagin (RPR) test. Several factors can cause biologically false-positive test results, such as collagen vascular disease, bacterial and viral infections, intravenous drug use, multiple blood transfusions, and pregnancy. Accordingly, a positive screening test must be confirmed by a specific treponemal assay such as the fluorescent treponemal antibody absorption test (FTA-ABS) or microhemagglutination assay (MHA-TP). Biologic false-positive treponemal tests have been reported in patients with Lyme disease, leprosy, malaria, mononucleosis, and collagen vascular disease.

Lumbar puncture is indicated when neurosyphilis is suspected and in all patients who are co-infected with syphilis and HIV. Cerebrospinal fluid abnormalities include a mononuclear pleocytosis (10 to 400 cells/mm^3), elevated protein (>45 mg/dl), and a positive VDRL test.[208-210]

Virtually all patients will have a positive serologic test within 4 weeks of their primary infection. With appropriate antibiotic treatment, quantitative nontreponemal tests usually decrease fourfold within 3 months in patients with primary or secondary syphilis. When this decline does not occur, patients should be reevaluated and considered for a second course of treatment. Antibody titers may decline more slowly in patients with more advanced stages of disease. Specific treponemal tests typically remain positive for life even after adequate treatment. Ideally, patients should be followed with quantitative titers for up to 12 to 18 months after their initial infection to determine if they become seronegative.

Perinatal Complications

Syphilis in pregnancy may be associated with an increased risk of fetal demise, IUGR, and preterm delivery.[211] It also may accelerate the course of HIV infection in pregnant women. However, the most frequent, and potentially ominous, complication of syphilis in pregnancy is congenital infection. *T. pallidum* can cross the placenta and infect the fetus *at any stage of gestation.* Up to one-third of fetuses with congenital syphilis are stillborn.[4] The frequency of vertical transmission varies primarily with the stage of maternal disease (Table 22-12). The many possible clinical manifestations of congenital syphilis are summarized in Table 22-13.

The prenatal diagnostic test with the greatest potential for identifying the severely infected fetus is ultrasound. Ultrasound findings suggestive of in utero infec-

Table 22-12   Frequency of Vertical Transmission of Syphilis

Stage of Maternal Infection	Approximate Frequency of Congenital Syphilis (%)
Primary	50
Secondary	50
Early latent	40
Late latent	10
Tertiary	10

Table 22-13   Clinical Manifestations of Congenital Syphilis

Early	Late
Maculopapular rash	Hutchinson teeth
Snuffles (syphilitic rhinitis)	Mulberry molars
Mucous patches	Interstitial keratitis
Hepatosplenomegaly	Deafness
Jaundice	Saddle nose
Pneumonia	Rhagades
Lymphadenopathy	Saber shins
Osteochondritis	Mental retardation
Chorioretinitis	Hydrocephalus
Iritis	Generalized paresis
	Optic nerve atrophy
	Clutton joints (hydrarthosis)

tion include placentomegaly, IUGR, microcephaly, hepatosplenomegaly, and hydrops.

Treatment

The treatment of syphilis in pregnancy is summarized in Table 22-14.[208-210] Clearly, penicillin is the drug of choice for this infection because of its proven ability to prevent congenital infection in most cases. Patients who have a previous history of an allergic reaction to penicillin should be skin tested to determine if their allergy persists.[208-210] Only approximately 10 percent of patients who report a history of severe allergy to penicillin remain allergic throughout life. They can be reliably identified by testing with major and minor penicillin determinants. If allergy is confirmed, patients should be desensitized with either oral or intravenous regimens.[206,210,213] Desensitization can usually be completed within 4 hours. It is best accomplished in consultation with an allergist and performed with immediate access to emergency resuscitative equipment. Alternative antibiotic regimens are not of proven value for prevention of congenital syphilis or treatment of advanced stages of disease. Accordingly, they should be used only if desensitization is unsuccessful.

Nearly half of the pregnant women receiving penicillin for treatment of syphilis may develop uterine contractions and decreased fetal movement as a result of a Jarisch-Herxheimer reaction. The reaction is particu-

Table 22-14 Recommendations for Treatment of Syphilis in Pregnancy

Stage of Disease	Principal Treatment	Alternate Treatment If Allergic to Penicillin[a]
Primary, secondary, or latent syphilis <1 year's duration	Benzathine penicillin G, 2.4 million units IM × 1[b]	Erythromycin, 500 mg PO qid × 15 days; ceftriaxone, 250 mg IM QD × 10 days
Latent syphilis >1 year's duration	Benzathine penicillin G, 2.4 million units IM weekly × 3	Erythromycin, 500 mg qid × 30 days
Neurosyphilis	Aqueous crystalline penicillin G, 2–4 million units q4h × 10–14 days, followed by benzathine penicillin G, 2.4 million units IM × 1	No regimen of proven value other than penicillin
	Aqueous procaine penicillin G, 2.4 million units IM daily with probenecid, 500 mg PO qid, both for 10–14 days, followed by benzathine penicillin G, 2.4 million units IM × 1	

[a] These regimens should be administered only if desensitization to penicillin is unsuccessful.

[b] In patients who are concurrently infected with HIV, treat as outlined below for late latent or tertiary syphilis. Patients also should have a lumbar puncture to determine if neurosyphilis is present.

larly likely in patients with primary and secondary syphilis. It usually appears 2 to 8 hours after treatment and resolves within 24 hours. There are no reliable clinical or laboratory tests that predict which patients will develop the Jarisch-Herxheimer reaction, and no specific treatment is available.

Toxoplasmosis

Epidemiology

Toxoplasma gondii is a protozoan with three distinct forms: trophozoite, cyst, and oocyst. The life cycle of *T. gondii* is dependent on wild and domestic cats, the only host for the oocyst. The oocyst is formed in the cat intestine and subsequently excreted in the feces. Mammals, such as cows, ingest the oocyst, which is disrupted in the animal's intestine, releasing the invasive trophozoite. The trophozoite then is disseminated throughout the body, ultimately forming cysts in brain and muscle.

Human infection occurs when infected meat is ingested or when food is contaminated by cat feces. Infection rates are highest in areas of poor sanitation and crowded living conditions. Stray cats and domestic cats that eat raw meat are most likely to carry the parasite. The cyst is destroyed by heat. For this reason, meat should be thoroughly cooked before consumption.[215]

Approximately 40 to 50 percent of adults in the United States have antibody to this organism. The frequency of seroconversion during pregnancy is 5 percent or less. Clinically significant congenital toxoplasmosis occurs in approximately 1/8,000 pregnancies.

Clinical Manifestations

The ingested organism invades across the intestinal epithelium and spreads hematogenously throughout the body. Clinical manifestations of infection are the result of direct organ damage and the subsequent immunologic response to parasitemia and cell death.

Most infections in humans are asymptomatic. Even in the absence of symptoms, however, patients may have evidence of multiorgan involvement, and clinical disease can follow a long period of asymptomatic infection. Symptomatic toxoplasmosis usually presents as an illness similar to mononucleosis.[215,216]

Diagnosis

The diagnosis of toxoplasmosis can be confirmed by serologic and histologic methods. Serologic tests that suggest an acute infection include detection of IgM-specific antibody, demonstration of an extremely high IgG antibody titer, and documentation of IgG sero-conversion from negative to positive.[215,216] Because serologic assays for toxoplasmosis are not well standardized, when initial laboratory tests indicate that an acute infection has occurred, repeat serology should be performed in a well-recognized reference laboratory.

Congenital Toxoplasmosis

Congenital infection can occur if a woman develops *acute* toxoplasmosis during pregnancy. Chronic or latent infection is unlikely to cause fetal injury except perhaps in an immunosuppressed patient. Approximately 40 percent of neonates born to mothers with acute toxoplasmosis show evidence of infection. Congenital infection is most likely to occur when maternal infection develops in the third trimester. Less than half of affected infants are symptomatic at birth. The clinical manifestations of congenital toxoplasmosis are quite varied.[216–218]

The most valuable tests for antenatal diagnosis of congenital toxoplasmosis are ultrasound, cordocentesis, and amniocentesis. Ultrasound findings suggestive of infection include ventriculomegaly, intracranial calcifications, microcephaly, ascites, hepatosplenomegaly, and IUGR. Fetal blood samples can be tested for IgM-specific antibody after 20 weeks' gestation. Fetal blood and amniotic fluid can be inoculated into mice, and the organism can subsequently be recovered from the blood of infected animals. *T. gondii* can also be identified in amniotic fluid using a polymerase chain reaction test.

Management

Toxoplasmosis in the immunocompetent adult is usually an asymptomatic or self-limited illness and does not require treatment. However, treatment is indicated when acute toxoplasmosis occurs during pregnancy. Treatment of the mother reduces the risk of congenital infection and decreases the late sequelae of infection.[217,218] Pyrimethamine is not recommended for use during the first trimester of pregnancy because of possible teratogenicity. Sulfonamides can be used alone, but single-agent therapy appears to be less effective than combination therapy. Spiramycin, a macrolide antibiotic, is available for use in the United States through the CDC.

In the management of the pregnant patient, *preven-*

tion of acute toxoplasmosis is of paramount importance. Pregnant women should be advised to avoid contact with stray cats or cat litter. They should always wash their hands after preparing meat for cooking and should never eat raw or rare meat. Fruits and vegetables also should be washed carefully to remove possible contamination by oocysts.

Varicella

Epidemiology

Natural varicella infection occurs primarily during early childhood. Less than 10 percent of cases occur in individuals over 10 years of age; however, older patients account for more than 50 percent of all fatalities due to varicella. Varicella is transmitted by direct contact and respiratory droplets. The virus is highly infectious, and approximately 95 percent of susceptible household contacts become infected following exposure. The incubation period is 10 to 14 days. Patients are infectious from 1 day before the outbreak of the rash until all of the cutaneous lesions have dried and crusted over. Immunity to varicella is usually lifelong.[221]

Herpes zoster infection occurs as a result of reactivation of latent virus infection in a patient who already has had varicella. Because of the presence in the host of virus-specific antibody, herpes zoster is usually a much less serious disorder than varicella and rarely poses a major risk to either the mother or her baby unless the former is immunocompromised.

Clinical Manifestations

The usual clinical manifestations of varicella are fever, malaise, and a skin rash. The characteristic skin lesions usually begin as pruritic macules, which appear in crops. The macules progress to papules, then to vesicles, and finally to crusts. The lesions initially appear on the trunk and then spread centripetally to the extremities.

In adults, two life-threatening sequelae may develop: encephalitis and pneumonia. The former occurs in 1 percent or less of pregnant women; the latter may develop in up to 20 percent of patients. Prior to the development of acyclovir, the mortality associated with varicella pneumonia in pregnancy approached 40 percent.[221,222]

Diagnosis

The diagnosis of varicella is usually made by clinical examination alone. Serologic assays are of primary value in assessing a patient's susceptibility to varicella immediately following exposure. The two most useful antibody assays are the fluorescent anti-membrane antibody test (FAMA) and the ELISA. Both assays show sustained elevations, usually lifelong, following natural infection.[221,223]

Management of Maternal Infection

The optimal approach to maternal varicella infection is *prevention*. All women of reproductive age should be assessed for immunity to varicella, ideally before they attempt pregnancy. Susceptible patients, particularly those who are likely to be exposed to varicella either at home or in the workplace, should be offered the new varicella vaccine. Vaccine recipients should use effective contraception for 3 months after immunization. The vaccine is contraindicated in patients who are pregnant.

Patients should be questioned about varicella immunity at the time of their first prenatal appointment. If uncertain about prior infection, an IgG varicella serology should be performed. If the serology is positive, the patient can be reassured that she is immune and that she and her fetus are not at risk should subsequent exposure occur. If the serology is negative, the patient should be counseled to avoid exposure to individuals who may have varicella or herpes zoster.

Unfortunately, however, the more common situation that the obstetrician encounters is a pregnant patient who has been exposed acutely to an individual who "may have had chickenpox." The clinician's first step is to verify that the index patient actually has varicella. If infection is confirmed, the pregnant woman should then be questioned about immunity to varicella. If immunity cannot be documented by history, an IgG varicella serology should be obtained, and the result should be reviewed within 24 to 48 hours of exposure. If the serology is positive, the patient can be reassured that her fetus is not at risk. If the serology is negative, the patient should receive varicella-zoster immune globulin (VZIG). This preparation is 60 to 80 percent effective in preventing infection if given within 96 hours of exposure. The dose of VZIG is one vial (125 units)/10 kg of actual body weight, up to a maximum of five vials. In problematic cases, if waiting for the varicella serology will delay administration of VZIG for more than

96 hours after exposure, the immunization should be given without confirmatory serology.[221,225,226]

Patients who receive VZIG, as well as those who present for care too late for passive immunoprophylaxis, should be counseled about the clinical signs and symptoms of varicella. In particular, they must be advised to report immediately if early manifestations of varicella encephalitis or pneumonia develop. If serious sequelae occur, the patient should be admitted to the hospital for intravenous therapy with acyclovir. The recommended dose of acyclovir is 500 mg/m^2 every 8 hours, and treatment should be continued until the patient's systemic symptoms have resolved and the cutaneous lesions have begun to crust.

Congenital Infection

Congenital varicella results primarily from hematogenous dissemination of virus across the placenta. Congenital infection may lead to spontaneous abortion, intrauterine fetal demise, and varicella embryopathy manifested by cutaneous scars, limb hypoplasia, muscle atrophy, malformed digits, psychomotor retardation, microcephaly, cortical atrophy, cataracts, chorioretinitis, and microphthalmia.[221] The frequency of varicella embryopathy associated with infection in the first 20 weeks of pregnancy is 1 to 2 percent.

Ultrasonography is the preferred diagnostic modality to detect fetal infection. Sonographic findings suggestive of fetal varicella include polyhydramnios; hydrops; hyperechogenic foci in the abdominal organs, particularly the liver; cardiac malformations; limb deformities; microcephaly; and IUGR.[221]

Neonatal Infection

The final major complication of varicella infection in pregnancy is neonatal varicella. Infection of the neonate occurs in 10 to 20 percent of infants whose mothers have acute varicella within the period from 5 days before to 2 days after delivery.[221] Infection usually results from hematogenous dissemination of virus across the placenta at a time when no maternal antibody is present to provide passive immunity to the fetus.

The clinical course of neonatal varicella can be variable in progression and severity. The infant usually becomes symptomatic within 5 to 10 days of delivery. Some neonates have only scattered skin lesions and no systemic signs of illness. Others have a more severe acute illness associated with extensive cutaneous lesions, visceral infection, and pneumonia. In reports published before the widespread availability of acyclovir, the mortality associated with neonatal varicella was 20 to 30 percent.[221]

To prevent neonatal varicella, an effort should be made to delay delivery until 5 to 7 days after the onset of maternal illness. If delay is not possible, the neonate should receive VZIG (one vial, 125 units) immediately after birth. An important additional preventive measure is isolation of the infant from the mother until all vesicular lesions likely to come in contact with the infant have crusted over.[221,226]

Key Points

- Vaginal infections occur commonly in pregnancy. Moniliasis is best treated with topical antifungal compounds such as miconazole, terconazole, or clotrimazole. Metronidazole is the only antibiotic with uniform efficacy against trichomonas. Oral metronidazole is the most cost-effective agent for treatment of bacterial vaginosis.

- Urinary tract infections in pregnancy are caused primarily by E. coli, K. pneumoniae, and Proteus species. Pyelonephritis is a particularly serious infection in pregnancy because it may be complicated by preterm labor, bacteremia, and ARDS.

- Chorioamnionitis and puerperal endometritis are caused by multiple aerobic and anaerobic organisms. Antibiotic therapy should be directed against group B streptococci, aerobic gram-negative bacilli, and Bacteroides and Prevotella species.

- Primary maternal CMV infection during pregnancy is associated with a 40 percent risk of fetal infection. Ten to 15 percent of infected infants are severely affected at birth. Ultrasonography and amniotic fluid viral culture are the best methods for diagnosing fetal infection.

- All pregnant women should be screened for hepatitis B infections. Infants delivered to seropositive mothers should receive both HBIG and HBV shortly after birth.

- HSV infection may be classified as *primary, nonprimary,* and *recurrent. Primary infection* poses the major risk of perinatal transmission. Women with prodromal symptoms or visible lesions should be delivered by cesarean; asymptomatic women may deliver vaginally.

- All pregnant women should be screened for HIV infection. All infected patients should be treated with antiviral chemotherapy to reduce the risk of perinatal transmission and slow the rate of disease progression in the mother.

- Maternal parvovirus infection may result in fetal hydrops. Intrauterine transfusion may be a lifesaving intervention for the hydropic fetus.
- Primary maternal toxoplasmosis poses a serious risk of fetal infection. Fetal infection is best diagnosed by DNA analysis of amniotic fluid. Spiramycin is effective in treating both maternal and fetal infection.
- Varicella in pregnancy presents serious risk to both the mother and her infant. Susceptible women exposed to varicella should be treated with VZIG. Neonates delivered to mothers with acute varicella also should receive immunoprophylaxis with VZIG. Following delivery, susceptible women should be vaccinated with the new live virus vaccine, provided they are willing to use effective contraception for 3 months.

Appendices: Obstetric Ultrasound Measurement Tables

With
Obstetric Doppler

Compiled by:

Pamela M. Foy, BS, RDMS

Clinical Coordinator of Ultrasound Services
Department of Obstetrics and Gynecology
The Ohio State University Hospitals
Columbus, Ohio

First Trimester

Appendix 1   Crown–Rump Length Measurement

Gestational Age (weeks)	Mean Predicted Crown–Rump Length (mm)	Gestational Age (weeks)	Mean Predicted Crown–Rump Length (mm)
6.3	6.7	10.1	34
6.4	7.4	10.3	35.5
6.6	8.0	10.4	36.9
6.7	8.7	10.6	38.4
6.9	9.5	10.7	39.9
7.0	10.2	10.9	41.4
7.1	11.0	11.0	43
7.3	11.8	11.1	44.6
7.4	12.6	11.3	46.2
7.6	13.5	11.4	47.8
7.7	14.4	11.6	49.5
7.9	15.3	11.7	51.2
8.0	16.3	11.9	52.9
8.1	17.3	12.0	54.7
8.3	18.3	12.1	56.5
8.4	19.3	12.3	58.3
8.6	20.4	12.4	60.1
8.7	21.5	12.6	62
8.9	22.6	12.7	63.9
9.0	23.8	12.9	65.9
9.1	25.0	13.0	67.8
9.3	26.2	13.1	69.3
9.4	27.4	13.3	71.8
9.6	28.7	13.4	73.9
9.7	30.0	13.6	76.0
9.9	31.3	13.7	78.1
10.0	32.7	13.9	80.2
		14.0	82.4

From Robinson HP, Fleming JEE: A critical evaluation of sonar crown-rump length measurements. Br J Obstet Gynaecol 82:702, 1975, with permission.

Appendix 2   Gestational Sac Measurement

Gestational Age (weeks)	Mean Predicted Gestational Sac (mm)	Gestational Age (weeks)	Mean Predicted Gestational Sac (mm)
5.0	10	8.8	36
5.2	11	8.9	37
5.3	12	9.0	38
5.5	13	9.2	39
5.6	14	9.3	40
5.8	15	9.5	41
5.9	16	9.6	42
6.0	17	9.7	43
6.2	18	9.9	44
6.3	19	10.0	45
6.5	20	10.2	46
6.6	21	10.3	47
6.8	22	10.5	48
6.9	23	10.6	49
7.0	24	10.7	50
7.2	25	10.9	51
7.3	26	11.0	52
7.5	27	11.2	53
7.6	28	11.3	54
7.8	29	11.5	55
7.9	30	11.6	56
8.0	31	11.7	57
8.2	32	11.9	58
8.3	33	12.0	59
8.5	34	12.2	60
8.6	35		

From Hellman LM, Kobayashi M, Fillisti L et al: Growth and development of the human fetus prior to the twentieth week of gestation. Am J Obstet Gynecol 103:789, 1969, with permission.

Second- and Third-Trimester

Appendix 3   Transverse Cerebellar Diameter

Gestational Age (weeks)	Cerebellum (mm) by Percentile				
	10	25	50	75	90
15	10	12	14	15	16
16	14	16	16	16	17
17	16	17	17	18	18
18	17	18	18	19	19
19	18	18	19	19	22
20	18	19	20	20	22
21	19	20	22	23	24
22	21	23	23	24	24
23	22	23	24	25	26
24	22	24	25	27	28
25	23	21.5	28	28	29
26	25	28	29	30	32
27	26	28.5	30	31	32
28	27	30	31	32	34
29	29	32	34	36	38
30	31	32	35	37	40
31	32	35	38	39	43
32	33	36	38	40	42
33	32	36	40	43	44
34	33	38	40	41	44
35	31	37	40.5	43	47
36	36	29	43	52	55
37	37	37	45	52	55
38	40	40	48.5	52	55
39	52	52	52	55	55

From Goldstein I, Reece EA, Pilu G et al: Cerebellar measurements with ultrasonography in the evaluation of fetal growth and development. Am J Obstet Gynecol 156:1065, 1987, with permission.

Appendix 4 Composite Biparietal Diameter (BPD)

BPD (mm)	Gestational Age (weeks)			BPD (mm)	Gestational Age (weeks)		
	10 %ile	50 %ile	90 %ile		10 %ile	50 %ile	90 %ile
20	12	12	12	61	22.6	24.2	25.8
21	12	12	12	62	23.1	24.6	26.1
22	12.2	12.7	13.2	63	23.4	24.9	26.4
23	12.4	13	13.6	64	23.8	25.3	26.8
24	12.6	13.2	13.8	65	24.1	25.6	27.1
25	12.9	13.5	14.1	66	24.5	26	27.5
26	13.1	13.7	14.3	67	25	26.4	27.8
27	13.4	14	14.6	68	25.3	26.7	28.1
28	13.6	14.3	15	69	25.8	27.1	28.4
29	13.9	14.5	15.2	70	26.3	27.5	28.7
30	14.1	14.8	15.5	71	26.7	27.9	29.1
31	14.3	15.1	15.9	72	27.2	28.3	29.4
32	14.5	15.3	16.1	73	27.6	28.7	29.8

(continued)

Appendix 4 (Continued)

BPD (mm)	Gestational Age (weeks)			BPD (mm)	Gestational Age (weeks)		
	10 %ile	50 %ile	90 %ile		10 %ile	50 %ile	90 %ile
33	14.7	15.6	16.5	74	28.1	29.1	30.1
34	15	15.9	16.8	75	28.5	29.5	30.5
35	15.2	16.2	17.2	76	29	30	31
36	15.4	16.4	17.4	77	29.2	30.3	31.4
37	15.6	16.7	17.8	78	29.6	30.8	32
38	15.9	17	18.1	79	29.9	31.1	32.5
39	16.1	17.3	18.5	80	30.2	31.6	33
40	16.4	17.6	18.8	81	30.7	32.1	33.5
41	16.5	17.9	19.3	82	31.2	32.6	34
42	16.6	18.1	19.8	83	31.5	33	34.5
43	16.8	18.4	20.2	84	31.9	33.4	35.1
44	16.9	18.8	20.7	85	32.3	34	35.7
45	17	19.1	21.2	86	32.8	34.3	36.2
46	17.4	19.4	21.4	87	33.4	35	36.6

47	17.8	19.7	21.6
48	18.2	20	21.8
49	18.6	20.3	22
50	19	20.6	22.2
51	19.3	20.9	22.5
52	19.5	21.2	22.9
53	19.8	21.5	23.2
54	20.1	21.9	23.7
55	20.4	22.2	24
56	20.7	22.5	24.3
57	21.1	22.8	24.5
58	21.5	23.2	24.9
59	21.9	23.5	25.1
60	22.3	23.8	25.5

88	33.9	35.4	37.1
89	34.6	36.1	37.6
90	35.1	36.6	38.1
91	35.9	37.2	38.5
92	36.7	37.8	38.9
93	37.3	38.8	39.3
94	37.9	39	40.1
95	38.5	39.7	40.9
96	39.1	40.6	41.5
97	39.9	41	42.1
98	40.5	41.8	43.1

From Kurtz A, Wapner R, Kurtz R et al: Analysis of biparietal diameter as an accurate indicator of gestation age. J Clin Ultrasound 8:319, 1980, with permission.

Appendix 5   Head and Abdominal Circumference: HC/AC Ratio

Gestational Age (weeks)	Head Circumference HC (mm)			Abdominal Circumference AC (mm)			HC/AC Ratio		
	− 2SD	Mean	+ 2SD	− 2SD	Mean	+ 2SD	− 2SD	Mean	+ 2SD
12	51	70	89	31	56	81	1.12	1.22	1.31
13	65	89	103	44	69	94	1.11	1.21	1.30
14	79	98	117	56	81	106	1.11	1.20	1.30
15	92	111	130	68	93	118	1.10	1.19	1.29
16	105	124	143	80	105	130	1.09	1.18	1.28
17	118	137	156	92	117	142	1.08	1.18	1.27
18	131	150	169	104	129	154	1.07	1.17	1.26
19	144	163	182	116	141	166	1.06	1.16	1.25
20	156	175	194	127	152	177	1.06	1.15	1.24
21	168	187	206	139	164	189	1.05	1.14	1.24
22	180	199	218	150	175	200	1.04	1.13	1.23
23	191	210	229	161	186	211	1.03	1.12	1.22

24	202	221	240	172	197	220	1.02	1.12	1.21
25	213	232	251	183	208	233	1.01	1.11	1.20
26	223	242	261	194	219	244	1.00	1.10	1.19
27	233	252	271	204	229	254	1.00	1.09	1.18
28	243	262	281	215	240	265	0.99	1.08	1.18
29	252	271	290	225	250	275	0.98	1.07	1.17
30	261	280	299	235	260	285	0.97	1.07	1.16
31	270	289	308	245	270	295	0.96	1.06	1.15
32	278	297	316	255	280	305	0.95	1.05	1.14
33	285	304	323	265	290	315	0.95	1.04	1.13
34	293	312	331	275	300	325	0.94	1.03	1.13
35	299	318	337	284	309	334	0.93	1.02	1.12
36	306	325	344	293	318	343	0.92	1.01	1.11
37	311	330	349	302	327	352	0.91	1.01	1.10
38	319	336	355	311	336	361	0.90	1.00	1.09
39	322	341	360	320	345	370	0.89	0.99	1.08
40	326	345	364	329	354	379	0.89	0.98	1.08

From Hadlock FP et al: Appl Radiol, 12:28, 1983, with permission.

Appendix 6   Normal Values for the Arm

Gestational Age (weeks)	Humerus (mm) by Percentile			Ulna (mm) by Percentile			Radius (mm) by Percentile		
	5	50	95	5	50	95	5	50	95
12		9			7			7	
13	6	11	16	5	10	15	6	10	14
14	9	14	19	8	13	18	8	13	17
15	12	17	22	11	16	21	11	15	20
16	15	20	25	13	18	23	13	18	22
17	18	22	27	16	21	26	14	20	26
18	20	25	30	19	24	29	15	22	29
19	23	28	33	21	26	31	20	24	29
20	25	30	35	24	29	34	22	27	32
21	28	33	38	26	31	36	24	29	33
22	30	35	40	28	33	38	27	31	34
23	33	38	42	31	36	41	26	32	39
24	35	40	45	33	38	43	26	34	42
25	37	42	47	35	40	45	31	36	41

26	39	44	49	37	42	47	32	37	43
27	41	46	51	39	44	49	33	39	45
28	43	48	53	41	46	51	33	40	48
29	45	50	55	43	48	53	36	42	47
30	47	51	56	44	49	54	36	43	49
31	48	53	58	46	51	56	38	44	50
32	50	55	60	48	53	58	37	45	53
33	51	56	61	49	54	59	41	46	51
34	53	58	63	51	56	61	40	47	53
35	54	59	64	52	57	62	41	48	53
36	56	61	65	53	58	63	39	48	54
37	57	62	67	55	60	65	45	49	57
38	59	63	68	56	61	66	45	49	53
39	60	65	70	57	62	67	45	50	54
40	61	66	71	58	63	68	46	50	55

From Jeanty P: Fetal limb biometry (letter). Radiology 147:602, 1983, with permission.

Appendix 7   Normal Values for the Leg

Gestational Age (weeks)	Femur (mm) by Percentile			Tibia (mm) by Percentile			Fibula (mm) by Percentile		
	5	50	95	5	50	95	5	50	95
12	4	8	13		7			6	
13	6	11	16		10			9	
14	9	14	18	7	12	17	6	12	19
15	12	17	21	9	15	20	9	15	21
16	15	20	24	12	17	22	13	18	23
17	18	23	27	15	20	25	13	21	28
18	21	25	30	17	22	27	15	23	31
19	24	28	33	20	25	30	19	26	33
20	26	31	36	22	27	33	21	28	36
21	29	34	38	25	30	35	24	31	37
22	32	36	41	27	32	38	27	33	39
23	35	39	44	30	35	40	28	35	42
24	37	42	46	32	37	42	29	37	45
25	40	44	49	34	40	45	34	40	45

26	42	47	51	37	42	47	36	42	47
27	45	49	54	39	44	49	37	44	50
28	47	52	56	41	46	51	38	45	53
29	50	54	59	43	48	53	41	47	54
30	52	56	61	45	50	55	43	49	56
31	54	59	63	47	52	57	42	51	59
32	56	61	65	48	54	59	42	52	63
33	58	63	67	50	55	60	46	54	62
34	60	65	69	52	57	62	46	55	65
35	62	67	71	53	58	64	51	57	62
36	64	68	73	55	60	65	54	58	63
37	65	70	74	56	61	67	54	59	65
38	67	71	76	58	63	68	56	61	65
39	68	73	77	59	64	69	56	62	67
40	70	74	79	61	66	71	59	63	67

From Jeanty P: Fetal limb biometry (letter). Radiology 147:602, 1983, with permission.

Appendix 8   Estimated Fetal Weight (g) Based on Biparietal Diameter (BPD) and Abdominal Circumference

BPD (mm)	Abdominal Circumference (mm)																
	155	160	165	170	175	180	185	190	195	200	205	210	215	220	225	230	235
31	224	234	244	255	267	279	291	304	318	332	346	362	378	395	412	431	450
32	231	241	251	263	274	286	299	312	326	340	355	371	388	406	423	441	461
33	237	248	259	270	282	294	307	321	335	349	365	381	397	415	433	452	472
34	244	255	266	278	290	302	316	329	344	359	374	391	408	425	444	463	483
35	251	262	274	285	298	311	324	338	353	368	384	401	418	436	455	475	495
36	259	270	281	294	306	319	333	347	362	378	394	411	429	447	466	486	507
37	266	278	290	302	315	328	342	357	372	388	404	422	440	458	478	496	519
38	274	286	298	310	324	337	352	368	382	398	415	432	451	470	490	510	532
39	282	294	306	319	333	347	361	376	392	409	426	444	462	482	502	523	545
40	290	303	315	328	342	356	371	386	403	419	437	455	474	494	514	536	558
41	299	311	324	338	352	366	381	397	413	430	448	467	486	506	527	549	572
42	308	320	333	347	361	376	392	408	424	442	460	479	498	519	540	562	585
43	317	330	343	357	371	387	402	419	436	453	472	491	511	532	554	576	600
44	326	339	353	367	382	397	413	430	447	465	484	504	524	545	567	590	614
45	335	349	363	377	393	408	425	442	459	478	497	517	538	559	581	605	629
46	345	359	373	386	404	420	436	454	472	490	510	530	551	573	596	620	644
47	355	369	384	399	415	431	448	466	484	503	524	544	565	588	611	635	660

48	366	380	395	410	426	443	460	478	497	517	537	558	580	602	626	650	676
49	376	391	406	422	438	455	473	491	510	530	551	572	594	617	641	666	692
50	387	402	418	434	451	468	486	505	524	544	565	587	610	633	657	683	709
51	399	414	430	446	463	481	499	518	538	559	580	602	625	649	674	699	726
52	410	426	442	459	476	494	513	532	552	573	595	618	641	665	690	717	744
53	422	438	455	472	489	508	527	547	567	589	611	634	657	682	708	734	762
54	435	451	468	485	503	522	541	561	582	604	627	650	674	699	725	752	780
55	447	464	481	499	517	536	556	577	598	620	643	667	691	717	743	771	799
56	461	477	495	513	532	551	571	592	614	636	660	684	709	735	762	789	818
57	474	491	509	527	547	566	587	608	630	653	677	701	727	753	780	809	838
58	488	505	524	542	562	582	603	625	647	670	695	719	745	772	800	829	858
59	502	520	539	558	578	598	619	642	664	688	713	738	764	792	820	849	879
60	517	535	554	573	594	615	636	659	682	706	731	757	784	811	840	870	900
61	532	550	570	590	610	632	654	677	700	725	750	777	804	832	861	891	922
62	547	566	586	606	627	649	672	695	719	744	770	797	824	853	882	913	945
63	563	583	603	624	645	667	690	714	738	764	790	817	845	874	904	935	967
64	580	600	620	641	663	686	709	733	758	784	811	838	867	896	927	958	991

(continued)

Appendix 8 *(Continued)*

BPD (mm)	Abdominal Circumference (mm)																
	155	160	165	170	175	180	185	190	195	200	205	210	215	220	225	230	235
65	597	617	638	659	682	705	728	753	778	805	832	860	889	919	950	982	1015
66	614	635	656	678	701	724	748	773	799	826	853	882	911	942	973	1006	1039
67	632	653	675	697	720	744	769	794	820	848	876	905	935	965	997	1030	1065
68	651	672	694	717	740	765	790	816	842	870	898	928	958	990	1022	1056	1090
69	670	691	714	737	761	786	811	838	865	893	922	952	983	1015	1048	1082	1117
70	689	711	734	758	782	807	833	860	888	916	946	976	1008	1040	1074	1108	1144
71	709	732	755	779	804	830	856	883	912	941	971	1002	1033	1066	1100	1135	1171
72	730	763	777	801	827	853	880	907	936	965	996	1027	1060	1093	1128	1163	1200
73	751	775	799	824	850	876	904	932	961	991	1022	1054	1087	1121	1156	1192	1229
74	773	797	822	847	874	901	928	957	987	1017	1049	1081	1114	1149	1184	1221	1259
75	796	820	845	871	898	925	954	983	1013	1044	1076	1109	1143	1178	1214	1251	1289
76	819	844	870	896	923	951	980	1009	1040	1072	1104	1137	1172	1207	1244	1281	1320
77	843	868	894	921	949	977	1007	1037	1068	1100	1133	1167	1202	1238	1275	1313	1352
78	868	894	920	947	975	1004	1034	1065	1096	1129	1162	1197	1232	1269	1306	1345	1385
79	893	919	946	974	1003	1032	1062	1094	1126	1159	1193	1228	1264	1301	1339	1378	1418
80	919	946	973	1002	1031	1061	1091	1123	1156	1189	1224	1259	1296	1333	1372	1412	1453

81	946	973	1001	1030	1060	1090	1121	1153	1187	1221	1256	1292	1329	1367	1406	1446	1488
82	974	1001	1030	1059	1089	1120	1152	1185	1218	1253	1288	1325	1363	1401	1441	1482	1524
83	1002	1030	1059	1089	1120	1151	1183	1217	1251	1286	1322	1359	1397	1436	1477	1518	1561
84	1032	1060	1090	1120	1151	1183	1216	1249	1284	1320	1356	1394	1433	1473	1513	1555	1599
85	1062	1091	1121	1151	1183	1216	1249	1283	1318	1355	1392	1430	1469	1510	1551	1594	1637
86	1093	1122	1153	1184	1216	1249	1283	1318	1354	1390	1428	1467	1507	1548	1589	1633	1677
87	1125	1155	1186	1218	1250	1284	1318	1353	1390	1427	1465	1505	1545	1586	1629	1673	1717
88	1157	1188	1220	1252	1285	1319	1354	1390	1427	1465	1504	1543	1584	1626	1669	1714	1759
89	1191	1222	1254	1287	1321	1356	1391	1428	1465	1503	1543	1583	1625	1667	1711	1756	1802
90	1226	1258	1290	1324	1358	1393	1429	1456	1504	1543	1583	1624	1666	1709	1753	1799	1845
91	1262	1294	1327	1361	1396	1432	1468	1506	1544	1584	1624	1666	1708	1752	1797	1843	1890
92	1299	1332	1365	1400	1435	1471	1508	1546	1586	1626	1667	1709	1752	1796	1841	1886	1936
93	1337	1370	1404	1439	1475	1512	1550	1588	1628	1668	1710	1753	1796	1841	1887	1934	1982
94	1376	1410	1444	1480	1516	1554	1592	1631	1671	1712	1755	1798	1842	1887	1934	1982	2030
95	1416	1450	1486	1522	1559	1597	1635	1675	1716	1758	1800	1844	1889	1935	1982	2030	2080
96	1457	1492	1528	1565	1602	1641	1680	1720	1762	1804	1847	1892	1937	1984	2031	2080	2130
97	1500	1535	1572	1609	1647	1686	1726	1767	1809	1852	1895	1940	1986	2033	2082	2131	2181
98	1544	1580	1617	1654	1693	1733	1773	1815	1857	1900	1945	1990	2037	2085	2133	2183	2234
99	1589	1625	1663	1701	1740	1781	1822	1864	1907	1951	1996	2042	2089	2137	2186	2237	2288
100	1635	1672	1710	1749	1789	1830	1871	1914	1958	2002	2048	2094	2142	2191	2241	2292	2344

(continued)

Appendix 8   (Continued)

BPD (mm)	Abdominal Circumference (mm)																
	240	245	250	255	260	265	270	275	280	285	290	295	300	305	310	315	320
31	470	491	513	536	559	584	610	638	666	696	726	759	793	828	865	903	943
32	481	502	525	548	572	597	624	651	680	710	742	774	809	844	882	921	961
33	493	514	537	560	585	611	638	666	693	725	757	790	825	861	899	938	979
34	504	526	549	573	596	624	652	680	710	740	773	806	841	878	916	956	996
35	517	539	562	587	612	638	666	695	725	756	789	823	858	896	934	975	1017
36	529	552	575	600	626	653	681	710	740	772	805	840	876	913	953	993	1036
37	542	565	589	614	640	667	696	725	756	788	822	857	893	931	971	1012	1056
38	554	578	602	626	654	682	711	741	772	805	839	874	911	950	990	1032	1076
39	568	592	616	642	669	697	727	757	789	822	856	892	930	969	1009	1052	1096
40	581	606	631	657	684	713	743	773	806	839	874	911	949	988	1029	1072	1117
41	595	620	645	672	700	729	759	790	828	857	892	929	968	1008	1049	1093	1138
42	609	634	660	688	716	745	776	807	841	875	911	948	987	1028	1070	1114	1159
43	624	649	676	703	732	762	793	825	859	893	930	968	1007	1048	1091	1135	1181
44	639	665	692	719	749	779	810	843	877	912	949	987	1027	1069	1112	1157	1204
45	654	680	708	736	765	796	828	861	896	932	969	1008	1048	1090	1134	1179	1226
46	670	696	724	753	783	814	846	880	915	951	989	1028	1069	1112	1156	1202	1249
47	686	713	741	770	801	832	865	899	934	971	1010	1049	1091	1134	1178	1225	1273

48	702	730	758	788	819	851	884	919	954	992	1031	1071	1113	1156	1201	1248	1297
49	719	747	776	806	837	870	903	938	975	1013	1052	1093	1135	1179	1225	1272	1322
50	736	765	794	824	856	889	923	959	996	1034	1074	1115	1158	1203	1249	1297	1347
51	754	783	812	843	876	909	944	980	1017	1056	1096	1138	1181	1226	1273	1322	1372
52	772	801	831	863	895	929	964	1001	1039	1078	1119	1161	1205	1251	1298	1347	1398
53	790	820	851	883	916	950	986	1023	1061	1101	1142	1185	1229	1276	1323	1373	1425
54	809	839	870	903	936	971	1007	1045	1084	1124	1166	1209	1254	1301	1349	1399	1452
55	828	859	891	924	958	993	1030	1068	1107	1148	1190	1234	1279	1327	1376	1426	1479
56	848	879	911	945	979	1015	1052	1091	1131	1172	1215	1259	1305	1353	1402	1454	1507
57	869	900	933	966	1001	1038	1075	1114	1155	1197	1240	1285	1332	1380	1430	1482	1535
58	889	921	954	989	1024	1061	1099	1139	1180	1222	1266	1311	1358	1407	1458	1510	1564
59	911	943	977	1011	1047	1085	1123	1163	1205	1248	1292	1338	1386	1435	1486	1539	1594
60	932	965	999	1035	1071	1109	1148	1189	1231	1274	1319	1366	1414	1464	1515	1569	1624
61	955	988	1023	1058	1095	1134	1173	1214	1257	1301	1346	1393	1442	1493	1545	1599	1655
62	977	1011	1046	1083	1120	1159	1199	1241	1284	1328	1374	1422	1471	1522	1575	1630	1686
63	1001	1035	1071	1107	1145	1185	1226	1268	1311	1356	1403	1451	1501	1552	1606	1661	1718
64	1025	1059	1096	1133	1171	1211	1253	1295	1339	1385	1432	1481	1531	1583	1637	1693	1751
65	1049	1084	1121	1159	1198	1238	1280	1323	1368	1414	1462	1511	1562	1615	1669	1725	1784
66	1074	1110	1147	1185	1225	1266	1308	1352	1397	1444	1492	1542	1594	1647	1702	1759	1817
67	1100	1136	1174	1213	1253	1294	1337	1381	1427	1474	1523	1574	1626	1679	1735	1792	1852
68	1126	1163	1201	1241	1281	1323	1367	1411	1458	1505	1555	1606	1658	1713	1769	1827	1887
69	1153	1190	1229	1269	1310	1353	1397	1442	1489	1537	1587	1639	1692	1747	1803	1862	1922
70	1181	1219	1258	1298	1340	1383	1427	1473	1521	1570	1620	1672	1726	1781	1839	1898	1959

(continued)

Appendix 8 (Continued)

BPD (mm)	Abdominal Circumference (mm)																
	240	245	250	255	260	265	270	275	280	285	290	295	300	305	310	315	320
71	1209	1247	1287	1328	1370	1414	1459	1505	1553	1603	1654	1706	1761	1817	1875	1934	1996
72	1238	1277	1317	1358	1401	1445	1491	1538	1586	1636	1688	1741	1796	1853	1911	1971	2044
73	1267	1307	1348	1390	1433	1478	1524	1571	1620	1671	1723	1777	1832	1890	1948	2009	2072
74	1297	1338	1379	1421	1465	1511	1557	1605	1655	1706	1759	1813	1869	1927	1987	2048	2111
75	1328	1369	1411	1454	1499	1544	1592	1640	1690	1742	1795	1850	1907	1965	2025	2087	2151
76	1360	1401	1444	1487	1533	1579	1627	1676	1727	1779	1833	1888	1945	2004	2065	2127	2192
77	1393	1434	1477	1522	1567	1614	1663	1712	1764	1816	1871	1927	1985	2044	2105	2168	2233
78	1426	1468	1512	1557	1603	1650	1699	1749	1801	1855	1910	1966	2025	2085	2146	2210	2275
79	1460	1503	1547	1592	1639	1687	1737	1787	1840	1894	1949	2006	2065	2126	2188	2252	2318
80	1495	1538	1583	1629	1676	1725	1775	1826	1879	1934	1990	2048	2107	2168	2231	2296	2362
81	1531	1575	1620	1666	1714	1763	1814	1866	1919	1975	2031	2089	2149	2211	2275	2340	2407
82	1567	1612	1657	1704	1753	1803	1854	1906	1960	2016	2073	2132	2193	2255	2319	2385	2462
83	1605	1650	1696	1744	1793	1843	1895	1948	2002	2059	2116	2176	2237	2300	2364	2431	2499

84	1643	1689	1735	1784	1833	1884	1936	1990	2045	2102	2160	2220	2282	2345	2410	2477	2546
85	1682	1728	1776	1825	1875	1926	1979	2033	2089	2146	2205	2266	2328	2392	2457	2525	2594
86	1722	1769	1817	1866	1917	1969	2022	2077	2134	2192	2251	2312	2375	2439	2505	2573	2643
87	1764	1811	1859	1909	1960	2013	2067	2122	2179	2238	2298	2359	2423	2488	2554	2623	2693
88	1806	1854	1903	1953	2005	2058	2113	2169	2226	2285	2346	2408	2472	2537	2604	2673	2744
89	1849	1897	1947	1998	2050	2104	2159	2216	2274	2333	2394	2457	2521	2587	2655	2725	2796
90	1893	1942	1992	2044	2097	2151	2207	2264	2322	2382	2444	2507	2572	2639	2707	2777	2849
91	1938	1988	2039	2091	2144	2199	2256	2313	2372	2433	2496	2559	2624	2691	2760	2830	2903
92	1984	2035	2086	2139	2193	2248	2305	2363	2423	2484	2547	2611	2677	2744	2814	2885	2958
93	2032	2083	2135	2188	2242	2298	2356	2414	2475	2536	2599	2664	2731	2799	2869	2940	3014
94	2080	2132	2184	2238	2293	2350	2407	2467	2527	2590	2653	2719	2786	2854	2925	2997	3070
95	2130	2182	2235	2289	2345	2402	2460	2520	2582	2644	2709	2774	2842	2911	2982	3054	3129
96	2181	2233	2287	2342	2398	2456	2515	2575	2637	2700	2765	2831	2899	2969	3040	3113	3188
97	2233	2286	2340	2396	2452	2510	2570	2631	2693	2757	2822	2889	2958	3028	3099	3173	3248
98	2286	2340	2395	2451	2508	2567	2627	2688	2751	2815	2881	2948	3017	3088	3160	3234	3309
99	2341	2395	2450	2507	2565	2624	2684	2746	2810	2874	2941	3009	3078	3149	3222	3296	3372
100	2397	2452	2507	2564	2623	2682	2743	2806	2870	2935	3002	3070	3140	3211	3285	3359	3436

(continued)

Appendix 8 (Continued)

BPD (mm)	Abdominal Circumference (mm)															
	325	330	335	340	345	350	355	360	365	370	375	380	385	390	395	400
31	985	1029	1075	1123	1173	1225	1279	1336	1396	1458	1523	1591	1661	1735	1812	1893
32	1004	1048	1004	1143	1193	1246	1301	1258	1418	1546	1615	1686	1761	1838	1920	
33	1022	1067	1114	1163	1214	1267	1323	1381	1441	1504	1570	1639	1711	1786	1865	1946
34	1041	1087	1134	1183	1235	1289	1345	1403	1464	1528	1595	1664	1737	1812	1891	1973
35	1061	1107	1154	1204	1256	1311	1367	1426	1488	1552	1619	1689	1762	1838	1918	2001
36	1080	1127	1175	1226	1278	1333	1390	1450	1512	1577	1645	1715	1789	1865	1945	2029
37	1101	1147	1196	1247	1300	1356	1413	1474	1536	1602	1670	1741	1815	1893	1973	2057
38	1121	1168	1218	1269	1323	1379	1437	1498	1561	1627	1696	1768	1842	1920	2001	2086
39	1142	1190	1240	1292	1346	1402	1461	1523	1586	1653	1722	1794	1870	1948	2030	2115
40	1163	1212	1262	1315	1369	1426	1496	1548	1612	1679	1749	1822	1898	1977	2059	2145
41	1185	1234	1285	1338	1393	1451	1511	1573	1638	1706	1776	1849	1926	2005	2088	2174
42	1207	1256	1308	1361	1417	1475	1536	1599	1664	1733	1804	1878	1954	2035	2118	2205
43	1229	1279	1331	1385	1442	1500	1562	1625	1691	1760	1832	1906	1984	2064	2148	2236
44	1252	1303	1355	1410	1467	1526	1588	1652	1718	1788	1860	1935	2013	2094	2179	2267
45	1275	1326	1380	1435	1492	1552	1614	1679	1746	1816	1889	1964	2043	2125	2210	2298
46	1299	1351	1404	1406	1518	1579	1641	1706	1774	1845	1918	1994	2073	2156	2241	2330
47	1323	1375	1430	1486	1545	1605	1669	1734	1803	1874	1948	2024	2104	2187	2273	2363

48	1348	1401	1455	1512	1571	1633	1697	1763	1832	1904	1976	2055	2136	2219	2306	2396
49	1373	1426	1482	1539	1599	1661	1725	1792	1861	1934	2009	2086	2167	2251	2339	2429
50	1399	1452	1508	1566	1626	1689	1754	1821	1891	1964	2040	2118	2200	2284	2372	2463
51	1425	1479	1535	1594	1655	1718	1783	1851	1922	1995	2071	2150	2232	2317	2406	2498
52	1451	1506	1563	1622	1683	1747	1813	1882	1953	2027	2103	2183	2266	2351	2440	2532
53	1478	1533	1591	1651	1713	1777	1843	1913	1984	2059	2136	2216	2299	2386	2475	2568
54	1506	1562	1620	1680	1742	1807	1874	1944	2016	2091	2169	2250	2333	2420	2510	2604
55	1534	1590	1649	1710	1773	1838	1906	1976	2049	2124	2203	2284	2368	2456	2546	2640
56	1562	1619	1678	1740	1803	1869	1938	2008	2082	2158	2237	2319	2403	2491	2582	2677
57	1591	1649	1709	1770	1835	1901	1970	2041	2115	2192	2272	2354	2439	2528	2619	2714
58	1621	1679	1739	1802	1866	1934	2003	2075	2150	2227	2307	2390	2475	2564	2657	2752
59	1651	1710	1770	1834	1899	1966	2037	2109	2184	2262	2342	2426	2512	2602	2694	2790
60	1682	1741	1802	1866	1932	2000	2071	2144	2219	2298	2379	2463	2550	2640	2733	2829
61	1713	1773	1835	1899	1965	2034	2105	2179	2255	2334	2416	2500	2588	2678	2772	2869
62	1745	1805	1868	1932	1999	2069	2140	2215	2291	2371	2453	2538	2626	2717	2811	2909
63	1777	1838	1901	1967	2034	2104	2176	2251	2328	2408	2491	2577	2665	2757	2851	2949
64	1810	1872	1935	2001	2069	2140	2213	2288	2366	2446	2530	2616	2705	2797	2892	2991
65	1844	1906	1970	2037	2105	2176	2250	2326	2404	2485	2569	2656	2745	2838	2933	3032
66	1878	1941	2006	2073	2142	2213	2287	2364	2443	2524	2609	2696	2786	2879	2975	3075
67	1913	1976	2042	2109	2179	2251	2326	2403	2482	2564	2649	2737	2827	2921	3018	3117
68	1949	2012	2078	2147	2217	2290	2365	2442	2522	2605	2690	2778	2869	2964	3061	3161
69	1985	2049	2116	2184	2255	2329	2404	2482	2563	2646	2732	2821	2912	3007	3104	3205
70	2022	2087	2154	2223	2295	2368	2444	2523	2604	2688	2774	2863	2955	3050	3149	3250

(continued)

Appendix 8 (Continued)

BPD (mm)	Abdominal Circumference (mm)															
	325	330	335	340	345	350	355	360	365	370	375	380	385	390	395	400
71	2059	2125	2193	2262	2334	2409	2485	2564	2646	2730	2817	2907	2999	3095	3193	3295
72	2098	2164	2232	2302	2375	2450	2527	2607	2689	2773	2861	2951	3044	3140	3239	3341
73	2137	2203	2272	2343	2416	2491	2569	2649	2732	2817	2905	2996	3089	3186	3285	3386
74	2176	2244	2313	2384	2458	2534	2612	2693	2776	2862	2950	3041	3135	3232	3332	3435
75	2217	2265	2354	2426	2501	2577	2656	2737	2821	2907	2996	3088	3182	3279	3380	3483
76	2258	2326	2397	2469	2544	2621	2700	2782	2866	2953	3042	3134	3229	3327	3428	3531
77	2300	2369	2440	2513	2588	2666	2746	2828	2912	3000	3090	3181	3277	3376	3477	3581
78	2343	2412	2484	2557	2633	2711	2792	2874	2959	3047	3137	3230	3326	3425	3526	3631
79	2386	2456	2528	2603	2679	2757	2838	2921	3007	3095	3186	3279	3376	3475	3576	3681
80	2431	2501	2574	2649	2725	2804	2886	2969	3056	3144	3235	3329	3426	3525	3627	3733
81	2476	2547	2620	2695	2773	2852	2934	3018	3105	3194	3286	3380	3477	3577	3679	3785
82	2522	2594	2667	2743	2821	2901	2983	3068	3155	3244	3336	3431	3529	3629	3732	3838

83	2569	2641	2715	2791	2870	2950	3033	3118	3206	3296	3388	3483	3581	3682	3785	3891
84	2617	2689	2764	2841	2920	3001	3084	3169	3257	3348	3441	3536	3634	3735	3839	3945
85	2665	2739	2814	2891	2970	3052	3135	3221	3310	3401	3494	3590	3688	3790	3894	4000
86	2715	2789	2864	2942	3022	3104	3188	3274	3363	3454	3548	3644	3743	3845	3949	4056
87	2765	2840	2916	2994	3074	3157	3241	3328	3417	3509	3603	3700	3799	3901	4005	4113
88	2817	2892	2968	3047	3128	3210	3295	3383	3472	3565	3659	3756	3855	3958	4063	4170
89	2869	2944	3021	3101	3182	3265	3351	3438	3528	3621	3716	3813	3913	4015	4120	4228
90	2923	2998	3076	3155	3237	3321	3407	3495	3585	3678	3773	3871	3971	4074	4179	4287
91	2977	3053	3131	3211	3293	3377	3464	3552	3643	3736	3832	3930	4030	4133	4239	4347
92	3032	3109	3187	3268	3350	3435	3522	3611	3702	3795	3891	3989	4090	4193	4299	4408
93	3089	3166	3245	3326	3409	3494	3581	3670	3761	3855	3951	4050	4151	4254	4361	4469
94	3146	3224	3303	3384	3468	3553	3641	3738	3822	3916	4013	4111	4213	4316	4423	4532
95	3205	3283	3362	3444	3528	3614	3701	3791	3884	3978	4075	4174	4275	4379	4486	4595
96	3264	3343	3423	3505	3589	3675	3763	3854	3946	4041	4138	4237	4339	4443	4550	4659
97	3325	3404	3484	3567	3651	3738	3826	3917	4010	4105	4202	4302	4404	4508	4615	4724
98	3387	3466	3547	3630	3715	3802	3890	3981	4074	4170	4267	4367	4469	4573	4680	4790
99	3450	3529	3611	3694	3779	3866	3956	4047	4140	4236	4333	4433	4536	4640	4747	4857
100	3514	3594	3676	3759	3845	3932	4022	4113	4207	4303	4400	4501	4603	4708	4815	4924

From Shepard MJ, Richards VA, Berkowitz RL et al: An evaluation of two equations for predicting fetal weight by ultrasound. Am J Obstet Gynecol 142:47, 1982, with permission.

Appendix 9 Estimated Fetal Weight (g) Based on Abdominal Circumference and Femur Length (FL)

FL (mm)	Abdominal Circumference (mm)																				
	200	205	210	215	220	225	230	235	240	245	250	255	260	265	270	275	280	285	290	295	300
40	663	691	720	751	783	816	851	887	925	964	1006	1048	1093	1139	1188	1239	1291	1346	1403	1463	1525
41	680	709	738	769	802	836	871	907	946	986	1027	1070	1115	1162	1211	1262	1315	1371	1429	1489	1551
42	697	726	757	788	821	855	891	928	967	1007	1049	1093	1138	1186	1235	1287	1340	1396	1454	1515	1578
43	715	745	776	808	841	875	912	949	988	1029	1071	1116	1162	1209	1259	1311	1365	1422	1480	1541	1605
44	734	764	795	827	861	896	933	971	1010	1051	1094	1139	1185	1234	1284	1336	1391	1448	1507	1568	1632
45	753	783	815	847	882	917	954	993	1033	1074	1118	1163	1210	1259	1309	1362	1417	1474	1534	1596	1660
46	772	803	835	868	903	939	976	1015	1056	1098	1142	1187	1235	1284	1335	1388	1444	1501	1561	1623	1688
47	792	823	856	889	924	961	999	1038	1079	1122	1166	1212	1260	1310	1361	1415	1471	1529	1589	1652	1717
48	812	844	877	911	947	984	1022	1062	1103	1146	1191	1237	1286	1336	1388	1442	1498	1557	1618	1681	1746
49	833	865	899	933	969	1007	1046	1086	1128	1171	1216	1263	1312	1363	1415	1470	1527	1585	1647	1710	1776
50	855	887	921	956	993	1031	1070	1111	1153	1197	1243	1290	1339	1390	1443	1498	1555	1615	1676	1740	1806
51	877	910	944	980	1016	1055	1095	1136	1179	1223	1269	1317	1367	1418	1471	1527	1584	1644	1706	1770	1837
52	899	933	967	1004	1041	1080	1120	1162	1205	1250	1296	1344	1395	1447	1500	1556	1614	1674	1737	1801	1868
53	922	956	992	1028	1066	1105	1146	1188	1232	1277	1324	1373	1423	1476	1530	1586	1645	1705	1768	1833	1900
54	946	981	1016	1053	1091	1131	1172	1215	1259	1305	1352	1401	1452	1505	1560	1617	1675	1736	1799	1865	1933
55	971	1005	1041	1079	1118	1158	1199	1242	1287	1333	1381	1431	1482	1535	1591	1648	1707	1768	1832	1897	1966
56	995	1031	1067	1105	1144	1185	1227	1271	1316	1362	1411	1461	1513	1566	1622	1679	1739	1801	1864	1931	1999
57	1021	1057	1094	1132	1172	1213	1255	1299	1345	1392	1441	1491	1544	1598	1654	1712	1772	1834	1898	1964	2033
58	1047	1084	1121	1160	1200	1242	1285	1329	1375	1422	1472	1523	1575	1630	1686	1744	1805	1867	1932	1999	2068
59	1074	1111	1149	1188	1229	1271	1314	1359	1406	1454	1503	1555	1608	1663	1719	1778	1839	1902	1966	2034	2103

(continued)

60	1102	1139	1178	1217	1258	1301	1345	1390	1437	1485	1535	1587	1641	1696	1753	1812	1873	1936	2002	2069	2139
61	1130	1168	1207	1247	1289	1331	1376	1421	1469	1518	1568	1620	1674	1730	1788	1847	1908	1972	2038	2105	2175
62	1160	1198	1237	1278	1319	1363	1408	1454	1501	1551	1602	1654	1709	1765	1823	1882	1944	2008	2074	2142	2212
63	1189	1228	1268	1309	1351	1395	1440	1487	1535	1585	1636	1689	1744	1800	1858	1919	1981	2045	2111	2180	2250
64	1220	1259	1299	1341	1384	1428	1473	1520	1569	1619	1671	1724	1779	1836	1895	1956	2018	2082	2149	2218	2289
65	1251	1291	1332	1373	1417	1461	1507	1555	1604	1655	1707	1760	1816	1873	1932	1993	2056	2121	2188	2256	2328
66	1284	1324	1365	1407	1451	1496	1542	1590	1640	1691	1743	1797	1853	1911	1970	2031	2094	2160	2227	2296	2367
67	1317	1357	1399	1441	1486	1531	1578	1626	1676	1728	1780	1835	1891	1949	2009	2070	2134	2199	2267	2336	2408
68	1351	1391	1433	1477	1521	1567	1615	1663	1713	1765	1819	1873	1930	1988	2048	2110	2174	2240	2307	2377	2449
69	1385	1427	1469	1513	1558	1604	1652	1701	1752	1804	1857	1913	1970	2028	2089	2151	2215	2281	2348	2418	2490
70	1421	1463	1506	1550	1595	1642	1690	1740	1791	1843	1897	1953	2010	2069	2130	2192	2256	2322	2391	2461	2533
71	1458	1500	1543	1588	1633	1681	1729	1779	1830	1883	1938	1994	2051	2110	2171	2234	2299	2365	2433	2504	2576
72	1495	1538	1581	1626	1673	1720	1769	1819	1871	1924	1979	2035	2093	2153	2214	2277	2342	2408	2477	2547	2620
73	1534	1577	1621	1666	1713	1761	1810	1861	1913	1966	2021	2078	2136	2196	2258	2321	2386	2453	2521	2592	2665
74	1573	1616	1661	1707	1754	1802	1852	1903	1955	2009	2065	2122	2180	2240	2302	2365	2431	2498	2566	2637	2710
75	1614	1657	1702	1749	1796	1845	1895	1946	1999	2053	2109	2166	2225	2285	2347	2411	2476	2543	2612	2683	2756
76	1655	1699	1745	1791	1839	1888	1939	1990	2043	2098	2154	2211	2270	2331	2393	2457	2523	2590	2659	2730	2803
77	1698	1742	1788	1835	1883	1933	1983	2035	2089	2144	2200	2258	2317	2378	2440	2504	2570	2638	2707	2778	2851
78	1741	1786	1833	1880	1928	1978	2029	2082	2135	2191	2247	2305	2365	2426	2488	2553	2618	2686	2755	2827	2899
79	1786	1832	1878	1926	1975	2025	2076	2129	2183	2238	2295	2353	2413	2474	2537	2602	2668	2735	2805	2876	2949
80	1832	1878	1925	1973	2022	2073	2124	2177	2232	2287	2344	2403	2463	2524	2587	2652	2718	2785	2855	2926	2999
81	1879	1926	1973	2021	2071	2121	2173	2227	2281	2337	2394	2453	2513	2575	2638	2702	2769	2837	2906	2977	3050
82	1928	1974	2022	2070	2120	2171	2224	2277	2332	2388	2446	2504	2565	2626	2690	2754	2821	2889	2958	3029	3102
83	1978	2024	2072	2121	2171	2223	2275	2329	2384	2440	2498	2557	2617	2679	2743	2807	2874	2942	3011	3082	3155

656 Appendices

Appendix 9 (Continued)

FL (mm)	Abdominal Circumference (mm)																			
	305	310	315	320	325	330	335	340	345	350	355	360	365	370	375	380	385	390	395	400
40	1590	1658	1729	1802	1879	1959	2042	2129	2220	2314	2413	2515	2622	2734	2850	2972	3098	3230	3367	3511
41	1617	1685	1756	1830	1907	1987	2071	2158	2249	2344	2442	2545	2652	2764	2880	3002	3128	3260	3397	3540
42	1644	1712	1783	1858	1935	2016	2100	2187	2279	2373	2472	2575	2683	2794	2911	3032	3159	3290	3427	3570
43	1671	1740	1812	1886	1964	2045	2129	2217	2308	2404	2503	2606	2713	2825	2942	3063	3189	3321	3458	3600
44	1699	1768	1840	1915	1993	2075	2159	2247	2339	2434	2533	2637	2744	2856	2973	3094	3220	3352	3488	3630
45	1727	1797	1869	1944	2023	2105	2189	2278	2370	2465	2565	2668	2776	2888	3004	3125	3251	3383	3519	3661
46	1756	1826	1898	1974	2053	2135	2220	2309	2401	2497	2596	2700	2807	2919	3036	3157	3283	3414	3550	3692
47	1785	1855	1928	2004	2084	2166	2251	2340	2432	2528	2628	2732	2840	2952	3068	3189	3315	3446	3582	3723
48	1814	1885	1959	2035	2115	2197	2283	2372	2464	2560	2660	2764	2872	2984	3100	3221	3347	3478	3613	3754
49	1845	1916	1990	2066	2146	2229	2315	2404	2497	2593	2693	2797	2905	3017	3133	3254	3380	3510	3645	3786
50	1875	1947	2021	2098	2178	2261	2347	2437	2530	2626	2726	2830	2938	3050	3166	3287	3412	3542	3677	3818
51	1906	1978	2053	2130	2210	2294	2380	2470	2563	2659	2760	2864	2972	3084	3200	3320	3445	3575	3710	3850
52	1938	2010	2085	2163	2243	2327	2413	2503	2597	2693	2794	2898	3006	3117	3234	3354	3479	3608	3743	3882
53	1970	2043	2118	2196	2277	2360	2447	2537	2631	2728	2828	2932	3040	3152	3268	3388	3513	3642	3776	3915
54	2003	2076	2151	2229	2311	2395	2482	2572	2665	2762	2863	2967	3075	3186	3302	3422	3547	3676	3809	3948
55	2036	2109	2185	2264	2345	2429	2516	2607	2700	2797	2898	3002	3110	3221	3337	3457	3581	3710	3843	3981
56	2070	2143	2220	2298	2380	2464	2552	2642	2736	2833	2933	3038	3145	3257	3372	3492	3616	3744	3877	4015
57	2104	2178	2254	2333	2415	2500	2587	2678	2772	2869	2970	3074	3181	3293	3408	3527	3651	3779	3911	4048
58	2139	2213	2290	2369	2451	2536	2624	2714	2808	2905	3006	3110	3218	3329	3444	3563	3686	3814	3946	4082
59	2175	2249	2326	2405	2488	2573	2660	2751	2845	2942	3043	3147	3254	3366	3480	3599	3722	3849	3981	4117

60	2211	2286	2363	2442	2525	2610	2698	2789	2883	2980	3080	3184	3292	3403	3517	3636	3758	3885	4016	4151
61	2248	2323	2400	2480	2562	2647	2736	2827	2921	3018	3118	3222	3329	3440	3554	3673	3795	3921	4052	4186
62	2285	2360	2438	2518	2600	2686	2774	2865	2959	3056	3157	3260	3367	3478	3592	3710	3832	3957	4087	4222
63	2323	2398	2476	2556	2639	2725	2813	2904	2998	3095	3195	3299	3406	3516	3630	3747	3869	3994	4124	4257
64	2362	2437	2515	2595	2678	2764	2852	2943	3037	3134	3235	3338	3445	3555	3668	3785	3906	4031	4160	4293
65	2401	2477	2555	2635	2718	2804	2892	2983	3077	3174	3274	3378	3484	3594	3707	3824	3944	4069	4197	4329
66	2441	2517	2595	2675	2759	2844	2933	3024	3118	3215	3315	3418	3524	3633	3746	3863	3983	4106	4234	4366
67	2481	2557	2636	2716	2800	2885	2974	3065	3159	3256	3355	3458	3564	3673	3786	3902	4021	4144	4271	4402
68	2523	2599	2677	2758	2841	2927	3016	3107	3200	3297	3397	3499	3605	3714	3826	3941	4060	4183	4309	4439
69	2564	2641	2719	2800	2884	2969	3058	3149	3242	3339	3438	3541	3646	3754	3866	3981	4100	4222	4347	4477
70	2607	2683	2762	2843	2927	3012	3101	3192	3285	3381	3481	3583	3688	3796	3907	4022	4140	4261	4386	4514
71	2650	2727	2806	2887	2970	3056	3144	3235	3328	3424	3523	3625	3730	3838	3948	4062	4180	4300	4425	4552
72	2694	2771	2850	2931	3014	3100	3188	3279	3372	3468	3567	3668	3772	3880	3990	4104	4220	4340	4464	4591
73	2739	2816	2895	2976	3059	3145	3233	3323	3416	3512	3610	3712	3816	3922	4032	4145	4261	4381	4503	4629
74	2785	2861	2940	3021	3105	3190	3278	3369	3461	3557	3655	3756	3859	3966	4075	4187	4303	4421	4543	4668
75	2831	2908	2987	3068	3151	3236	3324	3414	3507	3602	3700	3800	3903	4009	4118	4230	4344	4462	4583	4708
76	2878	2955	3034	3115	3198	3283	3371	3461	3553	3648	3745	3845	3948	4053	4161	4272	4387	4504	4624	4747
77	2926	3003	3081	3162	3245	3331	3418	3508	3600	3694	3791	3891	3993	4098	4205	4316	4429	4545	4665	4787
78	2974	3051	3130	3211	3294	3379	3466	3555	3647	3741	3838	3937	4039	4143	4250	4360	4472	4588	4706	4827
79	3024	3100	3179	3260	3343	3427	3514	3604	3695	3789	3885	3984	4085	4188	4295	4404	4515	4630	4748	4868
80	3074	3151	3229	3310	3392	3477	3564	3653	3744	3837	3933	4031	4131	4234	4340	4448	4559	4673	4790	4909
81	3125	3202	3280	3360	3443	3527	3614	3702	3793	3886	3981	4079	4179	4281	4386	4493	4604	4716	4832	4950
82	3177	3253	3332	3412	3494	3578	3664	3752	3843	3935	4030	4127	4226	4328	4432	4539	4648	4760	4875	4992
83	3230	3306	3384	3464	3546	3630	3716	3803	3893	3985	4080	4176	4275	4376	4479	4585	4693	4804	4918	5034

From Hadlock FP, Harrist RB, Carpenter RJ et al: Sonographic estimation of fetal weight. Radiology 150:535, 1984, with permission.

Appendix 10 Birth Weight for U.S. Single Live Births in 1991

Gestational Age (weeks)	Percentile (g)				
	5th	10th	50th	90th	95th
20	249	275	412	772	912
21	280	314	433	790	957
22	330	376	496	826	1023
23	385	440	582	882	1107
24	435	498	674	977	1223
25	480	558	779	1138	1397
26	529	625	899	1362	1640
27	591	702	1035	1635	1927
28	670	798	1196	1977	2237
29	772	925	1394	2361	2553
30	910	1085	1637	2710	2847

31	1088	1278	1918	2986	3108
32	1294	1495	2203	3200	3338
33	1513	1725	2458	3370	3536
34	1735	1950	2667	3502	3697
35	1950	2159	2831	3596	3812
36	2156	2354	2974	3668	3888
37	2357	2541	3117	3755	3956
38	2543	2714	3263	3867	4027
39	2685	2852	3400	3980	4107
40	2761	2929	3495	4060	4185
41	2777	2948	3527	4094	4217
42	2764	2935	3522	4098	4213
43	2741	2907	3505	4096	4178
44	2724	2885	3491	4096	4122

From Alexander GR, Himes JH, Kaufman RB et al: A United States national reference for fetal growth. Obstet Gynecol 87:163, 1996, with permission.

Appendix 11 Tenth Percentile Birth Weight by Gender for U.S. Single Live Births in 1991

Gestational Age (weeks)	Birth Weight (g)	
	Male	Female
20	270	256
21	328	310
22	388	368
23	446	426
24	504	480
25	570	535
26	644	592
27	728	662
28	828	760
29	956	889
30	1117	1047
31	1308	1234
32	1521	1447
33	1751	1675
34	1985	1901
35	2205	2109
36	2407	2300
37	2596	2484
38	2769	2657
39	2908	2796
40	2986	2872
41	3007	2891
42	2998	2884
43	2977	2868
44	2963	2853

From Alexander GR, Himes JH, Kaufman RB et al: A United States national reference for fetal growth. Obstet Gynecol 87: 163, 1996, with permission.

Appendix 12 Estimated Fetal Weight in Twin Gestations

Gestational Age (weeks)	Fetal Weight (g)			
	5th %	25th %	50th %	75th %
16	132	141	154	189
17	173	194	215	239
18	214	248	276	289
19	223	253	300	333
20	232	259	324	378
21	275	355	432	482
22	319	452	540	586
23	347	497	598	684
24	376	543	656	783
25	549	677	793	916
26	722	812	931	1049
27	755	978	1087	1193
28	789	1145	1244	1337
29	900	1266	1395	1509
30	1011	1387	1546	1682
31	1198	1532	1693	1875
32	1385	1677	1840	2068
33	1491	1771	2032	2334
34	1597	1866	2224	2601
35	1703	2093	2427	2716
36	1809	2321	2631	2832
37	2239	2540	2824	3035
38	2669	2760	3017	3239

From Yarkoni S, Reece EA, Holford T: Estimated fetal weight in the evaluation of growth in twin gestations: A perspective longitudinal study. Obstet Gynecol 69:636, 1987, with permission.

Appendix 13 Amniotic Fluid Index Values in Normal Pregnancy

	Amniotic Fluid Index Percentile Values (mm)					
Week	2.5th	5th	50th	95th	97.5th	n
16	73	79	121	185	201	32
17	77	83	127	194	211	26
18	80	97	133	202	220	17
19	83	90	137	207	225	14
20	86	93	141	212	230	25
21	88	95	143	214	233	14
22	89	97	145	216	235	14
23	90	98	146	218	237	14
24	90	98	147	219	238	23
25	89	97	147	221	240	12
26	89	97	147	223	242	11
27	85	95	146	226	245	17
28	86	94	146	228	249	25
29	84	92	145	231	254	12
30	82	90	145	234	258	17
31	79	88	144	238	263	26
32	77	86	144	242	269	25
33	74	83	143	245	274	30
34	72	81	142	248	278	31
35	70	79	140	249	279	27
36	68	77	138	249	279	39
37	66	75	135	244	275	36
38	65	73	132	239	269	27
39	64	72	127	226	255	12
40	63	71	123	214	240	64
41	63	70	116	194	216	162
42	63	69	110	175	192	30

From Moore TR, Cayle JE: The amniotic fluid index in normal human pregnancy. Am J Obstet Gynecol 171:218, 1990, with permission.

Obstetric Doppler

Appendix 14 Umbilical Artery Resistance Index (RI) and Systolic-to-Diastolic (S/D) Ratio

Gestational Age (weeks)	5th Percentile		50th Percentile		95th Percentile	
	RI	S/D	RI	S/D	RI	S/D
16	0.70	3.33	0.80	5.00	0.90	10.00
17	0.69	3.23	0.79	4.76	0.89	9.09
18	0.68	3.13	0.78	4.55	0.88	8.33
19	0.67	3.03	0.77	4.35	0.87	7.69
20	0.66	2.94	0.76	4.17	0.86	7.14
21	0.65	2.86	0.75	4.00	0.85	6.67
22	0.64	2.78	0.74	3.85	0.84	6.25
23	0.63	2.70	0.73	3.70	0.83	5.88
24	0.62	2.63	0.72	3.57	0.82	5.56
25	0.61	2.56	0.71	3.45	0.81	5.26
26	0.60	2.50	0.70	3.33	0.80	5.00
27	0.59	2.44	0.69	3.23	0.79	4.76
28	0.58	2.38	0.68	3.13	0.78	4.55
29	0.57	2.33	0.67	3.03	0.77	4.35
30	0.56	2.27	0.66	2.94	0.76	4.17
31	0.55	2.22	0.65	2.86	0.75	4.00
32	0.54	2.17	0.64	2.78	0.74	3.85
33	0.53	2.13	0.63	2.70	0.73	3.70
34	0.52	2.08	0.62	2.63	0.72	3.57
35	0.51	2.04	0.61	2.56	0.71	3.45
36	0.50	2.00	0.60	2.50	0.70	3.33
37	0.49	1.96	0.59	2.44	0.69	3.23
38	0.47	1.89	0.57	2.33	0.67	3.03
39	0.46	1.85	0.56	2.27	0.66	2.94
40	0.45	1.82	0.55	2.22	0.65	2.86
41	0.44	1.79	0.54	2.17	0.64	2.78
42	0.43	1.75	0.53	2.13	0.63	2.70

From Kofinas AD, Espeland MA, Penry M et al: Uteroplacental Doppler flow velocity waveform indices in normal pregnancy: a statistical exercise and the development of appropriate reference values. Am J Perinatol 9:98, 1990, with permission.

Index

Note: Page numbers in *italics* refer to illustrations; page numbers followed by b refer to boxed material, and those followed by t refer to tables.